Eye Diseases in Hot Climates

Eye Diseases in Hot Climates

John Sandford-Smith
Consultant Ophthalmologist
The Leicester Royal Infirmary, England

formerly
Ophthalmologist, the Christian Hospital,
Quetta, Pakistan, and
Senior Lecturer in Ophthalmology,
Ahmadu Bello University Hospital,
Kaduna, Nigeria

WRIGHT
Bristol
1986

Published by:
John Wright & Sons Ltd, Techno House, Redcliffe Way, Bristol BS1 6NX, England.

British Library Cataloguing in Publication Data

Sandford-Smith, John
    Eye diseases in hot climates.
    1. Eye—Diseases and defects—Tropics
    I. Title
    617.7'0913   RE48

ISBN 0 7236 0749 4
ISBN 0 7236 0750 8 Pbk

Typset from disc by
Avon Dataset Limited, Stratford-upon-Avon, Warwickshire

Printed in Great Britain by
J. W. Arrowsmith Ltd., Bristol

Preface

We all have a 'blind spot'. This is a small area in our field of vision where we cannot see anything at all. Surprisingly none of us is aware of this blind spot, even though we all have one.

There is unfortunately a large blind spot in the world-wide ophthalmic services. This is the problem of avoidable blindness and eye disease, especially in the rural areas of hot countries. There is apparently little awareness of this problem although it is by far the most important cause of avoidable blindness world-wide.

The medical profession is concerned with treating and preventing disease and yet most doctors, and particularly specialists, choose to work in those areas where people are most healthy. Each year many new ophthalmic textbooks are published, but most of them are written about those patients who are already receiving excellent eye care. Therefore avoidable blindness and eye disease in hot climates remains a blind spot both to the medical profession and to medical science.

I have tried to write this book particularly for the non-specialist—doctor, nurse or medical assistant—who has to see and treat eye patients without any specialist supervision, and often with limited equipment and facilities. I hope it will also be of value to the specialist, either as an introduction for the postgraduate in training or else for the specialist who has trained in the western world and is returning to or visiting the 'tropics'. I have tried to concentrate on common diseases and particularly on those which cause blindness and can be treated or prevented.

For many people who read this book, English may be their second or even third language. I am particularly grateful to Lyn Edwards, a language expert, for her help in writing this book. She has revised and often rewritten the entire text, to make both the language and the grammar more simple and direct. Dr Keith Waddell of Kuluva Hospital, Uganda, has very kindly read through the whole text, and made many valuable suggestions.

Any book about eye disease must have good clear pictures. With these the reader can recognise each disease and learn how to examine the eye. This book contains both colour plates and black and white pictures.

The colour plates have been placed in a separate section to save printing costs, and they are numbered separately from the pages of the book. For example, *Plate* 5a or 5b will be found on the 5th page of the colour plates.

The black and white pictures and diagrams are printed with the text in the appropriate chapters. They are referred to as 'figures'. For example, *Fig.* 5.2 is found in chapter 5 and is the second picture in that chapter.

Many textbooks are too expensive for those who work in poor countries. I am very grateful to the following organisations who have given very generous financial support so that this book can be reasonably priced.

Ulverscroft Foundation, Anstey, Leicester, UK
Christoffel Blindenmission, Bensheim, West Germany
Royal Commonwealth Society for the Blind, Haywards Heath, UK
CooperVision Ltd, Southampton, UK

I would also like to thank all the staff of the Audio Visual Aids Department of the Leicester Royal Infirmary, and in particular Georgean Lochhead, who have freely given their time and talents in producing many of the illustrations.

J.S.-S.

Acknowledgements

I would like to record my thanks to the following organisations and individuals who have very kindly provided some of the photographs in this book.

The World Health Organisation — *Cover photograph, Plate 3e, Plate 6 a,d, e and f, Plate 7c, Plate 12e, Plate 22 a,b,c, and d.*

Teaching Aids at Low Cost, London — *Plate 11e, Plate 12 a and b, Fig. 15.3, Fig. 15.4, Fig. 15.5, Fig. 15.8, Plate 22e.*

Professor Barrie Jones, London — *Fig. 7.3, Plate 6c, Plate 7d, Plate 21 c, e and f.*

Dr A. Sommer, Baltimore, USA — *Plate 11f.*

Mr E. Rosen, Manchester — *Plate 7e.*

Mr J. Talbot, Sheffield — *Plate 19a.*

Mr M. Kerr-Muir, London — *Plate 22f.*

Contents

1.   Introduction

What is special about eye diseases in hot climates?

Firstly, many countries with hot climates are also poor and less developed. They are usually called 'developing' countries. In these countries, there is a high incidence of disease caused by poor hygiene and poor nutrition. There is also a shortage of medical care and personnel.

Secondly, there are diseases which are specifically caused by hot climates. Other diseases are spread by insects or other carriers found only in hot climates. These are usually called 'tropical' diseases.

The eye is an external organ, and so it is particularly affected by the environment. This means that poor hygiene and nutrition, the climate and insect vectors all significantly affect the incidence and pattern of eye disease. Therefore eye disease in 'hot', 'tropical' 'developing' countries differs from that in other countries in four particular ways.

— The number of blind or partially blind people is high.
— Most of the blindness is either preventable or treatable.
— The pattern of tropical eye diseases varies from area to area.
— The medical resources are usually inadequate.

(The adjectives 'hot', 'tropical' and 'developing' do not have exactly the same meaning. I have tried to use whichever seems most appropriate rather than using just one or all three.)

1. The number of blind or partially blind people is high.

According to reports, between 0.1% and 0.2% of the population in most developed countries are blind. In developing countries, however, between 0.5% and 1% are blind — and there are good reasons to believe that the true figure may be even higher than this.

— First, blindness is such a handicap in poor and rural communities that blind people have a much shorter life expectancy.
— Second, nearly all blind people in developed countries are old people. (For example, in England, three-quarters of the people who register as blind each year are over 70.) However, developing countries with an expanding population of young people, and a shorter life expectancy have far fewer old people.
— Third, in most developed countries, there are good reasons for people to register as blind e.g. Social Security benefits etc. In developing countries, however, there are economic and cultural reasons for people to hide their

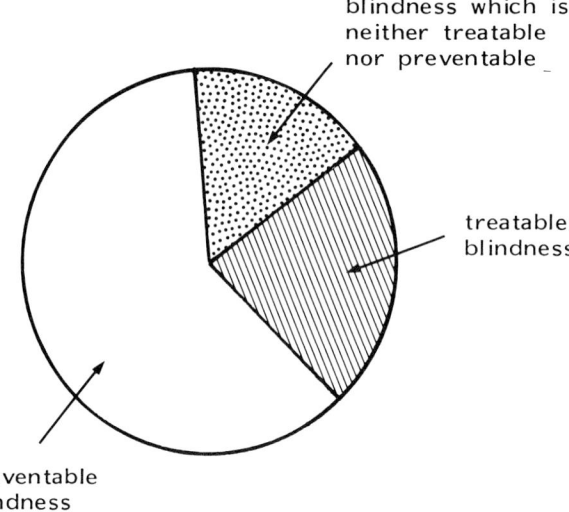

Fig. 1.1 The typical pattern of blindness in the tropics.

blindness. I once examined a young man who was totally blind. He asked me to write a note to explain his absence from work, and then said that he was a night watchman!

2. Most of the blindness is either preventable or treatable.

The main causes of blindness in the developed countries are untreatable — degenerative and vascular disorders of the retina in old people, and congenital abnormalities in children. These conditions are probably just as common in developing countries, but they are only a fraction of all cases of blindness (*Fig.* 1.1).

Most blindness in developing countries is the result of one of the following five conditions, which are all either preventable or treatable.

 - Trachoma. At least 2 million people in the world are blind from trachoma. Another 100 million people suffer severely.[1]
 - Malnutrition with xerophthalmia. In Asia alone, at least 100 000 children a year develop corneal ulcers from xerophthalmia. Half of these children may be left blind.[1]
 - Cataract. In India alone, there are about 5 million blind people waiting for a cataract operation. In Africa, there are another 3 million.[1]
 - Glaucoma. There are many people all over the tropics who are blind from glaucoma.
 - Onchocerciasis is only a problem in certain areas of the tropics. However, about half a million people are blind from onchocerciasis.

3. The pattern of tropical eye diseases varies from area to area.

The following are examples of this: −
 - Trachoma is common all over the tropics. However, it is much more severe

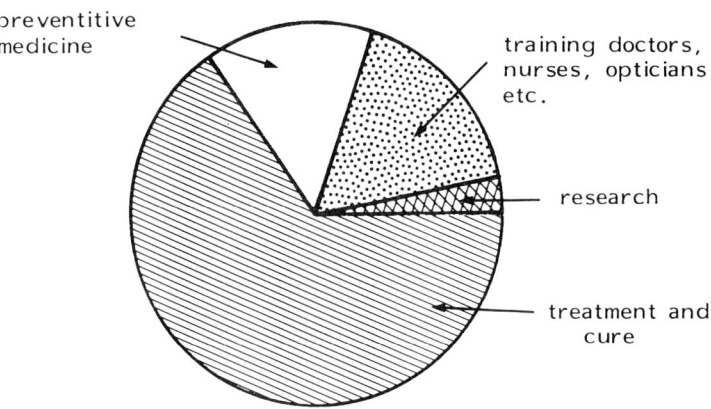

Fig. 1.2 The way most governments spend their money on eye care.

and disabling in dry, desert areas with many flies, than in the tropical rain forests.
- Xerophthalmia and corneal ulcers in children are caused by dietary deficiencies of vitamin A. However, there are many different factors which determine a child's diet. In one area, the staple food may be deficient in vitamin A. In another area, it may be the custom to wean children with foods deficient in vitamin A. In other areas, foods rich in Vitamin A may be too expensive for poor people to buy.
- Measles is a much more important cause of corneal ulceration in Africa than in Asia.

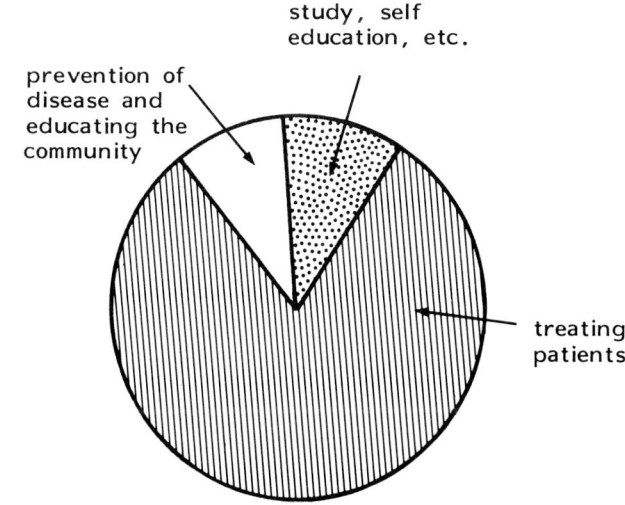

Fig. 1.3 The way most doctors spend their working time.

- Cataract is common all over the world, but it seems to be more common in certain areas, especially the Indian sub-continent.
- Onchocerciasis is very rare on the coast of West Africa. A few hundred miles inland, however, there are areas where almost everyone suffers, and many are blind.

Because eye diseases can vary so much from area to area, any plans for treatment and prevention must be imaginative and flexible. To take the example of corneal ulceration and blindness in young children. It may be appropriate to solve this problem by nutritional advice in one area, adding vitamin A to the food in another, and measles vaccination in yet another. In some areas, the pattern of disease does not fit the textbook pattern. This is especially difficult for a non-specialist, who must rely fairly heavily on textbooks to help diagnose and treat disease.

4. The medical resources are usually inadequate.

Eye diseases are a major health problem all over the tropics. Indeed in some areas, what is only a 'minor speciality' in the West may be the biggest health problem of all. Yet the medical resources to deal with this massive and diverse problem are usually inadequate. In many areas, there is only one eye specialist for a million or more people. (In Western Europe, there is 1 for every 50 000.) Often there is excellent specialist care in the big cities, but none at all in the rural areas.

The medical resources may exist, but are sometimes inappropriate. For example, ophthalmologists in the West have made great progress recently using complicated, sophisticated technology such as the following: –

- Fluorescein angiography, which helps to diagnose retinal disorders.
- Laser photocoagulation, which is used to photocoagulate localized areas of the retina.
- Vitrectomy, which makes vitreous surgery possible.

Instruments such as these are appropriate for North America and Western Europe, but inappropriate for most hot countries. They have many disadvantages: –

- They are very expensive, and therefore expensive for the patient.
- They break down easily, and are difficult to repair.
- They demand a lot of time, effort and skill from the doctor, but often give the patient only a small improvement in health. In other words, they are 'doctor intensive'.

Ophthalmologists are like all professional people. They want to be up to date with the most recent techniques. All too often, however, modern technology prevents the doctor from seeing the real needs of the community. This is especially true in many hot countries.

What are the basic needs for eye care in hot countries?

Unfortunately, it is much easier to define the problems of eye care in hot countries than to solve them! However, most blindness in these countries is either preventable or treatable. Some form of basic eye care therefore offers very real hope for the future. Clearly, this basic eye care will need certain features: –

- Careful planning, flexible enough to match the needs of the community.

- Methods and resources appropriate for even the poorest and least developed countries.
- A lot of effort and determination to succeed.

The exact details of a basic ophthalmic service will obviously vary from area to area. However, five features seem to be essential: –
- Training the right people for the right work
- Mobility
- Cost effectiveness
- Co-operation between different sciences
- An emphasis on prevention

1. Training the right people for the right work

Obviously it is necessary to train more workers in eye care in the tropics. However, it is not at all obvious who are the right people to train, and what are the right skills and knowledge for them to learn. At one extreme, there is the 'barefoot doctor', with very little formal training. The 'barefoot doctor' often mixes herbal and traditional medicine with modern science, but is very well integrated in the community. At the other extreme, there is the modern teaching hospital. Modern teaching hospitals are often called 'disease palaces', and with good reason. They are far too expensive for poor countries with only small health budgets. They also produce graduates who are not always interested in the major health problems of poor and rural communities.

There is an urgent need almost everywhere for some sort of primary health care worker in ophthalmology. The level of training and responsibility necessary for such health workers will vary according to the local situation. Obviously they will need the right incentives and the right motivation. They will also need supervision and encouragement in their work.

There is no need for a health care system to consist only of specialists. It is certainly much cheaper, and probably more effective, to have a few specialists supervising a large number of well-trained, primary health care ophthalmic assistants. The medical profession wishes to maintain high standards, and so is often unwilling to entrust the care of patients to unqualified staff. Unfortunately, this means that many people in the community either have no treatment at all, or must go to totally unqualified 'quacks' for help.

2. Mobility

A service which is mobile can make the most of limited resources and staff over a large area. It is obviously difficult for large numbers of blind (and often old) people to travel long distances. However, a small medical team can easily transport all the necessary equipment for examination and treatment. A mobile service also allows one specialist to supervise several primary health care workers in different outlying areas.

Many areas already operate mobile eye services to screen and assess patients. Some also give medical and surgical treatment, e.g. the mobile eye units which specialize in surgical treatment of cataract in India. These mobile eye units are a fine example of how one country has adapted modern technology to the needs of the community.

3. Cost effectiveness

People often think that cheap medical care is bad medical care. It is true that a few techniques need expensive equipment and take a long time to perform. However, it is possible to diagnose and treat most eye problems simply and quickly using fairly unsophisticated equipment. In other words, it should be possible to provide an eye care service which even the poorest people can afford. However, the greatest challenge in poor countries is how to lower the cost, but still maintain the effectiveness of medical treatment.

4. Co-operation between different sciences

Many of the major eye problems in the tropics need more than one scientific skill to solve them. For example, xerophthalmia is basically a disease of vitamin deficiency. An ophthalmologist is the best person to recognise xerophthalmia, but an expert in nutrition is the best person to solve it. Moreover the solution will only be effective in the community if other experts such as horticulturalists and health educators also lend their skills. The control of onchocerciasis and trachoma requires a similar co-operation between different sciences.

5. An emphasis on prevention

Only one of the five major causes of blindness in the tropics, cataract, is treatable. Blindness which results from the other four, trachoma, xerophthalmia, glaucoma and onchocerciasis is usually untreatable. The first priority in eye care in most tropical areas must therefore be prevention rather than cure.

Unfortunately, most government health spending goes towards curative rather than preventative medicine (*Fig.* 1.2). Also, most doctors and other medical workers spend nearly all their time and energy giving curative treatment (*Fig.* 1.3). There is therefore a huge difference between the health needs of the community and the work of both doctors and governments (Compare *Figs.* 1.1 – 3.)

Curative medicine attracts more interest than preventative medicine, mainly because it gives doctors satisfaction, status and success.
- Satisfaction comes from helping people in their needs, and from using the knowledge and the skills of modern science.
- Status comes from gaining the respect of the community.
- Success obviously comes because people will pay a lot of money for treatment.

In tropical countries there are few doctors available. These doctors are so busy treating patients in the big cities, that there is little interest in preventative or rural medicine.

Preventative medicine appears much less attractive than curative medicine. The clinical work is often repetitive and boring, and administration takes up a lot of time. There are no grateful patients or financial rewards. However, preventative medicine is the only way to solve the problem of unnecessary blindness.

Many people think that preventative medicine is the concern of governments, and that individuals can do little or nothing to prevent disease. It is true that government intervention is necessary to control onchocerciasis. However, the individual medical worker can do a lot to help prevent blindness from the other main blinding diseases, trachoma, xerophthalmia and glaucoma.

- Trachoma is a disease of bad hygiene, and the doctor can teach and encourage good hygiene.
- Xerophthalmia is a disease of poor nutrition, and a doctor can help to improve nutrition. A doctor can also encourage measles vaccination schemes, which are an important way to prevent nutritional blindness.
- Early detection can prevent glaucoma blindness.

In order to prevent unnecessary blindness, the doctor must be in close contact with the community. In this way the doctor becomes more aware of the health needs of the community. The community also becomes more aware how important hygiene and nutrition are in preventing blindness, and how important early diagnosis is. Unfortunately, it is all too easy to see the doctor as a superior and unapproachable person, who dispenses injections and medicines and performs operations.

The practice of preventative medicine is connected to the four other features of basic eye care in hot countries. The use of ophthalmic assistants and mobile clinics will give the greatest contact between the community and the ophthalmic services. Preventative medicine involves the whole community, and so must be cost effective to be of any value. Finally, preventative measures usually require co-ordination and co-operation between various different sciences and organisations.

Reference

1. The International Agency for the Prevention of Blindness (1980) *World Blindness and its Prevention*. Oxford, OUP.

Further reading

WHO (1984) *Strategies for the prevention of Blindness in National Programmes: A Primary Health Care Approach*. Geneva

2. Basic Anatomy and Physiology of the Eye

The eyeball

The eyeball consists of three layers of tissue (*Fig.* 2.1): –
– An outer protective layer.
– A middle layer of blood vessels, pigment cells and muscle fibres.
– An inner, light sensitive layer, called the 'retina'.

The outer layer — the sclera and cornea

The outer layer is tough and thick, and is made of collagen fibres. Most of this layer is opaque, and is called the sclera (which means tough). The anterior part is transparent, and so allows light to enter the eye. This transparent 'window' is called the cornea.

The cornea itself consists of three layers (*Fig.* 2.2): –
– The surface epithelium is five or six cells thick, and is continuous with the epithelium of the conjunctiva. These epithelial cells are constantly changing. The cells at the surface are shed, and are replaced by cell division.
– The inert stroma forms the main bulk of the cornea. This stroma consists of specialized collagen fibres which are arranged in a regular pattern to make them transparent.
  – The anterior layer of the stroma is called 'Bowman's membrane', and is a special supporting membrane for the epithelium.
  – The posterior layer of the stroma is called 'Descemet's membrane', and is a tough supporting membrane for the endothelium.
– The endothelium lining the inner surface of the cornea is a single layer of very active cells. These cells transfer fluid out of the stroma into the anterior chamber of the eye, and so keep the cornea dehydrated. If these cells do not function properly, the cornea swells up and becomes oedematous.

The middle layer — the iris, ciliary body and choroid

If the outer layer of the eyeball is peeled away, the middle layer appears black, soft and round like a grape. This middle layer is called the uvea (which means grape in Latin), and it consists of the iris, the ciliary body and the choroid.
– The iris (*Figs.* 2.1 *and* 2.2) is a diaphragm of mainly pigment cells and smooth muscle fibres. When it contracts, it regulates the light entering the eye.

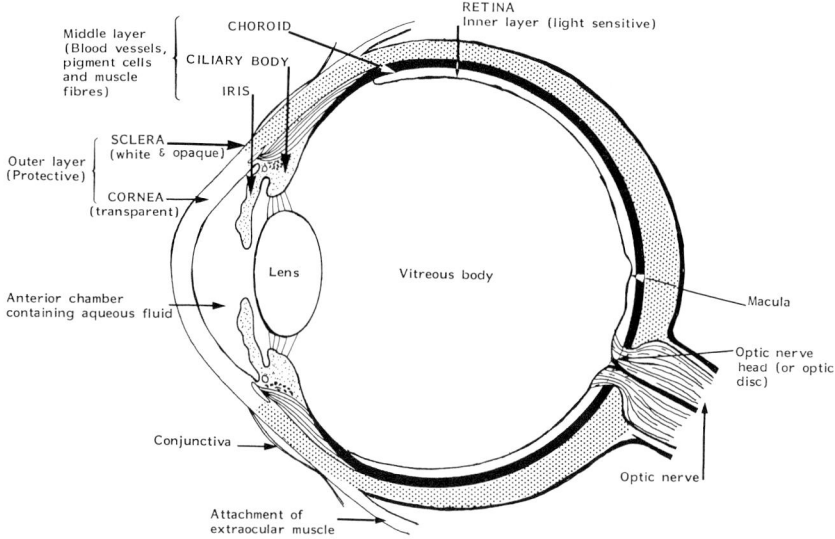

Fig. 2.1 The basic structure of the eye to show its three layers.

- The ciliary body (*Figs.* 2.1 *and* 2.2) is a ring of smooth muscle around the eye. Numerous fine fibres called the suspensory ligament pass from the ciliary

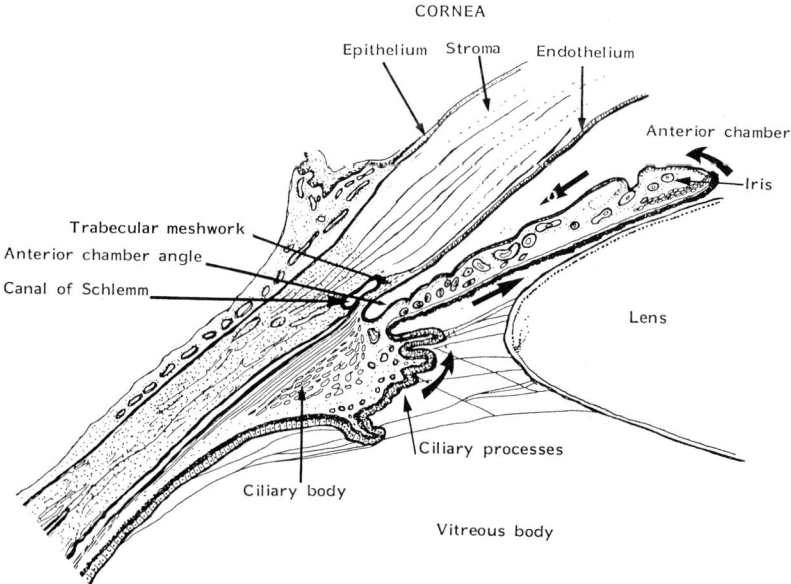

Fig. 2.2 An enlarged view of the angle of the anterior chamber. The thick black arrows show the direction of flow of the aqueous fluid.

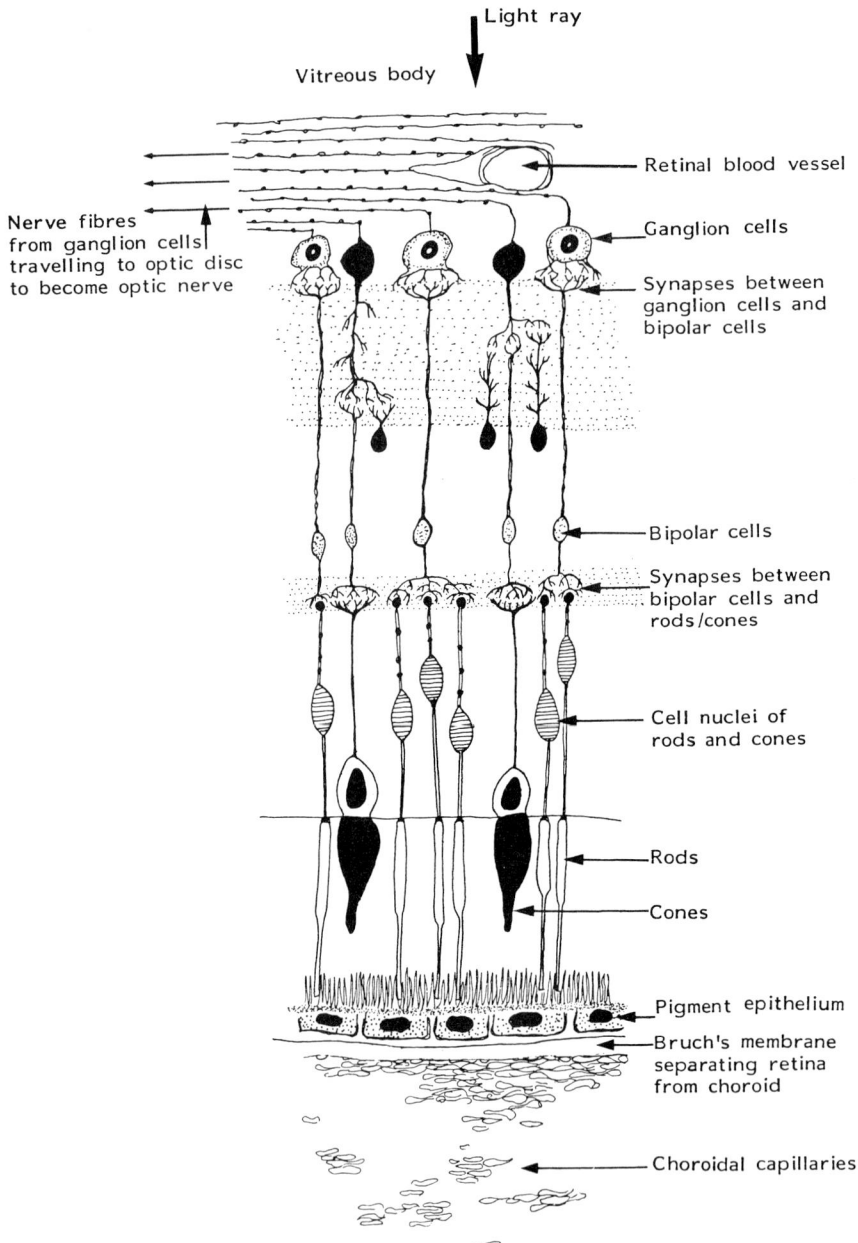

Fig. 2.3 An enlarged and diagrammatic view of the retina to show the arrangement of cells in it.

body to the lens. When the ciliary body contracts, the lens becomes more round in shape and therefore increases its focusing power. This change is called 'accommodation'.

- The choroid (*Figs.* 2.1 *and* 2.3) consists mainly of blood vessels and pigment cells. It lies next to the retina and is essential for the health of the retina. The pigment cells absorb light inside the eye, and so prevent unwanted reflections.

The inner layer — the retina

The retina is the light sensitive membrane at the back of the eye (*Figs.* 2.1 *and* 2.3). The cells of the retina are specialized, and have a very complex arrangement.
- On the outer surface, next to the choroid, is a single layer of pigment epithelial cells. The light sensitive cells, the rods and cones, rest on this layer. The rods are more sensitive in dim light, and these are found in the periphery of the retina. The cones are more sensitive in bright light, and these are found towards the centre of the retina. The very centre of the retina is called the 'macula'. The macula consists of closely packed cone cells.
- The inner layers of the retina consist of the bipolar and ganglion cells, as well as their nerve fibres and synapses (or junctions). Light entering the eye passes through the transparent retina to reach the rods and cones. These produce electrical impulses when they are exposed to light. The bipolar and ganglion cells and their synapses relay and modify these impulses.
- The nerve fibres from the ganglion cells travel to the optic disc, where they acquire a myelin sheath and unite to form the optic nerve. The optic nerve then passes backwards through the sclera. The retinal blood vessels which pass out from the optic disc to the retina run on the surface of the nerve fibre layer.

The lens and the vitreous body

The lens consists of closely packed transparent cells enclosed in a capsule (*Figs.* 2.1 *and* 2.2). It is attached to the fibres of the suspensory ligament. The lens and the cornea together focus the light on the retina. Four-fifths of the focusing power of the eye is in the cornea, and only one-fifth in the lens. The lens is the only solid structure inside the eye. Behind the lens is the vitreous body (*Fig.* 2.1). This is an inert, transparent jelly which fills most of the eye.

The aqueous fluid and the intraocular pressure (*see Fig.* 2.2.)

The aqueous fluid is secreted by the epithelial cells of the ciliary processes on the surface of the ciliary body. This fluid passes between the iris and the lens, and enters the anterior chamber of the eye. Here it circulates and controls the pressure in the eye.

The aqueous fluid is absorbed from the angle of the anterior chamber where the iris meets the back of the cornea. There is some specialized, sponge-like tissue here called the trabecular meshwork. The aqueous fluid passes through this meshwork into a collecting channel called the 'canal of Schlemm'. If the aqueous fluid does not drain away properly, there is a rise in the intraocular pressure. This causes a disease called 'glaucoma'.

The visual pathways (*Fig.* 2.4)

The visual pathways connect the optic nerve with the part of the brain concerned with vision. This is the occipital part of the cerebral cortex.

The optic nerve is not really a nerve, but a tract of the central nervous system. For this reason, it is surrounded by a sheath of dura which contains cerebrospinal fluid. It is also unable to regenerate after damage, because there are no Schwann cells or neurilemma around the individual fibres. (Schwann cells are responsible for the regeneration of damaged nerves.)

The optic nerve passes backwards from the eye to the apex of the orbit, then through the optic foramen into the skull. Inside the skull, the two optic nerves meet at the optic chiasm, just above the pituitary fossa, to form the optic tracts. The optic tracts then pass round the brainstem to the lateral geniculate body. Fibres from the optic tract synapse here with different nerve cells. The fibres from these cells then pass in the optic radiations to the occipital cortex at the posterior end of the cerebral hemisphere.

When both optic nerves meet at the chiasm, all the fibres from the nasal part of each retina cross over to the opposite side. In this way, everything in the left half

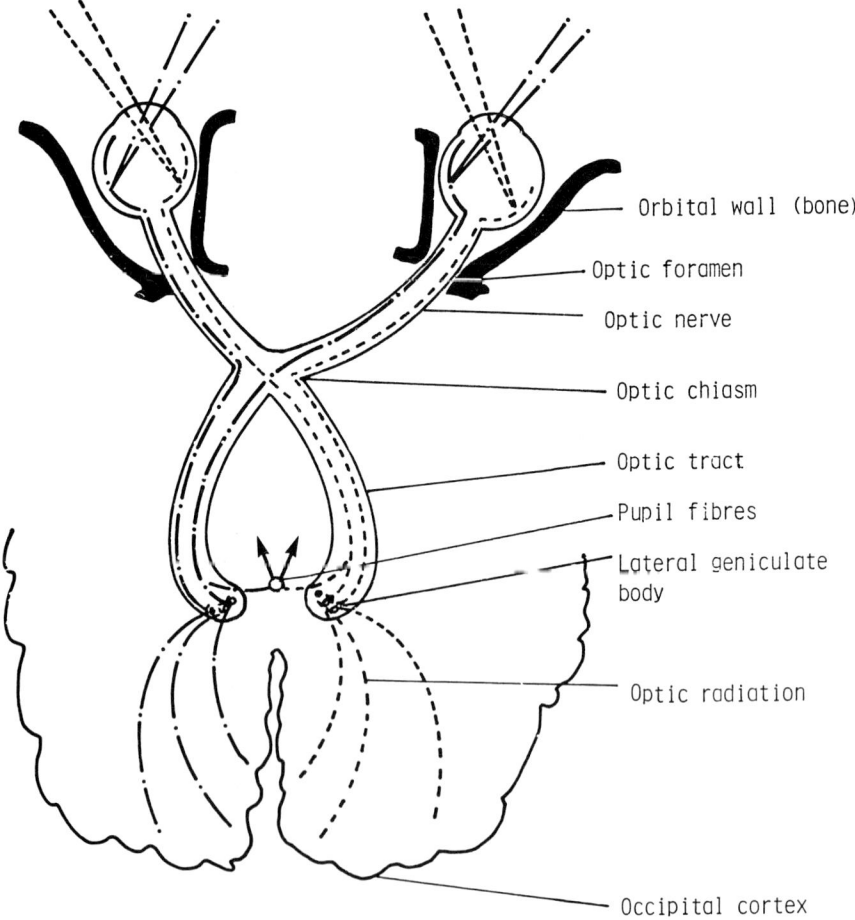

Orbital wall (bone)

Optic foramen

Optic nerve

Optic chiasm

Optic tract

Pupil fibres

Lateral geniculate body

Optic radiation

Occipital cortex

Fig. 2.4 The visual pathways from the retina to the brain.

of the field of vision in each eye is seen on the right side of each retina, and by the right side of the brain (see the dotted lines in *Fig.* 2.4). In the same way, everything in the right half of the field of vision in each eye is seen by the left side of the brain.

A few fibres in the optic nerve regulate the pupil size. These fibres pass to the brainstem. Here they connect with the nucleus of the third cranial nerve, which controls the size of the pupil. In this way, the pupil constricts when light is shone in the eye. Connections go to both sides, so that light shone in one eye causes both pupils to constrict equally.

The protection of the eye

The conjunctiva, the eyelids and the lacrimal apparatus protect the eye from injury and infection. They also keep the cornea healthy, moist and transparent.

The conjunctiva

The conjunctiva is a thin mucous membrane which lines the inner surface of the eyelids and the outer surface of the eyeball (*Fig.* 2.5). The part lining the eyelids is called the 'tarsal conjunctiva', and it is firmly attached to the underlying tarsal plate. The part lining the eyeball is called the 'bulbar conjunctiva', but it is only very loosely attached to the underlying sclera. The tarsal and bulbar conjunctiva are continuous with each other at the fornix.

The conjunctival epithelium is continuous with the corneal epithelium at the margin of the cornea. This is called the 'limbus'.

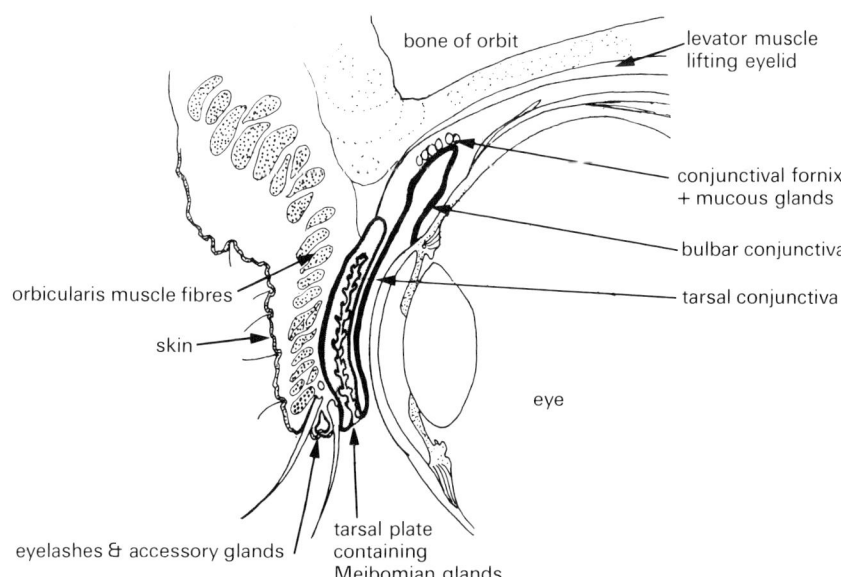

Fig. 2.5 The structure of the eyelids and conjunctiva.

Beneath the epithelial surface, the conjunctiva contains many small islands of lymphoid tissue, and many goblet cells which secrete mucus. Both of these are especially numerous in the fornix.

The main function of the conjunctiva is to protect the cornea: −

- When the eyelids are shut, the conjunctiva covers the cornea, and supplies some of its oxygen and metabolic needs.
- When the eyelids are open, it lubricates the cornea with tears.
- The conjunctiva also protects the exposed parts of the eye from infection. Conjunctival secretions contain antibodies and lymphocytes to fight against specific infections. The secretions also contain lysozyme, which is a non-specific, antibacterial substance. For these reasons the conjunctiva has been described as a 'lymph node, cut open and lined with epithelium'.

The eyelids

The eyelids protect the eye and keep the cornea healthy and moist. The upper eyelid is more important than the lower eyelid, and diseases of the upper eyelid are more likely to affect the cornea. *Fig.* 2.5 shows the basic structure of the eyelid.

- The tarsal plate is a fibrous structure which keeps the eyelids rigid, and which contains the Meibomian glands. These glands open out at the lid margin, and make a waxy secretion which helps to form the corneal tear film. The conjunctiva lines the posterior surface of the tarsal plate.
- The orbicularis oculi muscle fibres are in front of the tarsal plate. The seventh cranial (or facial) nerve stimulates this muscle to close the eyelids.
- The levator muscle is also attached to the tarsal plate of the upper lid. This muscle opens the eyelids, and is supplied partly by the IIIrd cranial nerve, and partly by the cervical sympathetic nerve.

The Lacrimal Apparatus

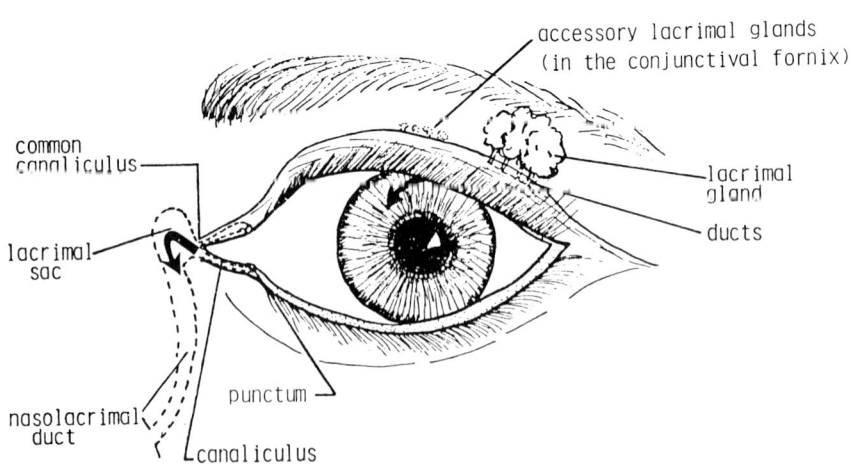

Fig. 2.6 The lacrimal apparatus. The arrows show the direction of tear flow.

The eyelids have a very rich blood supply, and the eyelid skin is very fine and very loose. The eyelashes are specialized hairs, and there are numerous sweat and sebaceous glands near their roots.

The lacrimal apparatus

The function of the lacrimal apparatus is to produce and drain the tears (*Fig.* 2.6). The tears form a thin film of fluid on the surface of the conjunctiva and cornea. This tear film is vital for the health and transparency of the cornea. It contains: –
– mucus which the conjunctival goblet cells secrete to keep the cornea moist,
– a waxy secretion from the Meibomian glands which prevents the tears from drying.

The lacrimal gland only produces excessive tears in response to injury, inflammation or emotional stress. Normally, the tears come almost entirely from the conjunctiva and small accessory glands in the conjunctival fornix.

The tears drain into the nose through the nasolacrimal passages. The tears drain into the punctum, which is a tiny opening at the inner end of each eyelid. A narrow canaliculus passes from the punctum to the lacrimal sac. Opening and closing the eyelids helps to 'milk' the tears into the lacrimal sac, and then down the nasolacrimal duct into the nose.

The extraocular muscles

There are six extraocular muscles which control eye movement (*Fig.* 2.7). They form a cone which passes backwards from the eye to the apex of the orbit. The actions of these muscles are rather complex. For a brief description, *see* Chapter 17.

The orbit

The orbit is a bony cavity which encloses the eye and the structures associated with the eye. The front of the orbit is thick, strong bone which protects the eye

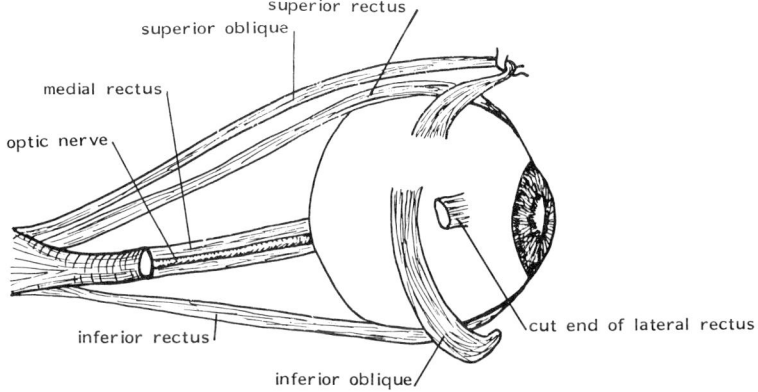

Fig. 2.7 The extraocular muscles seen from the lateral side of the orbit. The lateral rectus muscle has been partly removed to show the optic nerve and the medial rectus muscle.

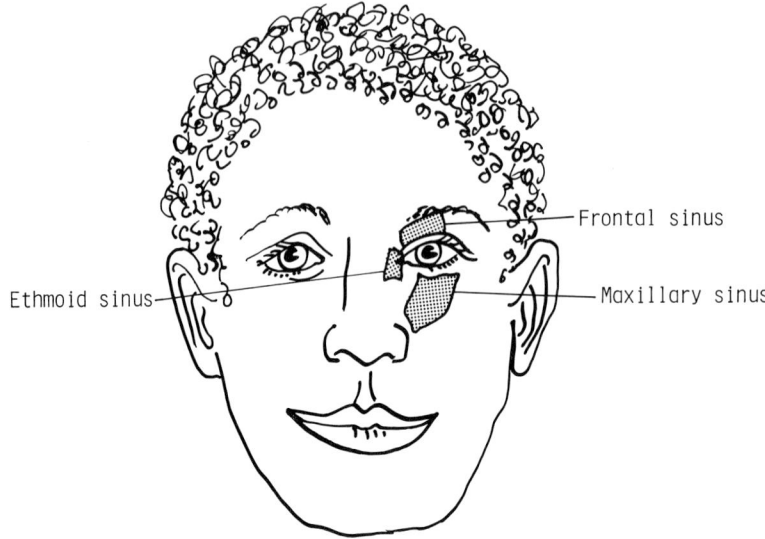

Fig. 2.8 The position of the nasal sinuses in relation to the eye and orbit.

from injury. It is easy to feel this bone under the skin of the cheek and the eyebrow. The walls of the orbit which separate the orbital contents from the nasal sinuses are, however, very thin bone. (*Fig.* 2.8) For this reason, nasal disease occasionally spreads into the orbit.

3. Clinical Methods —
History Taking and Eye Examination

To assess a patient with eye disease, it is necessary to take the patient's history, test the vision and examine the eye. There is usually no need for special investigations, such as X-rays and blood tests.
– History taking is usually fairly simple. The aim is to discover exactly what the patient's complaints are.
– Testing the vision is also fairly simple, except in young children.
– Examining the eye is the most important part of the assessment. It is also the most difficult.

History taking

It often helps to find out some background information about the patient e.g. age, sex, occupation and literacy. Such information will indicate what vision the patient needs for work and for personal satisfaction. It will also show if there is a risk of any particular environmental or occupational eye disease. The patient's diet, drinking and smoking habits are also sometimes relevant.

It is important to ask about previous treatment. In many areas where there are not enough doctors, the patient may have gone to a traditional healer, bought some medicine from the market, or used another person's medicine. Complications from such 'treatment' are quite frequent. It is true that traditional healers can give useful treatment for certain diseases. However, the eye is such a delicate organ that any interference is at best useless, and at worst very harmful.

The family history may also be important. Many eye diseases run in families, such as myopia and glaucoma. Members of the same family also share a common environment.

There are obviously many possible symptoms of eye disease, but they usually come under one of two headings: loss or alteration of vision, and discomfort or pain in the eye.

Loss or alteration of vision

Loss of vision is the most common visual symptom. Ask the patient if the onset was sudden or gradual, if there was any pain at first, and if there is any pain now. Visual loss is usually very obvious to the patient. However, the patient may not be

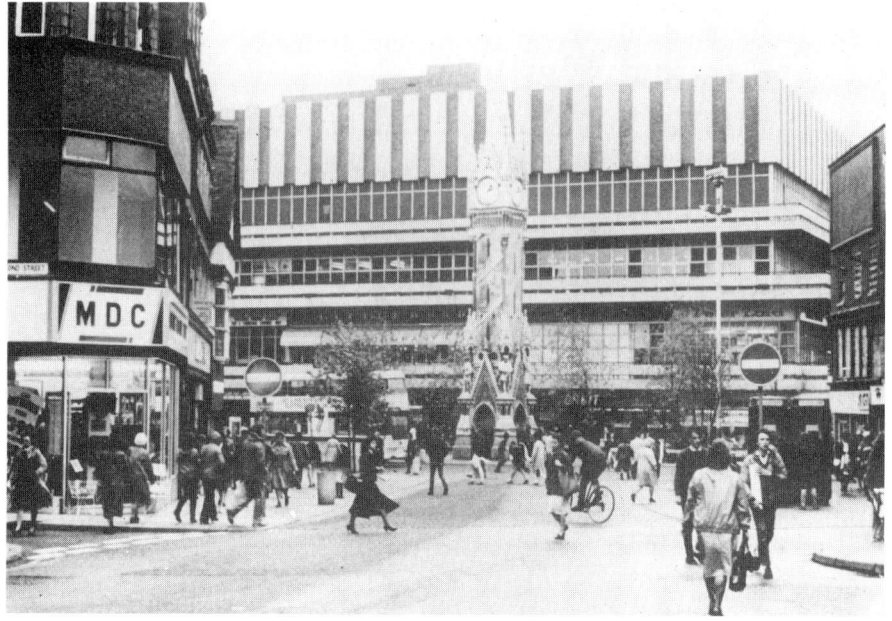

a — to someone with normal sight.

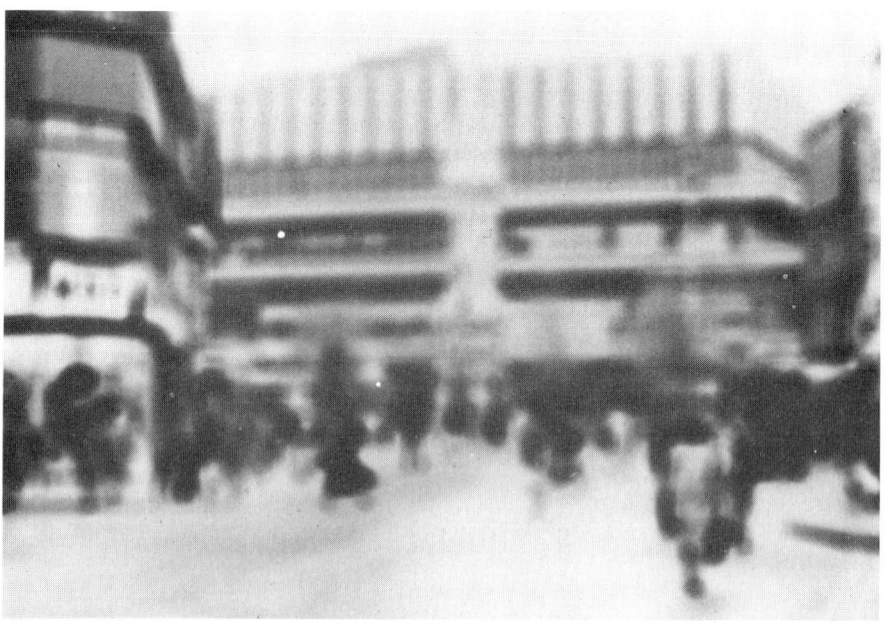

b — to someone with short sight.

Fig. 3.1 A street scene as it appears to four different people.

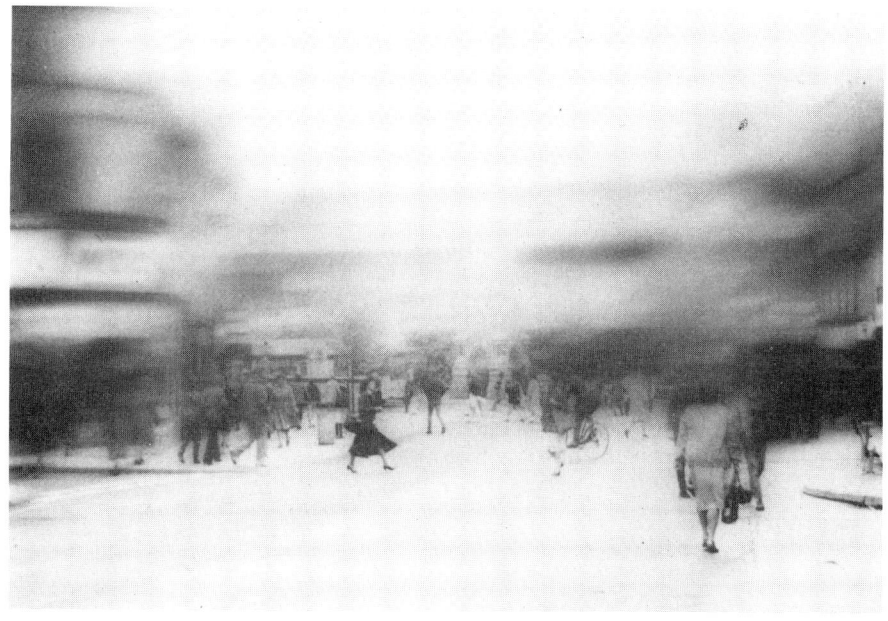

c — to someone with early cataract.

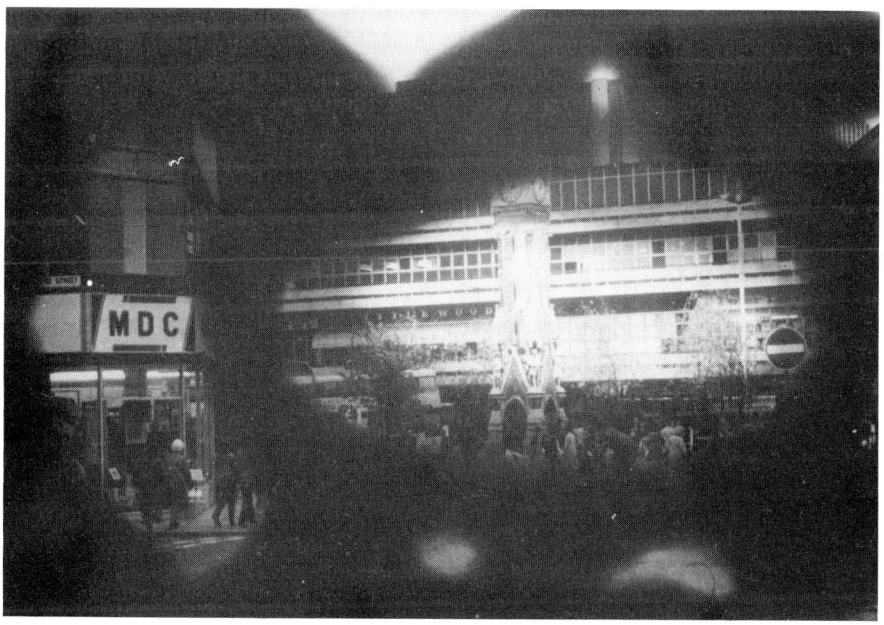

d — to someone with visual field defects, e.g. glaucoma.

Fig. 3.1 *cont.*

aware of a gradual loss of vision in one eye only, or gradual constriction of the visual field. Various alterations of vision may occur (*see also Fig.* 3.1): –

– Dazzling, or difficulty seeing in bright light may be caused by opacities in the cornea or lens.
– Photophobia is discomfort caused by bright light. It is usually a sign of inflammatory eye disease, especially a corneal ulcer.
– Distortion of shapes usually indicates a disturbance of the retina around the macula.
– Haloes, or rainbow-coloured rings around lights are caused either by early opacities in the lens, or by corneal oedema. Very small drops of fluid in the cornea split white light into the colours of the spectrum. Corneal oedema often indicates a rise in intraocular pressure.
– Visual field defects may be caused by various disorders in the retina, optic nerve or visual pathways.
– Spots which 'float' in front of the eyes (floaters) are usually caused by small opacities in the vitreous body, which cast a shadow on the retina.

Discomfort or pain in the eye

This is usually a symptom of inflammation of the eye, or of the structures surrounding the eye.

– The conjunctiva is not very sensitive to pain. Typically, conjunctivitis presents with discomfort, irritation or grittiness rather than pain.
– The iris and cornea are both very sensitive to pain. Iritis, corneal ulcers and acute glaucoma are three common eye conditions which are characterized by acute pain.
– Inflammation of the choroid (choroiditis) or optic nerve (optic neuritis) usually produces a sensation of dull pain behind the eye.

'Eye strain' and tiredness of the eyes are common complaints. Sometimes the extraocular muscles of both eyes are not equally balanced, and this causes eye strain. However, it is more likely that the cause is psychological rather than organic, and means that the patient cannot cope with the stresses of everyday life. Eye strain is very common among students who are having difficulties with their studies. (Many people think that eye strain is caused by refractive errors, and that the patient needs spectacles. However, refractive errors usually cause blurring of the vision rather than any specific discomfort or pain.)

Other symptoms

– Discharge, or watering of the eyes is common. It usually indicates conjunctivitis, or an obstruction in the lacrimal passages.
– Diplopia (double vision) is a feature of many types of squint. It will disappear when one eye is shut. Occasionally both the two images come from one eye only. This is usually caused by an opacity in the cornea or lens, which prevents the light rays from focusing clearly on the retina.
– A headache is a very common symptom, but it is not usually caused by eye disease. However, diseases such as hypertension and intracranial tumours cause headaches and may also produce eye changes.

Testing the vision

The human eye is an extremely complex organ, and there are many different ways to test the vision. In practice, however, only three types of test are used: —
— Visual acuity, which tests if the patient can see small objects or letters in good light directly ahead.
— The visual field, which tests the overall area of vision for each eye.
— Colour vision, which tests if the patient can discriminate between different colours.

Visual acuity

It is important to test the visual acuity in each eye separately, if possible. This is usually measured with a Snellen's chart (*Fig.* 3.2), showing either letters, or pictures for patients who cannot read. If the vision is very poor, other tests are usually more appropriate.

Unfortunately, the method for recording visual acuity is rather complicated. Near each line on the chart is a small number. This number is the distance (in metres) at which a person with normal sight should be able to see that line. For example, a normal person can see the top letter at 60 metres, the second line at 36 metres, and so on. The patient stands 6 metres away from the chart, and reads as much as he can.

If the patient can only see the top letter of the chart, his vision is 6/60. If he can see as far as the second line, his vision is 6/36, and so on. (The top number of the

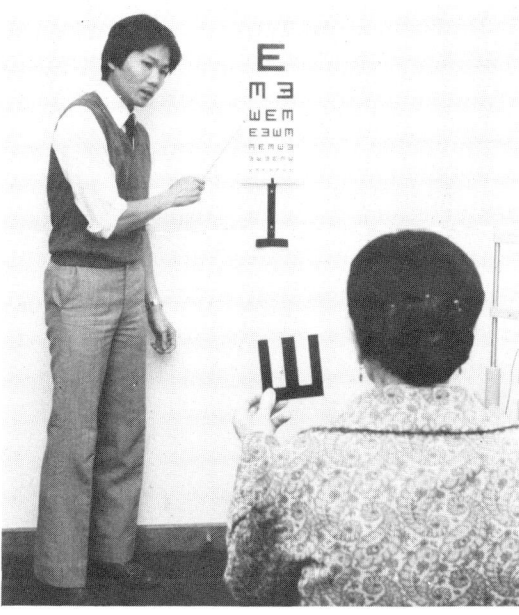

Fig. 3.2 A Snellen's chart used for patients who cannot read. The chart is identical for patients who can read, except that different letters are used.

fraction is the distance between the patient and the chart. The bottom number is the number of the smallest line of letters the patient can read.) A patient with normal sight should reach the line which is marked with a 6. This is 6/6 vision.

If the vision is below 6/60 and the patient cannot even see the top letter, he should come nearer the chart until he can see it. If he can see it at 2 metres, his vision is 2/60. If he can only see it at 1 metre, his vision is 1/60. Another method of testing people with poor vision is to ask the patient to count fingers. The human finger is about the same size as the top letter on the chart, and so counting fingers at 6 metres is about equal to 6/60 vision. Counting fingers (CF) at 1 metre distance is therefore the same as 1/60.

If the vision is below 1/60, the patient may still be able to detect the movement of a hand in front of his eye. If not, the final test is to shine a light into his eye.

There are therefore 3 more categories: −

HM   — Hand movements can be seen in front of the eye.

PL   — Perception of a light shone into the eye.

NPL — No perception of light, or total blindness.

If there is perception of light, it is also important to test if the patient can identify the direction the light is coming from. This is called projection of light. Good projection usually indicates that the retina and optic nerve are functioning normally. The defect is probably an opacity in the cornea, lens or vitreous body, and is treatable. Poor projection of light indicates retinal or optic nerve disease, and is probably untreatable.

It is necessary to re-test any patient with defective visual acuity through a pinhole (*Fig.* 3.3). This minimizes any refractive errors (page 48 explains how the pinhole test works). If the visual acuity improves when the patient looks through a pinhole, it indicates an error of refraction, which spectacles can usually correct. If there is no improvement, then the loss of vision is from eye disease.

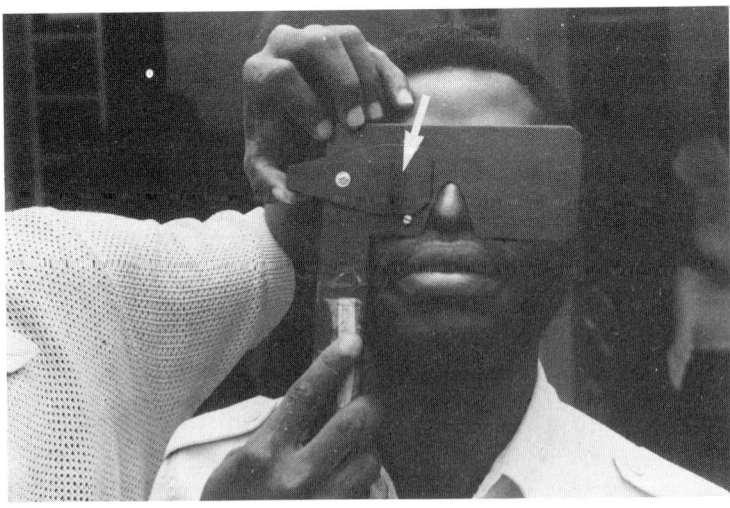

Fig. 3.3 Testing the vision through a pinhole. The white arrow points to several tiny holes in the black plastic screen.

If the patient is a young child, or an adult who cannot read, it will be necessary to use different symbols on the chart. These may be simple pictures of common objects, or a letter (usually either E or C) pointing in different directions. The patient holds a card with this letter on it, and must turn it so that it matches each symbol on the chart (*Fig.* 3.2). For testing very young children, it is best not to use a chart, but only show them a single picture or letter at a time. Showing them the whole chart will only confuse them. Testing the visual acuity of these, and indeed all patients, in both eyes takes time, but it is very important. It is also a task which an assistant can easily be trained to do.

6/6 vision is considered normal. A visual acuity of 6/12 is generally good enough to hold a driving licence, and 6/18 or better is adequate for most ordinary tasks in life. A patient with less than 3/60 vision will have great difficulty doing any work which requires vision, and is usually considered 'blind'. However, if the visual field is good, he may still be able to get around and lead an independent life.

The visual field

It is not routine to test the visual field in all patients. However, it is important to test any patients with suspected glaucoma, diseases of the optic nerves or visual pathways, and certain retinal diseases. Testing the visual field requires the patient to concentrate, and this is often difficult for children, and for old or unsophisticated people.

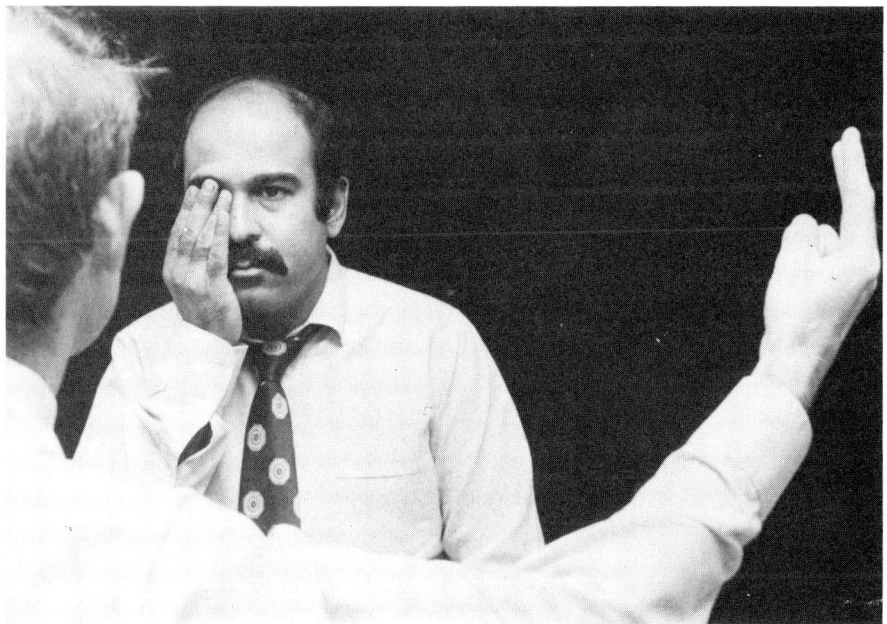

Fig. 3.4 Testing the visual field by confrontation.

In all visual field tests, each eye is tested separately, while the other eye is covered over. The patient must fix his gaze on a target or spot in front of him. The examiner then sees at what angle objects come into the patient's range of vision.

– The confrontation test (*Fig.* 3.4) requires no special equipment. It is very simple to perform, but will detect serious visual field defects. It works by comparing the patient's visual field with the examiner's.
– A calibrated black screen (the Bjerrum screen) and small white targets can be used to obtain a more accurate result (*Fig.* 3.5).
– Various instruments are available which can give a very detailed assessment of the visual field. These are used in specialist units, where technicians and assistants can be trained to use them. However, they are too expensive and take up too much time for general use.

Colour vision

It is usual to test the vision with special coloured charts called 'Ishihara charts'. However, specific colour vision defects are not very common, and so there is rarely any need for this test.

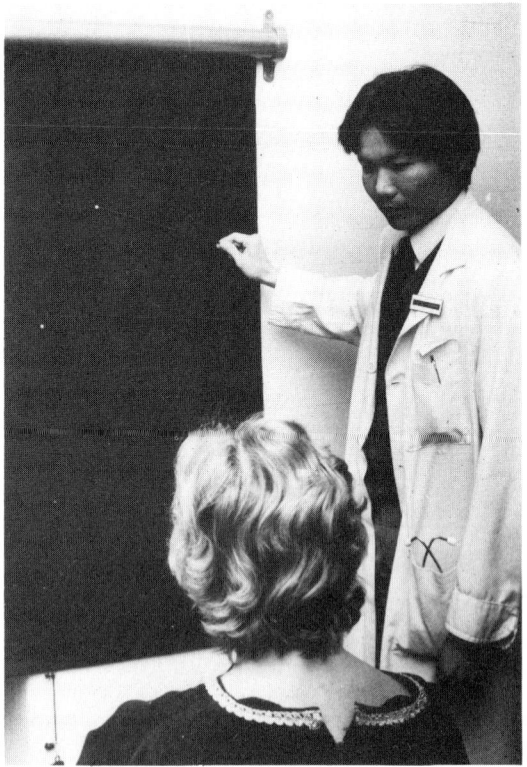

Fig. 3.5 Testing the visual field with a Bjerrum screen.

Examining the eye

Nearly all parts of the eye are visible either with the naked eye, or with the appropriate optical instrument. It is essential that anyone who cares for eye patients should know how to examine the eye. It is also essential to have the right instruments to make the examination. Some ophthalmic diagnostic instruments are very expensive, but a reasonable examination is possible with only a few simple instruments. There is indeed a great need for simple robust equipment, cheap to produce and distribute to small clinics in less developed countries all over the world.

It is possible to see all the parts of the eye with only two basic types of instrument: –

– An ophthalmoscope, to examine the back part of the eye. This is usually called the 'fundus', and it consists of the retina, choroid and optic nerve.
– Some form of magnification and illumination to examine the front part of the eye (the cornea, iris, anterior chamber and lens), and also the conjunctiva and eyelids.

Examining the fundus, and using the ophthalmoscope

Basically, the ophthalmoscope is a form of illumination which allows the examiner to look down the same axis as the rays of light. The patient's own cornea and lens act as a 'magnifying lens' to anyone looking into the eye, and so no extra magnification is necessary. To see the fundus clearly, the ocular media must be healthy and transparent. It is also necessary to dilate the pupil with mydriatic drops. The image of the fundus then appears through the ophthalmoscope about 15 times larger than its actual size. In a myopic patient, the magnification is greater, and in a hypermetropic patient it is less.

The standard instrument is called a 'direct ophthalmoscope'. It is important to hold it very close both to the examiner's and to the patient's eye. If the patient wears spectacles, it is best to remove them, and to use a correcting lens in the ophthalmoscope instead. If the examiner wears spectacles, he can either keep them on or use a lens of equal power in the ophthalmoscope. The procedure is then as follows (*Fig. 3.6*): –

– To examine the patient's right eye, hold the ophthalmoscope in the right hand, and hold the patient's head still with the left hand.
– Rest the right hand against the patient's cheek, so that the ophthalmoscope is just in front, but not touching the patient's eye.
– Bring one's own right eye up to the sight-hole, and look down into the patient's eye.
– To examine the patient's left eye, use the left hand and eye instead of the right, and vice versa.
– If the patient is myopic, it can be especially difficult to get a clear view of the fundus. In this case, hold the instrument as close as possible to the patient's eye.

Specialists sometimes use a different type of ophthalmoscope, called an 'indirect ophthalmoscope'. The examiner wears a special headlight, and holds a condensing lens in front of the patient's eye (*see Fig. 3.11*). To use an indirect ophthalmoscope requires both skill and practice, but it produces a very clear 3-dimensional view of a large area of the fundus. It is especially useful in assessing

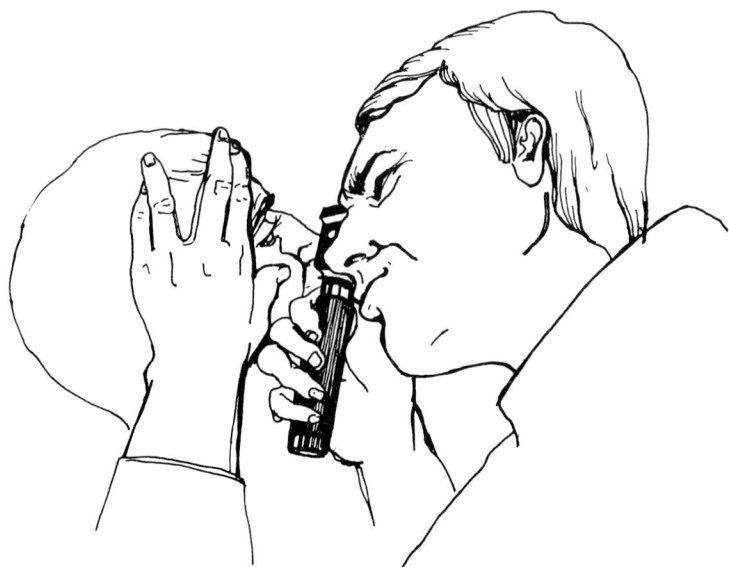

Fig. 3.6 Using a direct ophthalmoscope.

retinal detachments, examining myopic patients, or in looking through opacities in the ocular media.

The slit lamp can also be used for detailed examination of the fundus, but it needs a special mirrored contact lens.

Examining the front part of the eye

Obvious disorders in the front part of the eye can be seen without any special instruments. For a detailed examination, however, some form of magnification and illumination are both necessary. The best instrument for this is a slit lamp (*Fig.* 3.7). This is a binocular microscope with an adjustable beam of bright light. The disadvantage of the slit lamp is that it is very expensive and not portable. Fortunately, there are simpler ways to provide magnification and some illumination.

- Magnification. A hand-held magnifying lens (often called a 'loupe') is basically a strong convex lens which is held just in front of the eye (*Fig.* 3.8). The examiner will need to hold some sort of light source with his other hand. Many people do not realize that the ophthalmoscope can also be used as a magnifying lens, with a built-in light source. Hold the ophthalmoscope very close to the patient's eye, as in fundus examination, but using a very strong positive lens, e.g. +15 or +20 dioptres in the ophthalmoscope. It is now focused on the front part of the eye, and will give a clear, enlarged view of the conjunctiva, cornea, iris or lens. The focus can be adjusted either by moving it slightly nearer or further from the eye, or by using a different positive lens in the ophthalmoscope.
- Illumination. Good illumination is also necessary to see many of the delicate

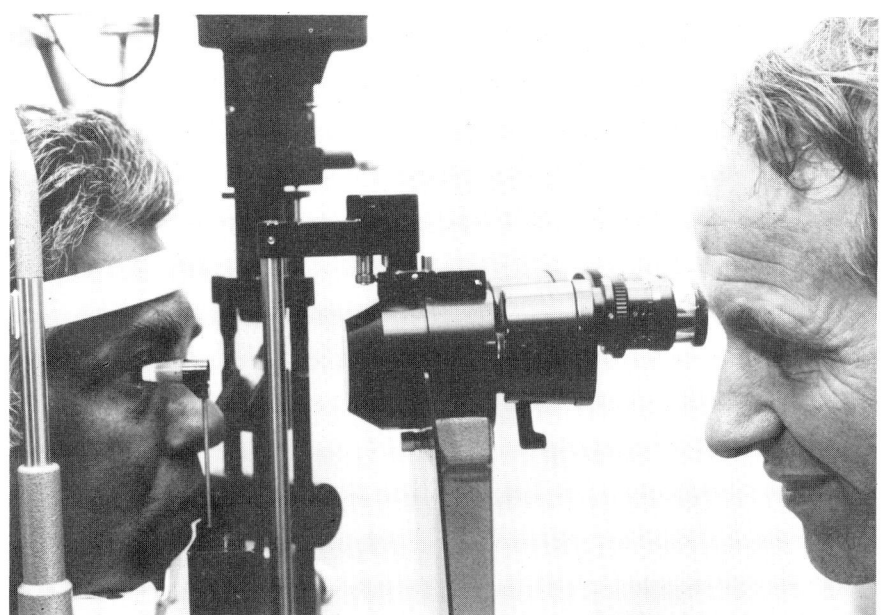

Fig. 3.7 A slit lamp, and an applanation tonometer.

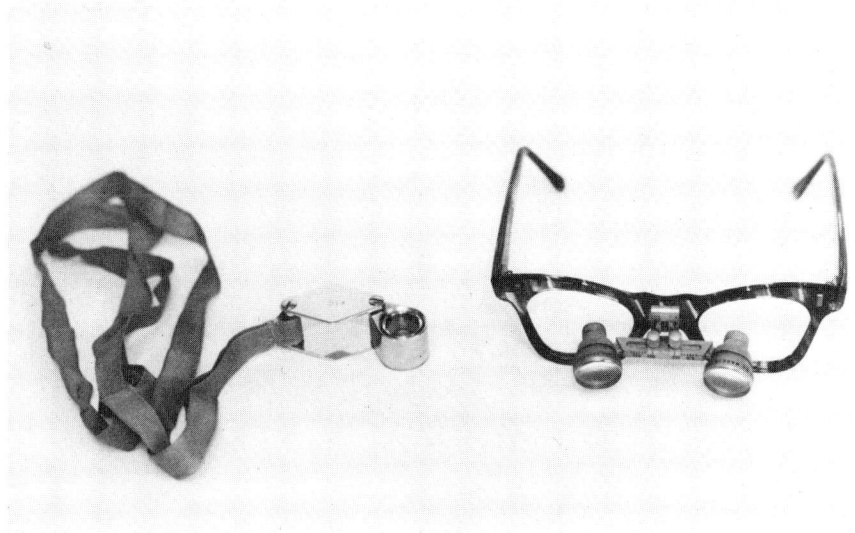

Fig. 3.8 Two different types of simple magnifying lenses. On the left a hand-held magnifying lens (X 10 magnification) for examining the front part of the eye. On the right binocular telescopic glasses (X 3 magnification). These are very useful for eye surgery.

pathological changes in the front of the eye and the transparent ocular media.
Three different types of illumination are used to examine the eye: –

1. Diffuse illumination (*Plate* 1a) means that the rays of light are travelling in all
directions. Normal daylight, electric light or torch light are examples of diffuse
illumination.

2. Focal illumination (*Plate* 1b) means that a small beam of light rays converge
upon a point. Examples of focal illumination are the slit lamp, and also some
hand torches for examining the eye which give a converging beam of light.

3. Coaxial illumination (*Plate* 1c) means that the examiner looks down the path
(or axis) of the light rays. An ophthalmoscope has this type of illumination.

Plate 1 shows a normal eye with these three types of illumination. Opaque
structures such as the sclera and iris appear much the same with all three types of
illumination. However, the transparent ocular media (that is the cornea, lens and
vitreous) look very different with these three different types of illumination.
– Focal illumination shows up any tiny defect or opacity which is not visible
  with diffuse illumination. An example of this is a room containing some
  smoke or dust. The smoke or dust is difficult to see with normal illumination.
  However, if a ray of sunlight enters the room through one small window, it
  will highlight the particles of smoke or dust. In the same way, focal
  illumination shows up cells or protein exudate in the anterior chamber. Focal
  illumination also shows up the structure of the cornea and the lens much more
  clearly. By looking at *Plate* 1b, it is possible to assess the thickness of the
  cornea and the lens, and also the depth of the anterior chamber. This is not
  possible with other types of illumination.
– Coaxial illumination from an ophthalmoscope can also be used to detect any
  small defect or opacity in the ocular media. It is necessary to dilate the pupil,
  so that a red glow of reflected light from the fundus is seen in the pupil. This is
  called the 'red reflex'. Against this red glow, any small opacity in the ocular
  media stands out as a small shadow. There are two ways of bringing these
  opacities into focus: –

1. To get a general view of the cornea, lens and vitreous, use a weak positive
lens (about + 5 dioptres) in the ophthalmoscope. Hold it close to your own
eye, but about 20 cm from the patient's eye. Then bring it slowly closer to the
patient's eye, looking through the ophthalmoscope all the time. In this way
first the cornea, then the lens, and then the vitreous will come into focus, and
any opacity in them can be seen.
2. To get a magnified view of the cornea and lens, use a strong positive lens
(about + 20 dioptres) in the ophthalmoscope. Hold it very close to your own
eye and very close to the patient's eye. The cornea and lens will come into
focus and any tiny opacity can be seen. This is an effective way of seeing
minute opacities in the cornea, such as keratic precipitates, and even the
microfilaria of onchocerciasis.

If the ocular media are completely opaque, then of course no red reflex at
all can be seen coming from the pupil.

It is not necessary to examine every part of the eye in detail in every patient. However, it is best to have a routine system, so that nothing is left out. The usual method is to start at the eyelids, and pass backwards to the fundus.

The eyelids

Most eyelid disorders are fairly obvious, and so do not require any special techniques to observe them. However, two particular disorders are not always obvious, a facial palsy and ingrowing eyelashes: –
– Check that the eyelids open and close properly. Poor eyelid closure from a facial palsy is a serious defect (*see Figs.* 16.2 *and* 16.3).
– Lift up and slightly evert the upper eyelid. Any ingrowing eyelashes will then become visible (*see Fig.* 7.1).

The conjunctiva

Diseases of the conjunctiva are so common in hot countries that examination is essential. Most of the common pathological changes in the conjunctiva are visible, either to the naked eye or with a simple magnifying lens.
– The bulbar conjunctiva (which lines the eyeball) is easy to see. Hold the eyelids open and ask the patient to look in different directions.
– The lower fornix and the conjunctiva which lines the lower eyelid are also easy to examine. Simply pull down the lower lid.
– The upper tarsal conjunctiva (which lines the upper lid) is more difficult to examine. However, it is a common site for foreign bodies, and for pathological changes, especially in trachoma. With a little practice, the following technique can be used to examine the upper tarsal conjunctiva without causing any discomfort to the patient (*Fig.* 3.9): –
  – Ask the patient to look down, and not squeeze the eyes shut.
  – Hold the upper lid eyelashes between the finger and thumb of one hand, and gently stretch the eyelid.

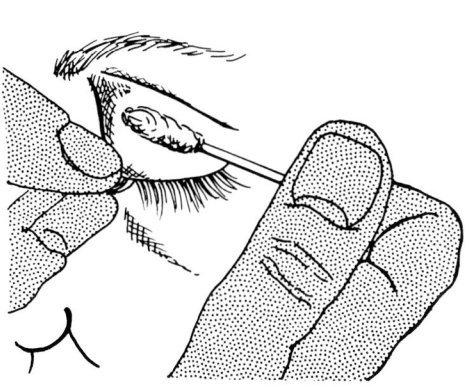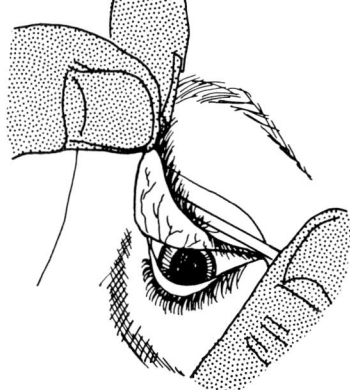

Fig. 3.9 Everting the upper eyelid.

— With the other hand, rest a cottonwool bud or glass rod on the upper
  margin of the tarsal plate, so that there is very slight pressure.
— Flick the tarsal plate inside out.
— The upper fornix is inaccessible, and so very difficult to examine.

The cornea

Diseases of the cornea are also very common in hot countries, and so examination
is essential. In theory, this should be easy, because the cornea is right at the front
of the eye. Indeed severe corneal disorders are usually obvious. However, many
diseases produce changes in the cornea which are small and faint, and so more
difficult to detect. Fortunately, it is possible to recognise most of these faint
corneal changes by using some form of magnification, focal illumination or even
an ophthalmoscope (*see above*).

An ulcer on the surface of the cornea is a common and important condition. A
shallow epithelial ulcer can be difficult to detect, but stains very easily with
fluorescein dye. It is therefore essential to put a drop of fluorescein into the
conjunctival sac of any patient with a painful red eye (*see Plates* 7e, 23b, c *and* d).

Opaque scars, blood vessels and other opacities may occur in the stroma. Cells
or debris may collect on the posterior surface of the cornea. These are called
'keratic precipitates', and indicate inflammation inside the eye. Corneal oedema
makes the cornea appear hazy rather than transparent, and is an important sign.

The cornea is very sensitive to touch. A loss of sensation is therefore an
important finding. It usually indicates either a lesion of the ophthalmic branch of
the fifth (trigeminal) nerve, or a present or past virus infection in the cornea. To
check for loss of sensation, touch the cornea lightly with a tiny piece of
cottonwool, and note if the patient can feel it or not.

The cornea is a bit like a glass window. It allows most of the light to pass
through, and helps focus it on the retina. However its shiny outer surface also
reflects some light. It is possible to use this fact to detect any irregularities in the
shape of the cornea. Hold a patterned disc, called a keratoscope, just in front of
the cornea and observe the reflection.

The anterior chamber

The normal anterior chamber contains only aqueous fluid, which is optically
clear. The most common abnormalities to occur in the aqueous fluid are white
blood cells and protein exudate. These are both found in inflammatory eye
disease. Less commonly, red blood cells may be present after an injury, and
microfilaria may occur in onchocerciasis. Very large numbers of red or white
blood cells will be visible to the naked eye. They fall to the bottom of the anterior
chamber, and form either a hyphaema (for red cells) or a hypopyon (for white
cells). If there are only a few cells in the anterior chamber, they will only be visible
with a slit lamp. Protein exudate in the aqueous fluid causes some reflection with
focal illumination. This is called 'aqueous flare'.

It is important to estimate the depth of the anterior chamber. This is only
possible with focal illumination, by comparing reflections from the cornea, iris
and lens (*Plate* 1b).

The iris

The iris can be seen without any special instruments, but magnification obviously helps to see details. It is especially important to inspect the pupil margin for any irregularity or any adhesions between the iris and the surface of the lens. These are called 'posterior synechiae'. These adhesions become much more obvious if one attempts to dilate the pupil with mydriatic drops.

Sometimes a penetrating ulcer or penetrating injury to the cornea causes adhesions between the iris and the back of the cornea. These are called 'anterior synechiae'.

The pupil

It is important to test the pupil reactions before using any mydriatic drops to dilate the pupil and examine the back of the eye. The two pupils should be equal in size, and a light shone into each eye should produce a brisk pupil constriction in the same eye. This is called the 'direct light reflex'.

Some of the nerve fibres controlling the pupil light reflex cross over in the brainstem (*see Fig.* 2.4). Therefore, a light shone in one eye causes the other pupil to constrict equally. This is called the 'consensual light reflex'.

If the direct light reflex is diminished or absent, it usually indicates retinal or optic nerve disease in that eye. (In other words, there is a defect in the sensory part of the reflex.) Occasionally, it can be due to a defect in the motor part of the reflex, such as a disease of the iris or the ocular motor nerve. As long as the other eye is normal, a comparison of the direct and consensual light reflexes will show whether the sensory or motor part is diseased.

The lens

The lens, like all transparent structures, looks very different under diffuse, focal and coaxial illumination (*Plate* 1). Lens opacities are very common, and it can be difficult to assess the opacity of the lens. For further details on how to examine the lens, *see* Chapter 11.

The vitreous body

The vitreous body is not an easy part of the eye to examine. Fortunately, it is not a very common site for significant pathological changes. The best instrument for detecting opacities is a direct ophthalmoscope with a +4 or +5 dioptre lens. It is possible to focus on the different layers of the vitreous body by gradually bringing the ophthalmoscope nearer to the patient's eye. The opacity is then seen against the red reflex. A large opacity, such as an extensive vitreous haemorrhage, will completely obscure the red reflex.

Two other instruments can be used to examine the vitreous body. These are the indirect ophthalmoscope, and the slit lamp using a special mirrored contact lens.

The fundus

The use of the ophthalmoscope has already been described (*see above*). It is possible to examine some parts of the fundus through a normal pupil. These are the optic nerve head and the retinal blood vessels emerging from it. However, for a full fundus examination, it is necessary to dilate the pupil with mydriatic drops. This reduces dazzle from reflected light and brings the periphery of the fundus into view. It is convenient to divide fundus examination into three parts: –

– The optic nerve head and the retinal blood vessels emerging from it. The optic nerve head is slightly nasal to the centre of the eye. The examiner must therefore hold the ophthalmoscope slightly temporal to the patient's visual axis, while the patient looks straight ahead. Another way to locate the optic nerve head is to follow one of the retinal blood vessels back to its origin.
– The macula is examined by asking the patient to look straight ahead at the ophthalmoscope light.
– The periphery of the fundus is examined by asking the patient to look in different directions.

Examining the eyes of young children

Examining the eyes of babies and young children is often very difficult. It requires patience and encouragement to gain the confidence of the child. If it is still difficult to get a good view, the following techniques may be helpful: –

1. Seat the baby on his mother's lap, so that her hands restrain his arms, and steady his head (*Fig.* 3.10).
2. Wrap the baby in a sheet or blanket, with his head on the examiner's lap, and

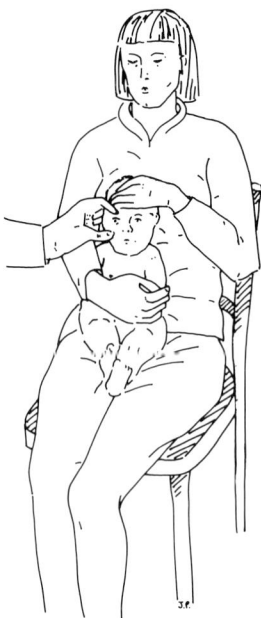

Fig. 3.10 Examining a baby.

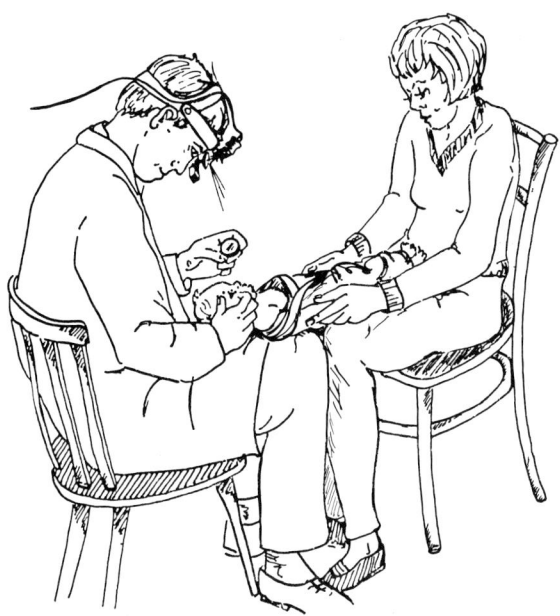

Fig. 3.11 Examining a baby with an indirect ophthalmoscope.

his body on his mother's lap. Gently hold open his lids with the fingers and thumb of one hand (*Fig.* 3.11). The other hand is then free to instill any eye drops, or hold a torch or condensing lens. This is probably the best way to get a satisfactory view of the eye, but it also provokes the greatest resentment from the baby.

3. In very difficult cases, it may be necessary to instill a drop of local anaesthetic, and use a speculum to hold open the eyelids. However, any type of speculum can seriously damage the cornea. It must be used with the greatest of care, and only by an experienced person.

The intraocular pressure

It is necessary to measure the intraocular pressure in any patient with suspected glaucoma. The risk of glaucoma increases in middle age, and so, ideally, this should be part of a routine eye examination in anyone over 40.

A very simple method of assessing the intraocular pressure is to place two fingers on the closed eyelid, and gently feel the eye. Unfortunately, this is not at all accurate. It is only really possible to feel the difference between a hard and a soft eye, and to say if one eye has a very different pressure from the other.

The intraocular pressure is measured with an instrument called a 'tonometer'. Most tonometers work in one of two ways: —

1. The Schiotz tonometer (*Fig.* 3.12) measures the intraocular pressure from the resistance of the cornea to indentation. The higher the pressure, the greater

the resistance. The Schiotz tonometer is reasonably cheap and robust, and is the most common tonometer in use, except in specialist units. It is fairly accurate (to 5 mm of mercury or less), if used correctly.

- Make sure the tonometer is very clean and dry. Even a tiny speck of dirt, or grease or moisture can cause friction in the plunger, and so give an inaccurate reading.
- Instill local anaesthetic drops into the patient's eye.
- Get the patient to lie flat, and ask him to look straight up.
- Add the lightest weight to the plunger.
- Hold the tonometer so that the footplate rests on the centre of the cornea.
- Look at the scale of the tonometer to find out the degree of indentation.
- If the weight is not enough to indent the cornea, use a heavier weight.
- Use the chart to calculate the intraocular pressure for that particular weight, and that degree of indentation.

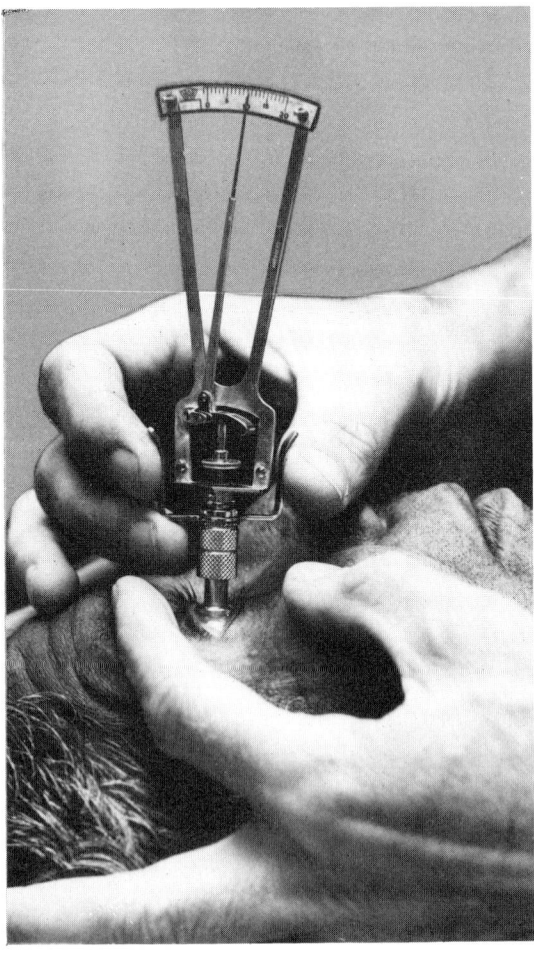

Fig. 3.12 The Schiotz tonometer.

- To check the accuracy of the tonometer, put a slightly heavier weight on the plunger. The indentation will increase, but the intraocular pressure (as calculated by the chart) should remain the same.

Unfortunately, a rise in intraocular pressure is not the only thing which helps the cornea to resist indentation. The rigidity of the cornea and sclera also affect the amount of indentation. Occasionally, patients have abnormal rigidity of the cornea and sclera, and this gives an inaccurate reading.

2. The applanation tonometer is a more accurate instrument. It works by pressing a flat, round surface against the cornea, and measuring the size of the circle it flattens. This method deforms the eye much less, and therefore gives a much more accurate result. Unfortunately, the standard applanation tonometer is expensive and must be used with a slit lamp (*Fig.* 3.7). However, the Perkins' applanation tonometer can be used without a slit lamp, and the 'Glaucotest' is a simple, cheap and portable type of applanation tonometer.

A full eye examination also includes the eye movements, the orbit and the lacrimal apparatus. These are all described in their specific chapters.

The following is a list of basic ophthalmic diagnostic equipment. Items in heavy type are for the non-specialist or for a rural eye clinic. The others are also recommended for a specialist: −

Snellen's chart and pinhole viewer
Ophthalmoscope
Hand torchlight (preferably with focal illumination) and magnifying lens
Schiotz tonometer, or portable applanation tonometer
Fluorescein, local anaesthetic and mydriatic eye drops
A room which can be darkened
Slit lamp
Applanation tonometer
Visual field testing screen or apparatus
Indirect ophthalmoscope
Retinoscope and trial set of lenses for refraction

4.   Principles of Treatment

There are three different types of treatment for disorders of the eye: medical treatment, surgical treatment and the correction of refractive errors. Ideally, only a trained specialist should give medical and surgical treatment (except for minor disorders), and only an optician should correct refractive errors. However, in many areas there so few specialists that anyone who sees patients with eye disorders should have a basic understanding of each type of treatment.

For many eye diseases there is a fourth type of 'treatment' which is even more important. This is prevention, and the importance of prevention has been discussed in Chapter 1.

Medical treatment and ocular pharmacology

There are two forms of medical treatment: local treatment and systemic treatment.

Local treatment

In local treatment, the drug is applied locally, and reaches the eye directly from the conjunctival sac. This form of treatment is more effective for the front of the eye — the conjunctiva, cornea, anterior chamber and iris. Local treatment can be given as drops, ointment or subconjunctival injections. Each method has particular advantages and disadvantages.
- Drops are the most convenient and common way of giving local treatment to the eye. However, the active drug is only in contact with the conjunctiva and cornea for a short time. If it is necessary to maintain high levels, the drops must be applied frequently, e.g. every hour or half hour. Some drops also contain substances such as methyl cellulose. This makes the solution more viscous, so that it stays longer in contact with the eye.
- Ointments stay longer in contact with the eye, and are often used at night just before sleep. Some patients also find ointments easier to apply than drops. However, in general, ointments blur the vision and are more messy than drops. Another disadvantage is that the active drug is usually dissolved in the oily part of the ointment. It is not always certain how quickly the active drug will pass out of the ointment into the tears, and then into the tissues.
- Subconjunctival injections can be painful, and so they are only used to maintain persistently high levels of a drug in serious diseases. The technique for a subconjunctival injection is as follows: –

- Anaesthetize the conjunctiva with local anaesthetic drops.
- Inject a small hypodermic needle into the conjunctival fornix, usually the lower fornix.
- Advance the needle a few millimetres just under the conjunctiva, and inject about 0.5 ml of the appropriate drug.

Unfortunately, local treatment sometimes produces side effects in the eye itself. There may be an allergic reaction to the drug, or even to the preservative in the drops or ointment. These reactions cause inflammation and irritation of the conjunctiva or the eyelids (*see Plate 5b*). Sometimes drops sting when they are applied to the eye. This is usually because excessive acid or alkali has been added to make the drug more stable.

Local treatment does not often produce systemic side effects. They may however occur, especially with mydriatics and drugs used for glaucoma.

Many patients need simple instructions on how to apply drops or ointment (*Figs. 4.1 and 4.2*). Most patients can apply their own drops or ointment, but it is easier if someone else does this for them.

Systemic treatment

Systemic treatment means that the drug is given by mouth or injection, and reaches the eye from the bloodstream. Systemic treatment is more effective for the back of the eye — the choroid, sclera, retina and optic nerve.

The following types of drugs are commonly used for eye treatment: –

1. Antibiotics

Most eye infections occur in the conjunctiva or cornea, and so antibiotics are usually applied locally to the eye. Because there are no problems from systemic side effects, a very wide range of antibiotics may be used for eye treatment.
- Chloramphenicol is the most popular antibiotic for local eye use. It has a wide range of activity, good penetration, and it is cheap.
- Tetracycline, penicillin, neomycin, gentamicin, polymyxin and sulfacetamide (or mixtures of these) are also commonly used as drops or ointment.

If the antibiotic is only available as powder for injection, it is possible in an emergency to dilute it to make a 1% solution in water. This can be used as eye drops.

Bacterial infections which threaten the sight (e.g. penetrating injuries and bacterial corneal ulcers) require subconjunctival antibiotic injections, if possible. Not all antibiotics are suitable for subconjunctival injection. However, the following list shows the doses of some antibiotics which are suitable. Most of these injections are painful, especially the penicillin derivatives.

Gentamicin	20 – 40 mg.
Colistin	10 – 20 mg.
Crystalline penicillin ⎫	
Methicillin ⎪	
Cephaloridine ⎬ 50 – 100 mg.	
Carbenicillin ⎭	

If there is infection inside the eye (endophthalmitis), then systemic antibiotics will also be necessary. In desperate cases of endophthalmitis, very small amounts

How to use your Eye Drops

FOLLOWING THESE STEPS WILL MAKE SURE YOU RECEIVE SAFE & EFFECTIVE TREATMENT

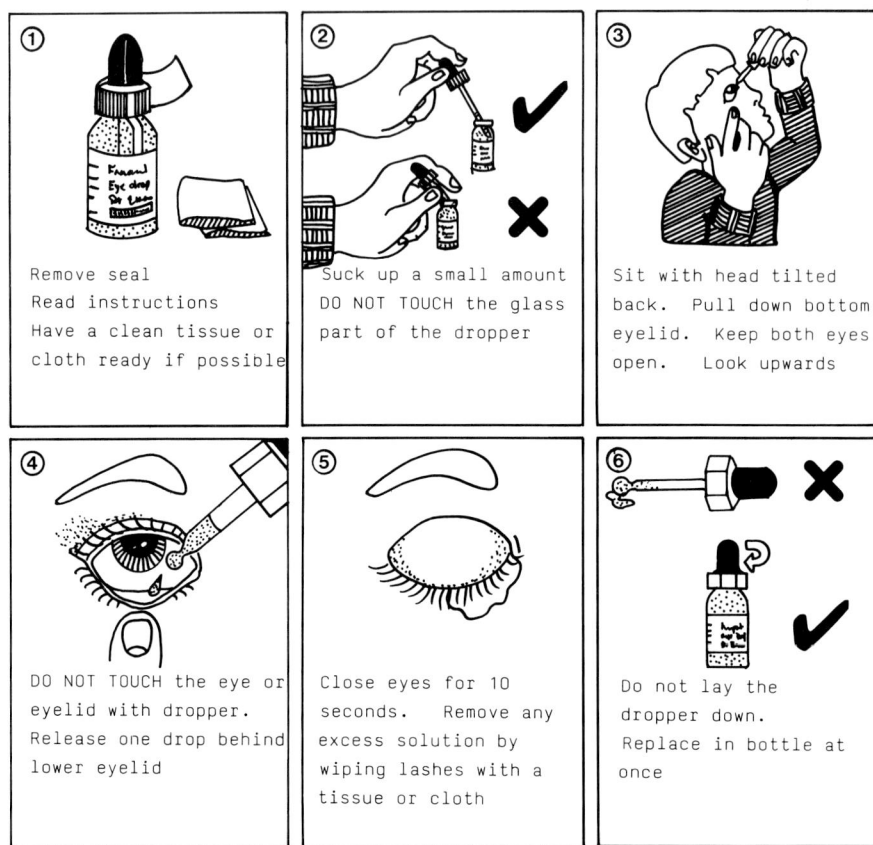

① Remove seal
Read instructions
Have a clean tissue or
cloth ready if possible

② Suck up a small amount
DO NOT TOUCH the glass
part of the dropper

③ Sit with head tilted
back. Pull down bottom
eyelid. Keep both eyes
open. Look upwards

④ DO NOT TOUCH the eye or
eyelid with dropper.
Release one drop behind
lower eyelid

⑤ Close eyes for 10
seconds. Remove any
excess solution by
wiping lashes with a
tissue or cloth

⑥ Do not lay the
dropper down.
Replace in bottle at
once

REMEMBER   Do not keep medicines when your treatment has finished
Store your drops upright, Tightly closed, In a cool place, Out of reach
of children

Fig. 4.1 A leaflet explaining how to use eye drops.

of antibiotic diluted in saline may be injected into the vitreous cavity.
(Gentamicin is usually used for this. 200 µg, that is 0.2 mg, are injected in 0.1 ml
of water.)

Antiviral drops and ointment are used to treat viral infections of the cornea
(*see* page 96). Similarly, antifungal drugs are used to treat fungal corneal
infections (*see* page 99). Several antifungal drugs are available, but unfortunately
they are usually sold as skin or vaginal creams.

To treat acute infections, antibiotic, antiviral or antifungal drops should be
applied every hour, and ointments every 2 hours until the infection resolves.

How to use your Eye Ointment

FOLLOWING THESE STEPS WILL MAKE SURE YOU RECEIVE SAFE & EFFECTIVE TREATMENT

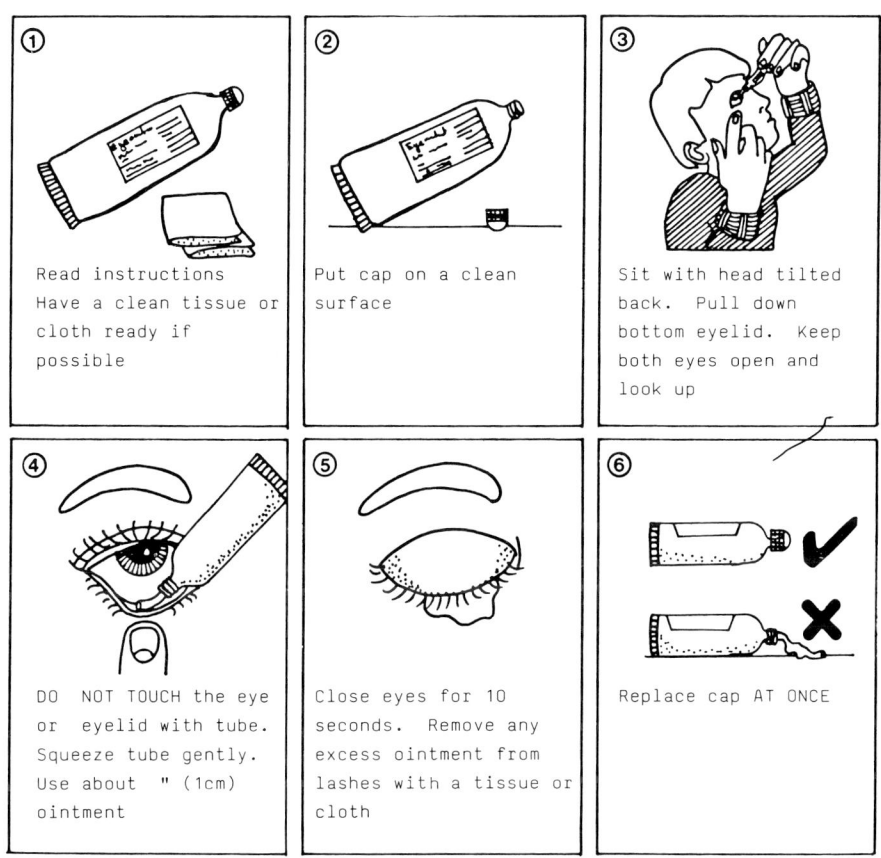

① Read instructions Have a clean tissue or cloth ready if possible

② Put cap on a clean surface

③ Sit with head tilted back. Pull down bottom eyelid. Keep both eyes open and look up

④ DO NOT TOUCH the eye or eyelid with tube. Squeeze tube gently. Use about " (1cm) ointment

⑤ Close eyes for 10 seconds. Remove any excess ointment from lashes with a tissue or cloth

⑥ Replace cap AT ONCE

REMEMBER Do not keep medicines when your treatment has finished
Store your ointment in a cool place, out of reach of children

Fig. 4.2 A leaflet explaining how to use eye ointment.

Antibiotic drops and ointments are also widely used to prevent bacterial corneal and conjunctival infections. These infections may occur after minor eye injuries, corneal foreign bodies and after eye surgery. In such cases it is only necessary to apply the drops or ointment 3 or 4 times a day.

2. Anti-inflammatory agents

The most powerful anti-inflammatory drugs are the corticosteroids. Hydrocortisone, prednisolone, betamethasone and dexamethasone are all used

extensively for both local and systemic eye treatment.
- Local steroid treatment is used for iridocyclitis, allergic types of conjunctivitis and keratitis, and after surgery. There are no systemic side effects, but unfortunately local steroids quite often cause serious side effects in the eye. Steroids act by suppressing the inflammatory responses in the tissues, but they also suppress the defences of the body to infection. Local steroid treatment therefore encourages any micro-organisms in the conjunctiva and cornea to multiply. The infection may continue to spread, but because the inflammatory responses are suppressed the patient's symptoms improve. This complication is especially serious if there is a herpes simplex viral infection of the cornea. The wrong treatment with local steroids will make the infection very severe and persistent.

   Patients who receive local steroid treatment over a long period of time are at risk from two particular side effects. Cataracts may form, or there may be a rise in intraocular pressure (steroid-induced glaucoma). The stronger the steroids, the greater the risk of both cataracts and glaucoma. These side effects are most common with dexamethasone, and least common with hydrocortisone. It is claimed that clobetasone, a recent steroid preparation, is less likely to raise the intraocular pressure.

   Local steroid preparations are more misused than any other eye treatment, and because of their serious side effects, the results can be disastrous. Unfortunately, it is both a common and a bad habit to treat an inflamed eye with a mixture of antibiotics and steroids, without trying to diagnose the cause. If the disease is caused by an infection, only antibiotics should be used; if it is caused by inflammation, without any infection, only steroids should be used.

   Steroids can also be given locally as a subconjunctival injection. This is especially useful for treating severe iridocyclitis.
- Systemic steroids are used to treat inflammations of the choroid, and occasionally the optic nerve. Unfortunately, systemic steroid treatment, especially when it is prolonged, may cause numerous side effects throughout the body. It may also cause lens opacities in the eye.

Other non-steroidal anti-inflammatory drugs can also be used in eye treatment, both locally and systemically. These drugs are less strong than steroids, but they do not have the same serious side effects. Cromoglycate (Opticrom) is used specifically to suppress allergic complications caused by IgE hypersensitivity reactions.

3. Mydriatics

Mydriatics are substances which dilate the pupil. There are two ways in which they act: –
- Most mydriatics act by blocking the parasympathetic system, and therefore make the pupil sphincter muscle relax. They also relax the ciliary muscle, which prevents the eye from accomodating and so causes blurring of near vision. This is called 'cycloplegia', and so these mydriatics are also cycloplegics. The most effective mydriatic and cycloplegic is atropine. The normal dose of atropine is one drop of a 1% solution once a day, and the effect may last for 2 weeks. Excessive use of atropine can cause systemic side

effects — drying of the mouth, loss of sweating and tachycardia. Old patients may become confused even with normal doses. Shorter acting mydriatics such as homatropine, cyclopentolate and tropicamide act in a similar way to atropine, but last only for a few hours.
- Some mydriatics stimulate the pupil dilator muscle which is controlled by the sympathetic nervous system. Phenylephrine 10% is the most effective drop for this. This does not cause cycloplegia.

There are two main uses for mydriatics: –
- They dilate the pupil, and so allow examination of the fundus. It is possible to use any of the short-acting mydriatics, or phenylephrine, or both.
- They relax the smooth muscle in the iris and ciliary body, and so are very important in the treatment of inflammatory eye disease. It is usual to prescribe atropine for this.

4. Miotics

Substances which constrict the pupil are called 'miotics'. They act by stimulating the parasympathetic system, and so make the iris sphincter muscle constrict. They also produce some contraction of the ciliary muscle which makes the eye accomodate involuntarily. This causes some blurring of distance vision, especially in young people.

Miotics are mainly used to treat glaucoma. Constricting the pupil opens up the angle of the anterior chamber (see page 167), which helps to relieve angle closure glaucoma. Miotics also increase the flow of aqueous through the trabecular meshwork, and so lower the intraocular pressure in open angle glaucoma as well. The most commonly used miotic is pilocarpine (1% – 4% drops), and its effect lasts for about 8 hours. Eserine and carbachol have similar actions.

The cholinesterase inhibitors are another group of powerful and long-acting miotics. However, they are not often used because of their possible side effects.

5. Other drugs used in glaucoma

- Adrenaline (1% drops) stimulates the sympathetic nerve endings, and lowers the intraocular pressure. The exact mechanism is uncertain, but it probably increases the drainage of aqueous fluid from the eye. Sometimes adrenaline causes eyebrow pain and vasodilatation of the conjunctiva. Recently, adrenaline has been combined with guanethidine to make it more effective (e.g. guanethidine 1% plus adrenaline 0.2%). Guanethidine is a sympathetic blocking agent which seems to make the eye more sensitive to adrenaline.
- Timoptol (timolol) (0.25% – 0.5% drops) is a beta sympathetic blocking drug which also lowers the intraocular pressure by decreasing the production of aqueous fluid. The most important side effect of Timoptol is that it may cause asthma in susceptible patients.
- Acetazolamide inhibits an enzyme, called 'carbonic acid anhydrase', which acts in the production of aqueous fluid. The effect is therefore to lower the intraocular pressure. Acetazolamide is usually taken as 250 mg tablets, once every 6 hours, and it seems to be more effective for short term treatment than long term treatment. Unfortunately, there are numerous side effects,

including tingling in the fingers, gastrointestinal discomfort and occasionally, after prolonged use, kidney stones.

– Osmotic agents draw fluid out of the extracellular spaces throughout the body. By drawing fluid out of the eye, they therefore lower the intraocular pressure. Unfortunately, osmotic agents also produce a rapid flow of urine, and often cause headaches, so that they are only used as a single dose in urgent and acute cases. The most convenient osmotic agent is glycerol, which can be given orally (1 g per kg body weight). Glycerol is usually diluted with fruit juice to make it taste better. Various osmotic agents can be given by intravenous injection, such as mannitol, urea, sucrose, or mixtures of these compounds.

6. Tear substitutes

Tear substitutes are viscous substances which help to maintain a thin film of fluid over the corneal surface. Tear substitutes are used in the following cases: –
– If the the patient has a lack of tears.
– If the eyelids will not close properly, and so cannot spread the tear film across the cornea.
– Tear substitutes are also added to some eye drops. This makes the preparation more viscous, so that it stays longer in the conjunctival sac.

Many preparations are sold as tear substitutes. The active substance is usually methyl cellulose (up to 1% solution), but other celluloses or polyvinyl alcohol or dextran may be used.

7. Local anaesthetics

Local anaesthetic drops are used to anaesthetize the cornea or conjunctiva in the following cases: –
– Before removing foreign bodies.
– Before surgery.
– Before any examination which involves touching the cornea, e.g. with a tonometer.

Benoxinate or amethocaine are the two most commonly used local anaesthetics. Cocaine is another very powerful local anaesthetic which also constricts the blood vessels. Local anaesthetics should never be used to treat painful eye conditions.

8. Other medicines

Most effective medicines belong to one of the above groups. However, other types of eye medicine are often very popular. Most of these are not very effective, but fortunately have no side effects. The following are examples: –
– Vasoconstrictor or astringent drops constrict the blood vessels, and so make a red eye look white. They usually contain zinc sulphate and dilute solutions of adrenaline (or other vasoconstrictors). Unfortunately, they do not treat the cause of the vasodilatation, and their effect wears off after frequent use.
– Antiseptic agents like mercuric oxide or boric acid are often used in minor eye infections.

– Several preparations containing mixtures of amino acids and vitamins claim to prevent the onset of cataract, and other degenerative changes in the eye. They are probably useless.

Most eye medicines are manufactured and distributed by pharmaceutical companies. However, many drops and ointments can be prepared much more cheaply in a small hospital pharmacy (*see reference on* p. 50).

Many drugs which are taken systemically for general diseases can cause complications in the eye. The problem is especially common when people take drugs excessively without proper supervision. Two drugs in particular can cause permanent damage to the sight, if taken excessively: –

– Chloroquine, which is used against malaria, can damage the retina.

– Ethambutol, which is used against tuberculosis, can damage the optic nerve.

Drugs which block the parasympathetic system are sometimes used systemically for intestinal disorders, Parkinson's disease and depression. Rarely, these may cause acute glaucoma.

Principles of ophthalmic surgery

Surgical skills are learned not from a textbook, but from an apprenticeship training (*Fig.* 4.3). The purpose of this section is therefore only to outline the basic principles of eye surgery. Very brief details of common important operations also appear in the appropriate chapters.

In many areas, but especially in parts of Africa, there are far too few eye surgeons. The only way of meeting the present needs of the community is to train other medical workers to perform certain operations. There is a great range of possible eye operations, but three are particularly important in preventing or curing blindness: –

– The correction of ingrowing eyelashes (trichiasis), following trachoma. If left untreated, these patients will develop corneal ulcers, scars and blindness.

– Cataract extraction. This is by far the most important treatable cause of blindness.

– Glaucoma surgery. This can prevent blindness in patients with early glaucoma.

The eye and its accessory structures are small, and so some magnification is essential for many eye operations.

– Telescopic operating spectacles (*see Fig.* 3.8) magnify from 2 – 4 times. This is adequate for most eye surgery.

– Operating microscopes give better magnification and illumination, and are an advantage for very fine surgery. Operating microscopes have improved the quality and range of eye surgery. Unfortunately, they are very expensive, require better anaesthesia and make operating slower.

Anaesthetizing the eye

Local anaesthesia is suffcient for most eye surgery in adults. The method of anaesthetizing the eye for surgery is as follows: –

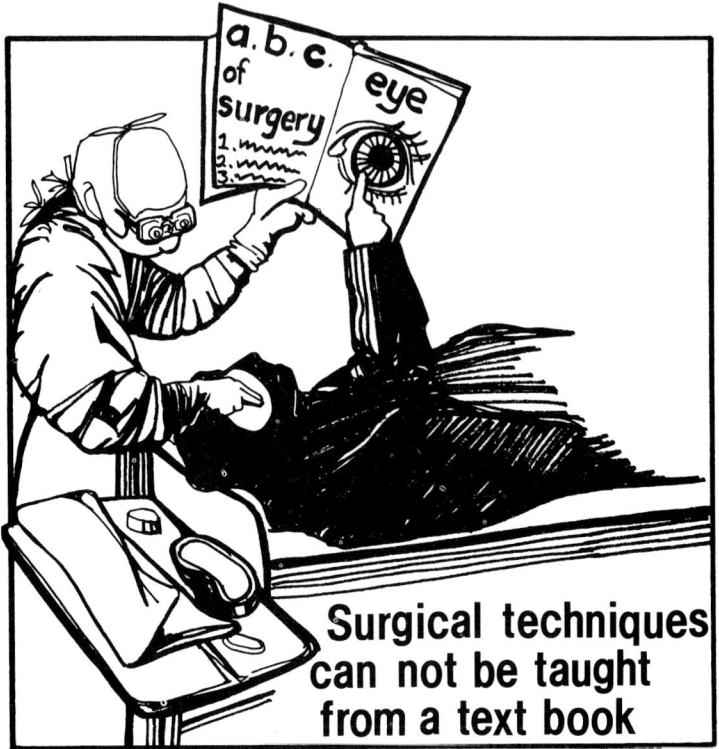

Fig. 4.3

1. Instill local anaesthetic drops into the conjunctival sac.
2. It is necessary to block the facial nerve which supplies the orbicularis oculi muscle, so that the patient cannot squeeze the eyelids, or close the eyes. Inject local anaesthetic either where the nerve winds around the neck of the mandible, or over the bone of the lateral orbital margin.
3. Inject 2 ml. of local anaesthetic (e.g. 2% xylocaine) into the retrobulbar space behind the eye. This will paralyse the eye muscles and block the sensory nerve supply to the eye. It will also block the optic nerve, so that the light of the operating lamp cannot dazzle the patient. The injection may contain hyaluronidase to help the anaesthetic diffuse, but not adrenaline. It is usual to give the injection through the outer part of the lower lid. Direct the needle backwards, but slightly upwards and inwards, so that the tip penetrates 2 − 3 cm (*Fig.* 4.4).

(For patients with a permanently blind and painful eye, a retrobulbar injection of alcohol will relieve the pain. The alcohol destroys the fine nerve fibres which transmit the sensation of pain.
− Inject 1 ml. of local anaesthetic into the retrobulbar space.
− With the same needle, inject 1 − 2 ml. of absolute alcohol.)
For eyelid surgery, injection of the tissues with local anaesthetic and dilute adrenaline (e.g. xylocaine 1% with adrenaline 1/200 000) is all that is necessary.

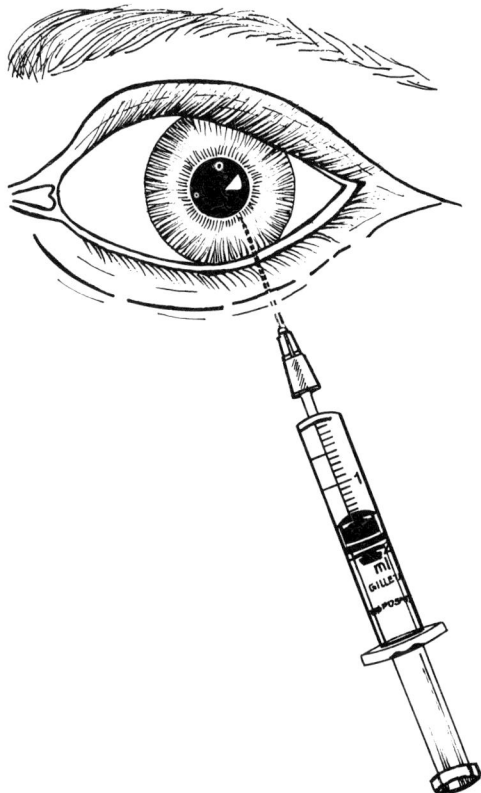

Fig. 4.4 A retrobulbar injection.

The techniques of eye surgery

It is convenient to divide the techniques of eye surgery into two groups: extraocular surgery and intraocular surgery.

- Extraocular surgery is surgery of the eyelids, extraocular muscles, lacrimal passages, orbit etc. The principles of extraocular surgery are the same as most other types of surgery. The surgery itself is usually straightforward. This is because most of the extraocular tissues are easily accessible and have a good blood supply. There is good healing with a low risk of infection.
- Intraocular surgery is surgery inside the eye, which carries three particular risks: —

  1. Intraocular infection. Bacteria will multiply very easily in the aqueous and vitreous fluid inside the eye. Any intraocular infection usually causes permanent destruction of the eye. It is therefore essential to make sure that no potentially infected material enters the eye. Unfortunately, it is impossible to sterilize the eyelids and conjunctival sac completely before surgery, but the eye should be cleaned as thoroughly as possible. All the instruments should be scrupulously sterilized, and the surgeon should use a good 'no touch' surgical technique.

2. The delicate intraocular tissues are very susceptible to physical or chemical damage. Therefore it is extremely important not to touch the inside of the eye any more than necessary in any intraocular manoeuvre. The endothelial cells lining the inner surface of the cornea are especially at risk. Even just touching these cells may cause permanent damage. This may produce permanent corneal oedema which causes pain and loss of vision. The lens is also extremely sensitive to surgical trauma, and just touching it may cause a lens opacity. It is also important not to introduce any fluids into the eye, apart from pure sterile isotonic saline or Ringer's solution free from any added preservatives.

3. It is important to make and suture the incision correctly, so that complications do not occur. Incisions into the eye are usually made at the limbus. (Scleral incisions often bleed, while corneal incisions are slow to heal and may distort the curvature of the cornea.) If the incision is made under a flap of conjunctiva, it will help to protect the wound. It is necessary to use very fine suture material to close a surgical incision into the eye securely. These fine sutures inevitably act as foreign bodies, but cause very little discomfort or irritation. There are a number of different suture materials: –

– The most popular suture material is 8/0 gauge virgin silk, catgut or a synthetic absorbable material.
– 9/0 or 10/0 monofilament nylon or polypropylene is even finer and can be used as a continuous stitch. This gives excellent wound closure, and does not irritate the eye at all.
– Even sterilized human hair can be used as a suture material. It is certainly cheap and non-antigenic, but is rarely used nowadays.

Some years ago it was usual to advise patients to have long periods of bedrest after intraocular surgery. However, with better wound closure, there is now no need for this. It is even possible to do most eye surgery on an outpatient basis.

Padding an eye increases the bacterial content of the conjunctival sac. However, it is usually adivsable to pad eyes for a few days after intraocular surgery. This will protect the eye from contamination, injury or irritation.

The complications of intraocular surgery

There are many possible complications after intraocular surgery. Most of these are the result of bad surgical technique, and should therefore be rare in skilled hands. The most common complications are as follows: –

1. Poor closure of the incision may be a problem, especially after cataract surgery. This is because a large incision is necessary to remove the lens. There may be a leak of aqueous fluid, producing a soft eye, and a shallow or absent anterior chamber. Alternatively, the iris or vitreous may prolapse through the wound or adhere to its edges.

2. Intraocular infection is a disastrous complication which should be very rare with good surgical technique. Any intraocular infection requires immediate treatment, using intensive antibiotic drops, subconjunctival injections of antibiotic, and also systemic antibiotics. Unfortunately, it is nearly always too late to save the eye. It is usual to apply antibiotic drops or ointment after any intraocular surgery. However, most infections enter the eye at the time of the

operation, and not afterwards.

3. Intraocular haemorrhage sometimes occurs. Slight bleeding during the operation is quite common, but normally the blood absorbs very quickly. If the incision has been poorly closed, however, small blood vessels will bridge the gap in the wound. Any slight movement may rupture these blood vessels and cause bleeding into the eye. It is best to remove a massive clot which obscures the iris completely, and then resuture the wound.

4. Intraocular inflammation or uveitis always occurs to some extent after any intraocular surgery. It is usual to give mydriatics and corticosteroids for a week or two after the operation. Severe cases require more prolonged and intensive treatment.

5. Corneal oedema may occur after damage to the corneal endothelial cells.

6. Post-operative glaucoma may also occur. The intraocular pressure often rises for a short time after any surgery. This is because the red blood cells and the plasma proteins obstruct the flow of aqueous fluid out of the eye. Persistent post-operative glaucoma is caused by damage or obstruction to the aqueous drainage pathways.

Recent advances in eye surgery

There have been several important recent advances in eye surgery. Unfortunately, most of these involve expensive and sophisticated equipment which may not be appropriate for the basic health needs of developing countries. The most important of these advances are cryosurgery, photocoagulation and vitrectomy.

– Cryosurgery uses a small probe to freeze tissues down to $-50\,°C$. It is a very effective instrument for removing cataracts. It is also used in retinal detachment surgery, and can remove misplaced eyelashes. A cryoprobe is quite expensive, but is a very useful instrument even for small surgical units.

– Photocoagulation uses a very bright light (usually from an argon laser) to produce localized burns on the choroid and retina. It prevents complications from diabetic retinopathy, and may help to treat other retinal conditions, such as sickle cell disease and senile macular degeneration. Laser-photocoagulators have recently been successful in treating glaucoma.

– Vitrectomy machines are tiny probes which can cut and remove tissue inside the eye. They are mainly used inside the vitreous, but can also remove the lens.

Both laser-photocoagulators and vitrectomy machines are very expensive, and need highly skilled maintenance. Most of the diseases which they treat are not common problems in the tropics. Therefore at present they are only really useful in highly specialized clinics.

Ophthalmic optics and the correction of refractive errors

The study of the eye as an optical instrument is called ophthalmic optics. Any defect in the focusing or refracting mechanism of the eye is called a refractive error. It is possible to correct most refractive errors with spectacles. The ordering and fitting of spectacles is the work of an optician. However, anyone who deals with eye diseases should have a basic understanding of ophthalmic optics, especially in areas where there are no opticians.

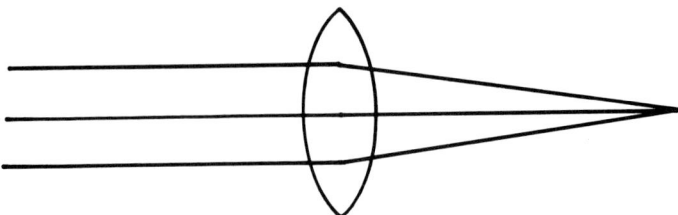

Fig. 4.5 A convex lens.

Ophthalmic optics

A convex (or converging) lens will bring parallel rays of light to a point focus (*Fig.* 4.5). The eye acts as a convex lens, and the normal healthy eye at rest will focus the light rays from a distant object onto the retina (*Fig.* 4.6). Rays of light from a distant object (e.g. a tree or a house) are assumed to run parallel to each other. The light rays are focused partly by the cornea, and partly by the lens.

The power of lenses is measured in dioptres. A 1 dioptre lens focuses parallel rays of light to a point 1 metre from the lens. A 2 dioptre lens focuses parallel rays of light to a point 1/2 metre from the lens, and a 10 dioptre lens focuses parallel rays of light to 1/10 metre from the lens. (In mathematical terms, this means that the power of a lens in dioptres is the reciprocal of its focal length.) The length of the eye from front to back is about 2 cm, or 1/50 of a metre. Therefore the total refractive power of the eye is about 50 dioptres. 40 dioptres of this comes from the curved corneal surface, and 10 dioptres from the lens.

Rays of light from an object close to the eye (e.g. a page of a book) will be diverging when they reach the eye (*Fig.* 4.7). These light rays are focused behind the retina, and so the image on the retina is blurred. The focusing power of the eye must therefore increase in order to see near objects clearly (*see* the dotted rays in *Fig.* 4.7). To do this, the lens becomes more spherical. This is called 'accommodation', and the mechanism is as follows: – The ciliary body forms a ring of smooth muscle around the lens, and it is attached to the lens by many tiny fibres, called the 'suspensory ligament'. These fibres constantly pull on the equator of the lens, causing it to flatten slightly. When the ciliary body contracts, the ring becomes smaller, so that the fibres of the suspensory ligament become loose. The lens then relaxes into a more spherical shape, and thus becomes a stronger lens.

Refractive errors

If there is any refractive error in the eye, the rays of light cannot come to a focus on the retina, and the object appears blurred. People with refractive errors often see better in bright light when the pupil constricts, and sometimes screw up their eyelids to see better. This is called the 'pinhole effect' (*Fig.* 4.8). By narrowing the beam of light entering the eye, the blurred area on the retina becomes smaller (see the dotted rays in *Fig.* 4.8), and the object appears clearer. The pinhole test is a simple way to detect refractive errors (*see Fig.* 3.3). If the patient has better vision through a pinhole, it indicates a refractive error.

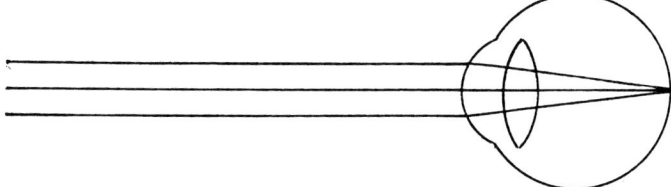

Fig. 4.6. To show how light rays from a distant object are focused on the retina.

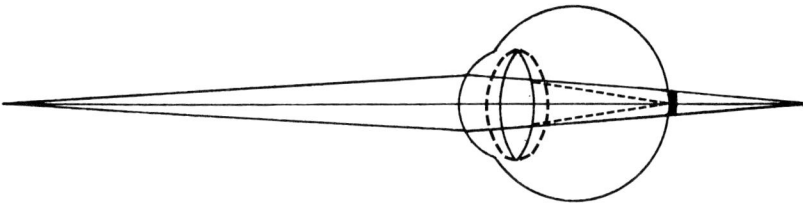

Fig. 4.7. Accommodation. The change in shape of the lens allows light rays from a near object to focus on the retina.

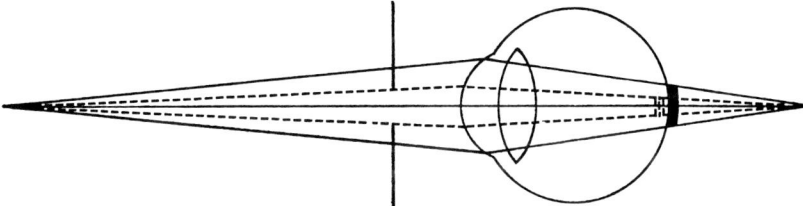

Fig. 4.8. The pinhole effect. Only the dotted rays pass through the pinhole.

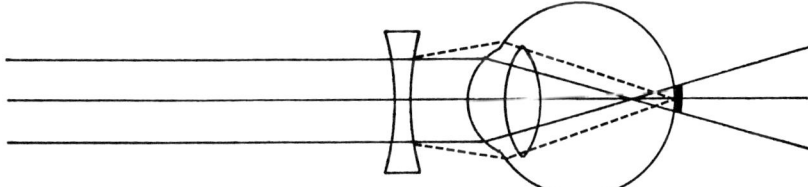

Fig. 4.9. Myopia.

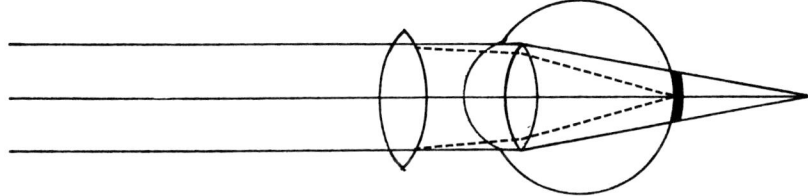

Fig. 4.10 Hypermetropia.

Most refractive errors can be corrected with spectacles. The purpose of the spectacle lens is to help focus the light rays on the retina.

The most common refractive errors are as follows: −
− Presbyopia means that the lens in the eye has become harder with age, and is therefore less able to change its shape. The eye can still see distant objects clearly, but cannot focus on near objects. This explains why most old people need spectacles with a convex lens for close work or reading.
− Myopia (or short-sight) means that the refractive power of the eye is too great. Parallel rays of light are therefore focused in front of the retina, and not on the retina itself (*Fig.* 4.9). Therefore distant objects appear blurred. A negative (or concave) spectacle lens will help to focus parallel rays of light onto the retina, and so correct myopia (*see* the dotted rays in *Fig.* 4.9). However, myopic people can see near objects clearly without the eye having to focus.
− Hypermetropia (or long-sight) is the opposite of myopia. Parallel rays of light are focused behind the retina (*Fig.* 4.10). A convex spectacle lens will focus the rays of light onto the retina, and so correct hypermetropia (*see* the dotted rays in *Fig.* 4.10). However, young children can increase the power of their own lens by accomodation, and so overcome hypermetropia themselves. With age, the power of accomodation decreases. Therefore as hypermetropic people get older, they have increasing need for spectacles, first for near vision, and later for distance vision also.
− Aphakia means that the patient's own lens has been removed, which makes the eye extremely hypermetropic. The patient needs a strong spectacle lens of + 10 dioptres to compensate for the loss of his own lens.
− Astigmatism means that the eye has a different focus in different planes. For example, vertical rays of light may be focused on the retina, while horizontal rays are focused behind the retina. A cylindrical lens with power in only one axis is used to correct astigmatism. Astigmatism often occurs combined with either myopia or hypermetropia.

A retinoscope and a set of lenses of different power are used to measure refractive errors. The correct lenses are then fitted into a spectacle frame. Obviously, everyone who needs spectacles should be tested so that they receive the correct lens. However, in areas where there are no opticians, it is useful to note that the most common refractive error is presbyopia. It occurs in all normal-sighted people who are over 40 or 50, and can be corrected with lenses of + 2 or + 3 dioptres. Aphakia is another common refractive error, and can be corrected with lenses of approximately + 10 dioptres. It may help to have a supply of such spectacles when working in isolated areas.

Reference

Taylor J. *The Local Production of Eye Drops*. A booklet available from the Christoffel − Blindenmission, Nibelungstrasse 124, D 6140 Bensheim 4, W. Germany.

5. The Eyelids and the Lacrimal Apparatus

The structure and function of the eyelids are described in Chapter 2 (*see also Fig.* 2.5). Most eyelid disorders are fairly easy to recognise, and can be divided into three main groups: –
– inflammations
– abnormalities of the function and position of the eyelids
– tumours

Inflammations

The eyelids are exposed and contain numerous glands. They are therefore prone to infection and inflammation. Fortunately, the eyelids have a very rich blood supply, and so most of these infections either heal or remain localized. Because the eyelid skin is thin and loose, oedema and swelling of the eyelids may develop very easily in any inflammation. Sometimes inflammation in another site, such as the nose, scalp or orbit, causes oedema of the eyelids (*see Figs.* 15.10 *and* 18.8).

Styes

A stye is an infection either of an eyelash follicle, or of the sebaceous glands near the eyelash roots. Such infections are common, and are usually caused by staphylococci. The traditional treatment is to apply antibiotic ointment as well as local heat and compresses (hot spoon bathing). However, even without any treatment, the small abscess soon discharges itself through the skin and the stye heals.

Inflammation of the Meibomian glands

The Meibomian glands are embedded in the tough tarsal plate, and each gland opens at the eyelid margin. Quite often, the mouths of these glands become blocked, causing a retention cyst called a 'Meibomian cyst' (*see Figs* 5.1 *and* 5.2). There may be chronic inflammation in or around these cysts which may contain Meibomian secretion, granulation tissue or pus. These cysts are common; sometimes there may be more than one of them, and they may recur.

Occasionally, an acute bacterial infection develops in a Meibomian gland. These infections can be quite severe, because the pus cannot easily drain away.

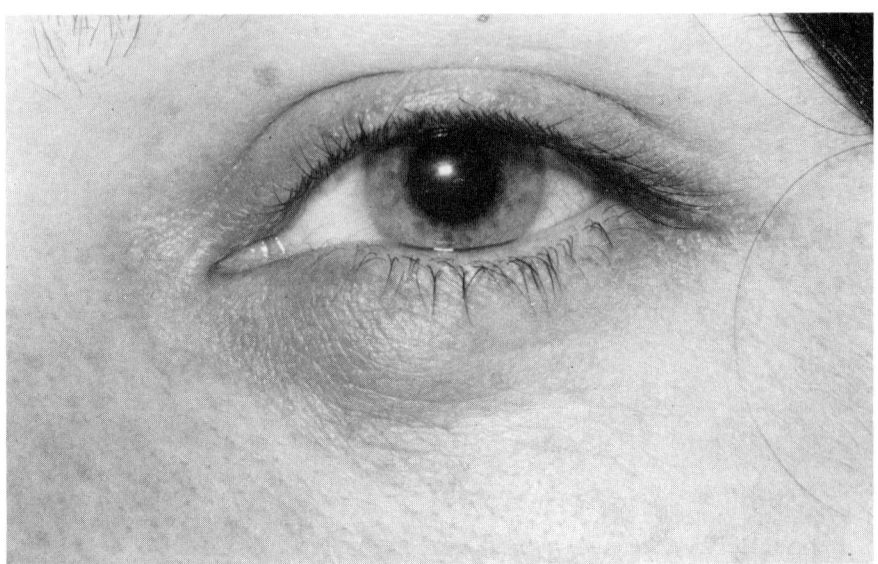

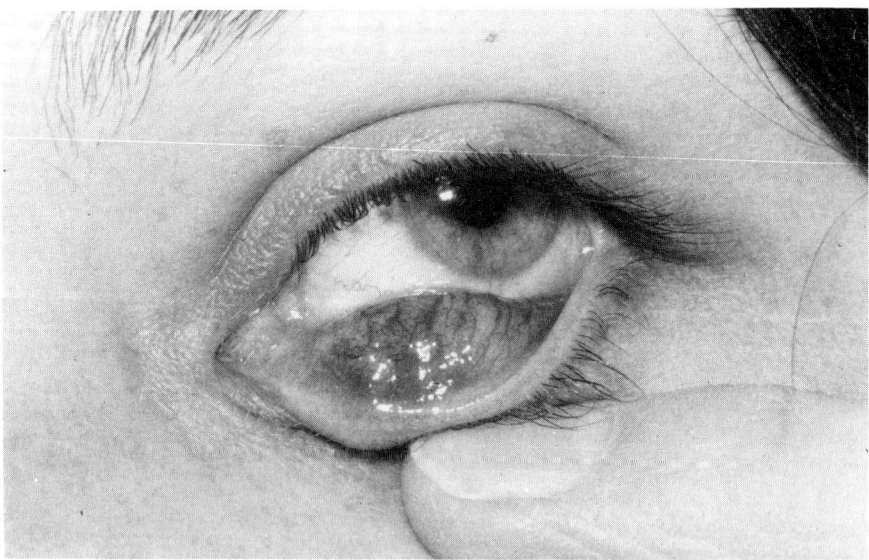

Fig. 5.1 *and* 5.2 A Meibomian cyst. It is sometimes easier to see the cyst and the surrounding inflammation from the conjunctival surface of the eyelid.

There may be some general malaise and fever as well as an inflamed eyelid. Eventually, the abscess either bursts through the skin or conjunctiva, or settles down to leave a Meibomian cyst.

The treatment of an acute infection is to give antibiotics locally, and possibly

systemically. Any abscess should be drained surgically. Meibomian cysts are usually treated as follows: –
1. Inject local anaesthetic with adrenaline into the eyelid, and instill local anaesthetic drops in the conjunctiva.
2. Evert the eyelid with a small eyelid clamp.
3. Incise through the conjunctiva into the tarsal plate over the cyst.
4. Curette out the contents of the cyst and apply antibiotic ointment.

Blepharitis

Blepharitis is the name for any generalized inflammation of the eyelids.
– Seborrhoeic blepharitis is a common form of blepharitis. This is a chronic or recurrent inflammation associated with over-active sebaceous glands. Crusts and scales form on the lid margins and lashes (*Plate* 2a). The crusts and scales irritate the eye and may cause secondary chronic staphylococcal infections of the eyelid margin. Because seborrhoeic blepharitis is basically a constitutional disease, effective treatment is difficult. However, it sometimes helps to clean the lid margins carefully and remove all the crusts. It is then possible to apply an ointment or cream containing a mixture of local antibiotics and corticosteroids.
– Shingles is caused by the herpes zoster/varicella virus, which also causes chickenpox. The virus infection only involves one sensory nerve on one side of the body. The ophthalmic branch of the fifth nerve is a common site for it. There is a rash on the forehead and scalp, and often iritis and keratitis also

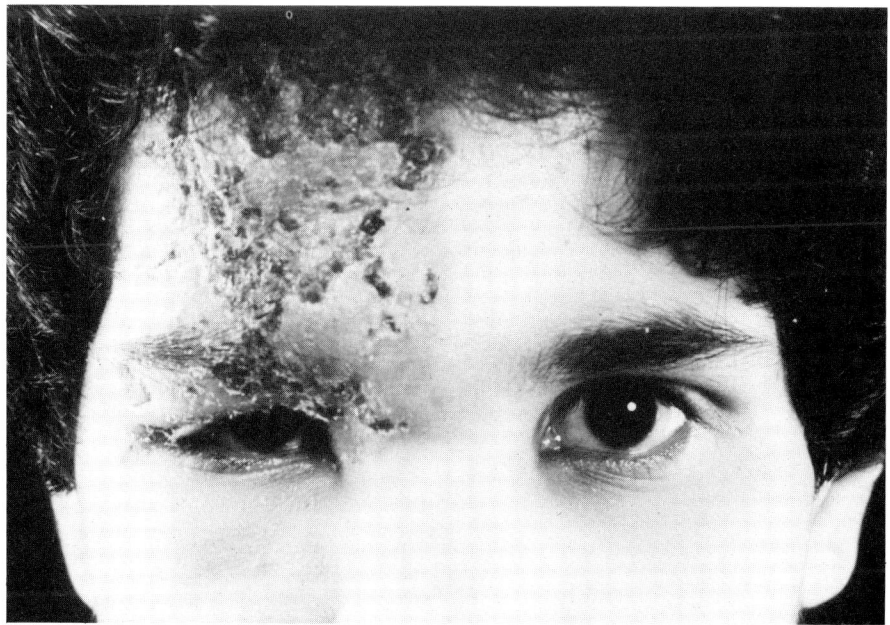

Fig. 5.3 Ophthalmic herpes zoster. Note how the rash only affects one side of the forehead.

(*Fig.* 5.3). The simplest treatment for the rash is to encourage the formation of a firm dry scab to prevent secondary infection. The iritis and keratitis may also need treatment.
– Allergies to eye drops or eye cosmetics occasionally cause blepharitis (*Plate* 5*b*).

Infections of the eyelids caused by 'tropical' diseases

The eyelids are exposed, and are therefore prone to various infections which occur only, or mainly, in the tropics. Most of these infections are caused by insect vectors, the climate, poor hygiene or malnutrition. It is often possible to make the correct diagnosis from a careful examination and a good knowledge of common local diseases. However, it is sometimes necessary to ask for laboratory investigations, such as a bacterial culture or a histological examination.
– Cutaneous leishmaniasis is common in many desert areas of the world. It is caused by a protozoan parasite which is spread by the bite of certain sandflies. The disease usually occurs in young children, who first develop a granulomatous nodule, and later a localised chronic necrotic ulcer where the sandfly has bitten (*Fig.* 5.4). A histological examination at the base of the ulcer will show macrophages containing large numbers of the parasite. Secondary infection is very common, and probably causes most of the scarring and contracture which occurs when the ulcer eventually heals. The contracture may develop on, or near the eyelids (*Plate* 2b). The most effective treatment for these ulcers is to try to prevent secondary infection by applying antiseptic or antibiotic dressings. At a later stage, skin grafting may be necessary.

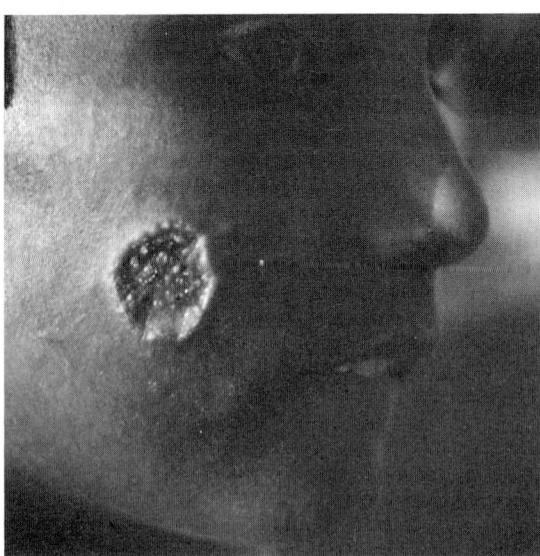

Fig. 5.4 Active cutaneous leishmaniasis of the face.

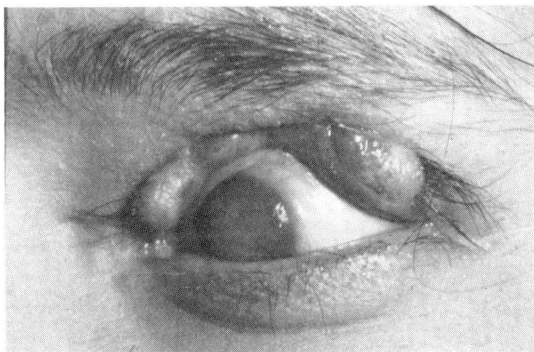

Fig. 5.5 Old cancrum which has destroyed the upper eyelid. Note the secondary corneal scarring.

- Cancrum is a poorly understood condition which occurs in malnourished young children, usually following a severe generalized infection. In cancrum, there is gangrene and necrosis of the facial skin, especially around the lips and cheeks, and sometimes on the eyelids (*Plate* 2c *and Fig.* 5.5). There is no known specific causative organism, but it may be due to a severe herpes simplex infection. The basis of treatment in the acute stage is to improve the nutrition, treat the primary disease and prevent secondary infection in the skin. Complex plastic surgical reconstruction may be possible later.
- Leprosy is an important cause of eyelid abnormalities. For a full discussion *see* Chapter 16.

Various other infections with bacteria, fungi or parasites may rarely involve the eyelid, and cause chronic inflammation, granuloma formation, ulcers, scars etc. The most important of these infections are: –

- Chronic bacterial infections, such as actinomycosis, tuberculosis and yaws.
- Anthrax is a bacterial infection spread by spores on animal skins. Anthrax of the face is found among people who handle the skins of animals, or people who sleep on infected sheep skins. The disease presents acutely with one or more small raised spots on the surface of the skin, and severe oedema and tissue reaction. It can then progress rapidly to gangrene and generalized illness. It can be treated with penicillin.
- Lice may infect the eyelids.
- Flies may lay their eggs under the surface of the eyelids of young or debilitated patients. As the larvae develop, they cause a chronic infection.
- Various insect bites and stings are common around the eyelids.
- Onchocerciasis and loaisis are both caused by parasitic worms, and may involve the eyelids. For a full discussion *see* Chapter 15.

Abnormalities of the function and position of the eyelids

Facial palsy (see Fig. 16.2 – 16.4, p. 190)

Paralysis of the VIIth cranial (or facial) nerve prevents the eyelid from closing properly. The defect is usually unilateral, and the diagnosis is obvious because the whole face appears lop-sided. However, if the facial palsy is incomplete or bilateral, the face is still symmetrical, and so the defect is much less obvious. Patients with facial palsy often complain of a watering eye. This is because the loss of the blink reflex and the sagging lower eyelid prevent the tears from draining properly.

When the eyelids cannot close properly, the cornea is at risk from exposure damage and infection. Fortunately, any attempt to close the eyelids causes a reflex action which turns the eye up under the protection of the upper eyelid. This often preserves the cornea.

Facial palsy may have many causes. The most important of these are: –
– Intracranial damage, e.g. from a tumour causing pressure atrophy of the nerve.
– Disease of the middle ear, damaging the nerve in the facial canal.
– Bell's palsy is the name given to a sudden facial palsy whose cause is unknown, but which often follows a mild upper respiratory infection. It is probably due to oedema of the nerve in the facial canal, and there is often partial or complete recovery of function some months later.
– Leprosy is the most important cause of superficial damage to the facial nerve. If it is bilateral, the facial palsy is often not recognised.

Facial palsy and its treatment are also described in Chapter 16.

Ptosis

Ptosis means that the upper eyelid droops, usually because the levator muscle is weak. Mild cases are only a cosmetic problem, but in severe cases the vision may be affected. There are many causes of ptosis, but the more common are as follows: –
– Congenital ptosis is quite common and may be unilateral or bilateral. If the drooping eyelid completely covers the pupil, the eye may develop amblyopia (*see* page 200).
– Third cranial (or oculomotor) nerve palsy. If the palsy is complete, it will cause a total ptosis, a dilated pupil, and limitation of all eye movements except abduction (*see* page 201). If the palsy is only partial, not all of these signs may be present.
– Cervical sympathetic nerve palsy causes only a partial ptosis. It usually also causes the pupil to constrict, and prevents sweating on the affected side of the face. This condition is called 'Horner's syndrome'. The cervical sympathetic fibres may be affected anywhere from the thoracic spinal cord to the eye. In most cases, it is impossible to find a specific cause.
– Myasthenia gravis is a complex disorder which affects the neuromuscular junction between the motor nerve and the muscle. It is sometimes associated with tumours of the thymus gland. One of the first signs is ptosis which is usually bilateral, and which comes on when the patient is tired. It is often associated with weakness of other muscles, causing double vision or difficulty in swallowing. The condition rapidly improves with a small dose of a drug which strengthens neuro-muscular transmission such as neostigmine.
– Senile ptosis occurs in old people. It is usually due to stretching of the fibrous aponeurosis where the levator muscle is inserted into the tarsal plate.
– Trachoma sometimes causes ptosis. This is because the extra thickness and

weight of the chronically scarred upper eyelid causes it to sag.

The treatment of ptosis is basically surgical. Unfortunately, the correction of ptosis is often difficult, and so under- and over-corrections are both common. If the problem is only cosmetic, there is no urgency for surgery. Surgical treatment should not usually be given for ptosis from a third nerve palsy, or from myasthenia gravis.

Eyelid retraction

Eyelid retraction is the opposite of ptosis. It is caused by overaction of the levator muscle and the smooth muscle fibres in both the upper and lower eyelid. It is nearly always associated with thyrotoxicosis or thyroid eye disease (*see* page 212).

Ectropion

If the eyelid turns outwards, exposing some of the tarsal conjunctiva, this is called 'ectropion'. There are two main types: –
- Cicatricial ectropion is caused by scarring and contracture of the eyelid skin which makes the eyelid turn outwards (*Plate* 2b *and Fig.* 5.6). This usually occurs after chronic skin infections or burns.
- Atonic ectropion means that the lower lid is too loose to rest against the eyeball. It is caused either by senile stretching of the tissues or by a facial palsy. The exposed conjunctiva is likely to become chronically inflamed and hypertrophic. This in turn will cause further eversion of the eyelids (*Fig.* 5.7).

The treatment for both types of ectropion is surgical. However, it may help to give a short course of local antibiotic and steroid ointment before surgery to suppress the inflammation in the exposed conjunctiva.
- In cicatricial ectropion, excise the scar and fill up the defect with a skin graft. It is usual to take a partial thickness graft from a limb, or a full thickness graft

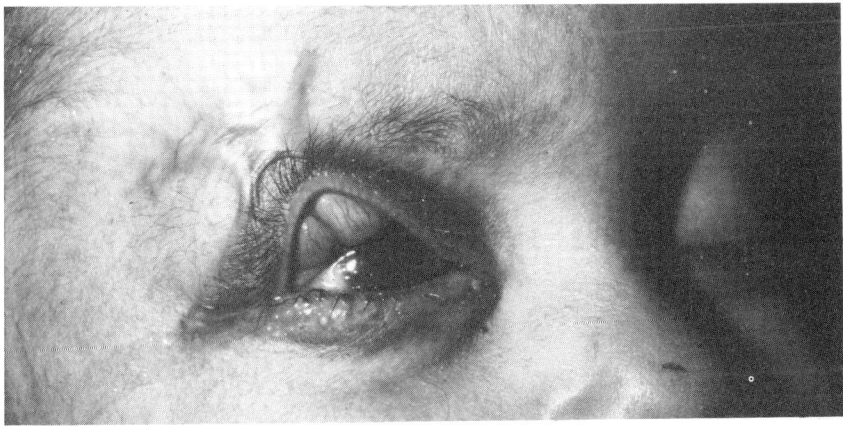

Fig. 5.6 Severe ectropion of the upper eyelid following a burn.

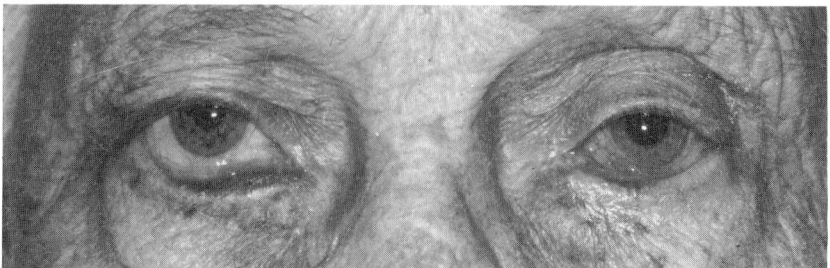

Fig. 5.7 Atonic ectropion of the lower eyelids.

from behind the ear.
- In atonic ectropion, excise a V-shaped wedge from the lateral end of the lower eyelid. This will tighten the eyelid.

Entropion

Entropion means that the eyelid turns inwards, so that the eyelashes irritate and inflame the cornea. The upper eyelashes irritate the cornea much more than the lower lashes. In severe and prolonged cases, this may lead to corneal scarring and eventual blindness. There are two main types of entropion: –
- Cicatricial entropion is caused by scarring and contracture of the conjunctiva and tarsal plate, which makes the eyelid turn in. This may occur after any chronic conjunctival infection or inflammation, but the most common is chronic trachoma (*see Plate* 7b). Cicatricial entropion is more common in the upper lid.
- Senile (or atonic) entropion occurs only in the lower lid in old patients. The tarsal plate becomes weak and floppy, and the connective tissue in the eyelid stretches. This means that when the orbicularis oculi muscle contracts to close the eyelid, the lower lid rolls in. It is possible to restore the lower lid to its normal position by gently pulling it down. However, closing the eyes will invert it again.
  The treatment of both cicatricial and senile entropion is surgical.
- The treatment of cicatricial entropion is described in Chapter 7, page 88).
- To treat senile entropion, there are many different surgical procedures. Most of these try to tighten up the tarsal plate, or prevent the orbicularis oculi muscle from rolling the eye inwards. It is possible to correct senile entropion temporarily by applying adhesive strapping to the lower lid.

Tumours

Eyelid tumours are quite common. The eyelids have a fairly complex structure, and so there are many different types of tumour. It can be difficult to distinguish clinically between a tumour and some chronic inflammatory conditions in the eyelid.

Benign tumours of the eyelid

These may originate in the skin or the connective tissue. A papilloma is a common benign tumour of the skin which is usually found near the eyelid margin. Occasionally, several papillomas may be present. Connective tissue tumours like haemangiomas or neurofibromas may also occur in the eyelids.

Often chronic inflammatory conditions such as warts may occur in the eyelid and appear like tumours. Sebaceous and other cysts are also common.

Malignant tumours of the eyelid

– Rodent ulcers (basal cell carcinomas) are the most common malignant tumours of the eyelids. They are found especially in fair-skinned people who have been exposed to excessive sunlight (*see Plate* 2d *and* 2e). They are therefore common in rural communities in the desert areas of the Middle East and Central Asia, but are almost unknown in blacks.

A rodent ulcer may occur anywhere around the eye, but it is most common on the lower lid. Typically, there is a central ulcerated area with a raised, irregular, nodular edge. Sometimes, the tumour may look like a cyst, or there may be diffuse inflammatory changes without any ulceration. The tumour is only locally malignant, and so does not spread to other parts of the body. However, it continues to grow and spread locally on the face. Any chronic ulcer or inflammation of the eyelid skin in a patient over 40 is suspicious of a rodent ulcer, especially if the patient is fair-skinned and has been exposed to excessive sunlight.

Other malignant tumours of the eyelids are less common.

– Squamous cell carcinomas are also caused by over-exposure to sunlight. They may spread through the local lymph nodes to other parts of the body.

– Malignant melanomas of the eyelids are highly malignant, but fortunately very rare.

– Carcinomas arising from the eyelid conjunctiva occasionally occur.

– Malignant tumours which develop from the connective tissue structures of the eyelid are rare.

The treatment of eyelid tumours

Most eyelid tumours can be treated surgically by local excision. Benign tumours, warts and cysts are usually easy to excise. It is possible to excise at least a quarter of the eyelid margin as a V-shaped wedge, and to close the wound edges with direct sutures. A larger excision may require a skin graft. Fortunately, skin grafts take very well on the eyelids because of their good blood supply. If a more extensive excision is necessary, various plastic surgical procedures can be used to reconstruct the eyelid (*Plate* 2f). If the tumour is possibly malignant, and especially if it is a rodent ulcer, it is important to excise a wide margin of healthy skin. It is better to leave the patient with an ugly scar than with active tumour cells still present in the wound.

Many malignant tumours, especially rodent ulcers, can also be treated with radiotherapy. It is sometimes unclear from a clinical examination whether the eyelid mass is a benign or malignant tumour, or even some type of chronic inflammation. In this case, it is best to take a small biopsy for histological examination before planning any definite treatment.

The lacrimal apparatus

The structure and function of the lacrimal apparatus are described in Chapter 2 (*see also Fig.* 2.6).

The lacrimal gland

Diseases of the lacrimal gland are not common. Occasionally, however, the lacrimal gland is the site of inflammation, or of a benign or malignant tumour. Because the lacrimal gland lies in the orbit, any swelling of the gland will behave like an orbital mass, and cause forward displacement of the eye (proptosis).

Destruction of the lacrimal gland has little effect on the eye. This is because the lacrimal gland only produces the reflex watery tears. The accessory lacrimal gland tissue under the conjunctiva produces the normal resting tear secretion. If this is diseased, the result will be a dry eye and chronic conjunctivitis (See page 74).

The nasolacrimal passages

Disorders of the nasolacrimal passages are common, and produce excessive watering of the eye (epiphora). A watering eye means that there is either some inflammatory eye disease, or an obstruction of the nasolacrimal passages. There are two ways to find if the nasolacrimal passages are obstructed: –
– A simple and quite effective method is to instill a drop of fluorescein into the conjunctival sac. After one or two minutes, ask the patient to blow his nose. Any dye on the handkerchief means that the tears are passing from the conjunctival sac into the nose.
– It is possible to syringe the nasolacrimal passages to see if any fluid passes down into the nose. This will also help to discover the exact site of the obstruction.

There are three common sites where the nasolacrimal passages may become blocked: the punctum, the common canaliculus and the nasolacrimal duct (*see Fig.* 2.6).

1. The punctum. Most of the tears pass through the lower punctum and the lower canaliculus. (The upper punctum and canaliculus are not so important). The punctum may become narrowed, occluded or everted, so that it no longer rests against the eye. A careful examination will detect defects of the punctum. An occluded or everted punctum can be corrected with a simple surgical procedure, such as slitting open the punctum with scissors.

2. The common canaliculus is one of the narrowest parts of the nasolacrimal passages. After an infection, or sometimes in old age, it may become obstructed. Obstructions anywhere in the canaliculus or the punctum will cause only epiphora without any secondary conjunctivitis.

3. The nasolacrimal duct is the commonest site for obstruction. This may be a congenital abnormality, or develop in adults. If the nasolacrimal duct is blocked, the lacrimal sac usually fills up with stagnant tears and becomes infected. This is

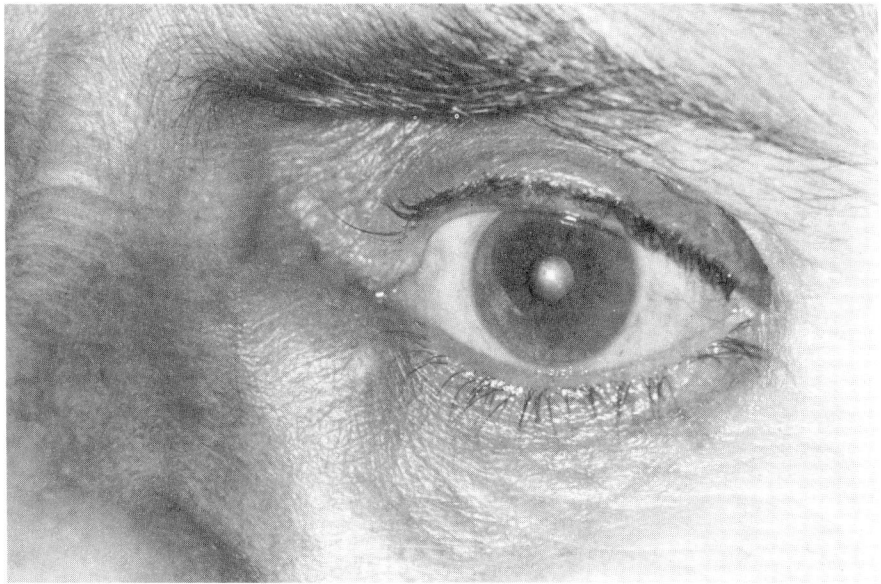

Fig. 5.8 An enlarged lacrimal sac in a patient with dacrocystitis.

called 'dacrocystitis' (*Fig.* 5.8). The infection usually spreads to the conjunctiva, so that there is a chronic mucopurulent conjunctivitis as well as the epiphora. The enlarged lacrimal sac can be seen or felt between the eye and the nose.

By gently pressing over the lacrimal sac, it is usually possible to massage the mucopurulent material in it back through the punctum to the conjunctival sac. It is helpful to teach the patient or the parents to massage the lacrimal sac, and so keep it empty while waiting for permanent surgical treatment. Local antibiotic drops are also helpful.

Sometimes an acute infection develops with pain, redness and inflammation over the sac. In this case, the patient should be given systemic antibiotics to help the inflammation subside. However, if the abscess bursts through the skin, this may leave a permanent fistula, so that tears pass out of the fistula and run down the cheek.

The treatment of nasolacrimal duct obstruction is different in children and adults. In children, the duct may spontaneously open within the first year. If not, the duct should be probed under a general anaesthetic. This will usually rupture the thin membrane at the bottom of the duct which is causing the obstruction.

In adults, it is not normally possible to treat nasolacrimal duct obstruction just by probing. It is necessary to construct a new drainage pathway from the lacrimal sac to the nose. There are various ways to do this: —

— A dacryocystorhinostomy is quite a complex operation. First, remove the bone between the lacrimal sac and the nose, and then suture flaps from the nasal mucous membrane to flaps from the lacrimal sac. Sometimes, the common canaliculus is also obstructed. In this case, thread a thin silicone tube

through both the upper and lower canaliculus and down into the nose at the same time.
- A much simpler method is to insert a short flanged plastic tube straight through the floor of the lacrimal sac and into the nose, using a trochar. The operation only takes a few minutes under local anaesthetic. Unfortunately, the long term results are not quite so satisfactory, because the flanged tube may fall out.

An alternative treatment is to excise the chronically infected lacrimal sac. This will cure the infection, but will still leave the patient with a watering eye.

6.   Diseases of the Conjunctiva

The anatomy of the conjunctiva is described in Chapter 2.

Conjunctivitis

Conjunctivitis is the general word for any infection or inflammation of the conjunctiva. Because the eyes are normally open, the conjunctiva is the most exposed mucous membrane in the body, and is especially prone to infection and inflammation.

Conjunctivitis is by far the most important disease of the conjunctiva, and it is also the most common of all tropical eye diseases. It is both more common and more serious in hot countries for the following reasons: –

- Warm and humid climates are ideal for micro-organisms to survive and multiply.
- Dust and solar radiation in desert climates constantly irritate the conjunctiva. Smoke from indoor wood fires is another common source of chronic irritation.
- Insect vectors, especially flies, may carry infection from eye to eye.
- Overcrowding, poor ventilation and poor hygiene in homes all help to spread micro-organisms from person to person.

Conjunctivitis usually recovers spontaneously. However, it is sometimes quite uncomfortable, and its complications occasionally cause visual loss.

The symptoms and signs of conjunctivitis

The conjunctiva has comparatively few sensory nerve endings and so conjunctivitis does not cause any real pain. There is usually a sensation of irritation, itching or discomfort in the eye. However, viral conjunctivitis may cause slight pain or photophobia. This is because viruses may also infect the epithelium of the cornea which is a very sensitive structure. If there is any significant pain, it is likely that some other disease is present instead of, or as well as, conjunctivitis.

The vision should be normal in conjunctivitis. Sometimes excess secretions may form a film across the cornea and blur the vision. This blurring usually improves when the patient blinks away this film. Viral conjunctivitis may cause a very slight blurring of the vision because it can affect the epithelium of the cornea also. However, any significant visual loss, just like significant pain, means that some other disease is present instead of, or as well as, conjunctivitis.

The signs vary very much according to the type of conjunctivitis, but will always include some of the following features. Most of them are visible to the naked eye, or only need a simple magnifying hand lens or magnifying spectacles to see them.

1. Vasodilatation is always part of any inflammatory response, and it makes the eye look red (*Plate* 3). For this reason conjunctivitis is sometimes called 'pink eye'. It is only the superficial vessels which are dilated, and the redness is either spread all over the conjunctiva, or is most obvious towards the fornices. Conjunctival vasodilatation which is only found around the limbus strongly indicates corneal or intraocular disease. In certain very acute infections, petechial conjunctival haemorrhages may also be visible (*Plate* 3c). In chronic conjunctivitis, the vasodilatation may be much less noticeable and confined to certain areas, such as the inner canthus or the upper fornix.

2. Increased secretions are a feature of most types of conjunctivitis. There are two causes. First, irritation of the inflamed conjunctiva provokes a reflex increase in tear production. Second, as a result of the inflammation, protein exudate and inflammatory cells leak from the blood vessels and add to the secretions. The character of these secretions often helps to diagnose the cause of the conjunctivitis: –

– Purulent or mucopurulent secretions are usual in acute bacterial infections (*Plate* 3b).

– Watery (serous) secretions are more typical of virus infections (*Plate* 3a).

– Thick sticky mucus is usually a sign of chronic allergic conjunctivitis (*Plate* 3f).

At night, when the eyelids are closed, the secretions usually dry. A crust then forms which makes it difficult to open the eye. The symptoms of conjunctivitis are also sometimes worse early in the morning. This is because the temperature behind the closed eyelid increases, and encourages the micro-organisms to multiply.

3. Oedema of the conjunctiva (chemosis) is sometimes visible in severe cases (*Plate* 3b). However, it does not usually indicate any specific cause. Oedema of the eyelids may also be present in severe cases.

4. Follicles are nodules of lymphoid tissue beneath the surface of the conjunctival epithelium. These follicles enlarge, especially in virus infections. (*see Plates* 3d, 6a, b *and* c). It is important to be able to recognize these enlarged follicles clinically. They are small, slightly pale nodules just visible to the naked eye under the conjunctival surface. They are usually most numerous in the fornices, and may also appear on the inside of the upper eyelid, especially in trachoma. The upper fornix is difficult to examine, and so it is easier to identify follicles in the lower fornix.

The lymphatic drainage from the conjunctiva passes to the preauricular node, which is just between the temporomandibular joint and the front of the ear. This preauricular node is sometimes enlarged and tender in conjunctivitis.

5. Papillae are raised areas on the surface of the epithelium and are caused by blood vessels and inflammatory cells growing in the subconjunctival tissues. This occurs in response to any chronic inflammation. Papillae are found especially in the conjunctiva lining the upper tarsal plate (*Plates* 3f, 4a and 6e), and occasionally near the corneal limbus (*Plate* 4b). At these two places the conjunctiva is bound firmly to the underlying tissues. To the naked eye, the papillae make the conjunctival surface appear rough and velvety rather than smooth and glistening. The conjunctiva also loses its normal transparency, so that it is difficult to see the underlying blood vessels very clearly. The individual papillae are not usually visible to the naked eye. However, with a slit lamp, and

especially in green light, it is possible to see each papilla with its small central blood vessel. Occasionally, the individual papillae are very large and can be seen with the naked eye (*Plate* 4a). This is called 'cobble-stone' hypertrophy, and is a characteristic feature of vernal conjunctivitis.

It can be difficult to distinguish between follicles and papillae without a slit lamp. They are both features of chronic conjunctivitis, and are often present together, especially in trachoma. However, it helps to remember that follicles are found beneath the conjunctival surface and are most numerous in the fornix. Papillae are found on the conjunctival surface, and especially in the upper tarsal conjunctiva.

6. Keratinization (*see Plates* 4d *and* 12a). Keratin is a hard protein which skin cells produce to resist wetting. In certain diseases, the conjunctival epithelium produces keratin, and so becomes hard and unwettable. The most important of these diseases is vitamin A deficiency. However, keratinization is also a feature of various rather rare types of 'endogenous' conjunctivitis.

7. Membrane formation is rare, and only occurs in acute streptococcal infections or diphtheria. It is more common for a pseudomembrane to form which looks like a membrane but cannot be peeled off. A pseudomembrane is sometimes found in the upper fornix in a common viral disease called 'epidemic keratoconjunctivitis'.

8. Scarring (fibrosis) can be the end result of any inflammatory process in the conjunctiva. It is especially common in trachoma (*see Plate* 6f). Usually, fibrous tissue appears as white opaque lines or patches under the tarsal conjunctiva. These opaque areas make it impossible to see the blood vessels underneath. Fibrous tissue always contracts. As it contracts, it either distorts the eyelid, or causes the conjunctiva to shrink and pull away from the fornix (*Plate* 4d). Sometimes the eyelid adheres to the eyeball, and this is called a 'symblepharon'. If the scars are severe, the conjunctiva will be unable to lubricate and protect the cornea properly, and so secondary corneal damage may occur.

9. Increased pigmentation can be the result of any chronic conjunctivitis in a dark-skinned person, and especially in a child. These changes are most noticeable around the limbus and in the exposed conjunctiva between the eyelids (*see Plates* 4b *and* c *and* 11f). The two most common conditions which present clinically with increased pigmentation are vitamin A deficiency xerophthalmia and vernal conjunctivitis. These pigmentary changes are characteristically diffuse and do not have well-defined margins. It is important not to confuse them with a quite normal pigmentation which is often found around the limbus but which is in irregular patches and has well-defined margins.

Causes of conjunctivitis

The list of possible causes of conjunctivitis is very large (*Table* 6.1). However, most cases of conjunctivitis come from one of four basic causes. These are bacterial infection, viral infection, trachoma or vernal conjunctivitis.

Bacterial conjunctivitis

Bacterial conjunctivitis is common. The bacteria may invade a normal, healthy conjunctiva to produce a primary bacterial conjunctivitis. In this case, the

Table 6.1. The main causes of conjunctivitis

Infective	*Bacterial infections* (common)	*Trachoma* (common)
	Staphylococcus	
	Haemophilus influenzae	*Viral infections* (common)
	Gonococcus	Adenoviruses
	Pneumococcus	Picornaviruses
	Meningococcus	Measles
	Streptococcus	Molluscum contagiosum
	Moraxella lacunata	Herpes simplex
	Proteus	etc.
	Pseudomonas	
	etc.	
	Granulomatous infections (rare)	
	(The granuloma may be caused by bacterial, fungal, viral or parasitic infections or foreign bodies)	
	Tuberculosis	
	Syphilis	
	Tularaemia	
	Actinomycosis	
	Sporotrichosis	
	Lymphogranuloma venereum	
	Parasitic worms	
	Myiasis (the larvae of flies)	
	Foreign bodies etc.	
Allergic	Vernal conjunctivitis (common) Hay fever Phlyctenular conjunctivitis Allergies to drugs and cosmetics	
Physical and chemical irritants	Foreign bodies Dust and smoke Ultraviolet light Snake venom etc.	
Nutritional	Xerophthalmia (vitamin A deficiency)	
Endogenous	Keratoconjunctivitis sicca (dry eyes) Ocular pemphigoid Rosacea etc.	
Secondary conjunctivitis (Following lacrimal or eyelid disease)	Dacrocystitis Trichiasis Entropion Ectropion Facial palsy etc.	
Others	Psychological Artefacta	

organisms are often quite virulent, and the inflammation is acute, severe and often bilateral. The disease lasts for 1 − 2 weeks, and then resolves spontaneously, usually without any significant scarring. Occasionally, primary bacterial conjunctivitis is caused by less virulent organisms with a more mild clinical course.

Sometimes, the bacteria may invade because the defences of the conjunctiva against infection are weakened. This is called 'secondary bacterial conjunctivitis', and the disease is often chronic or recurrent. The conjunctival defences may be weakened for many reasons: from disorders of the eyelids, the lacrimal apparatus or the conjunctiva itself. Some common examples are: −

- Eyelid abnormalities, e.g. ectropion, entropion, trichiasis, facial palsy, chronic blepharitis.
- Lacrimal abnormalities, e.g. dacryocystitis, keratoconjunctivitis sicca (dry eyes).
- Conjunctival abnormalities, e.g. xerophthalmia, severe scarring, foreign bodies.

Many different bacteria can cause conjunctivitis. Staphylococcus can cause an acute primary conjunctivitis, and is a very common cause of secondary conjunctivitis. Haemophilus influenzae is important because it causes seasonal epidemics of conjunctivitis in hot, dusty climates. Gonococcus usually comes from contact with genital discharges, and causes a particularly severe conjunctivitis. Pneumococcus, meningococcus and streptococcus are other bacteria which may cause acute conjunctivitis. *Moraxella lacunata* causes a more mild conjunctivitis. It is called 'angular conjunctivitis' because the inflammation is in the inner and outer canthus.

The clinical appearance of bacterial conjunctivitis will depend on how severe it is. There is always a mucopurulent discharge (*Plate* 3b). This is the characteristic feature of bacterial conjunctivitis. In severe cases, this is like yellow pus; in mild cases the eyelids may be stuck together on waking. There is always vasodilatation of the conjunctiva. In severe cases there may be chemosis of the conjunctiva, oedema of the eyelids and some general malaise.

It is not possible to identify particular bacteria by clinical examination. To identify the causative organism of any bacterial conjunctivitis requires a Gram stain of conjunctival smear, or a culture. However, even where such facilities are available, it is usually unnecessary to identify the causative organism. This is because there is a wide range of local antibiotic treatment available, and the condition nearly always resolves without any complications.

The standard treatment for acute infections is to give antibiotic drops every hour in the day, and ointment at night. Milder infections require drops or ointment 3 or 4 times a day. Many different antibiotic preparations are available commercially as either drops or ointment (*see* page 37).

It is important not to pad an eye with conjunctivitis. Padding will only encourage micro-organisms to multiply. Moist cottonwool swabs can be used to clean any discharge or dried secretions from the eyelids, especially in the morning. Acute bacterial conjunctivitis normally resolves after 3 or 4 days of antibiotic treatment.

Trachoma

Trachoma is the most common micro-organism to infect the eye in most hot countries. However, it is such an important disease that it needs a whole chapter to itself (*see* Chapter 7).

Viral conjunctivitis

Because so many viruses cause conjunctivitis, the symptoms vary very much. The disease may be so mild that it is impossible to recognize it clinically. At the other extreme, viral conjunctivitis may be a severe and disabling condition.

Unlike bacteria, all viruses live inside the body cells. For this reason they are all immune to antibiotics, and there is no specific treatment for most viruses. Viruses which affect the conjunctiva live in the epithelial cells and often invade the epithelial cells of the cornea also.

The typical symptoms and signs of a viral conjunctivitis are as follows: –
– There is a gritty foreign body sensation, and often there is slight photophobia because the virus may invade the corneal epithelium.
– The secretions are watery (serous), not purulent (*Plate* 3a).
– The blood vessels of the conjunctiva are dilated, and there is hypertrophy of the lymphoid follicles. There may be some papillary hypertrophy on the upper tarsal conjunctiva also.
– Conjunctival scrapings show lymphocytes and a few monocytes.

Adenovirus conjunctivitis

Adenovirus conjunctivitis is the most common viral infection of the conjunctiva. There are many different strains of the adenovirus. The more virulent strains (usually type 8 adenovirus) cause a disease called 'epidemic keratoconjunctivitis'. The more mild strains cause pharyngoconjunctival fever.
– Epidemic keratoconjunctivitis. The virus is transmitted from eye to eye by infected droplets or direct contact. The disease is common where people live close together in unhygienic conditions, and usually occurs in epidemics. It may be transmitted from patient to patient by tonometers or other such instruments in eye clinics.

Epidemic keratoconjunctivitis is usually bilateral, but often affects one eye more severely than the other. There are two specific signs: –
1. There are numerous fine punctate areas of inflammation in and under the epithelium of the cornea. These opacities are only visible with focal illumination and good magnification (*see Plate* 4e). They are called 'superficial punctate keratitis'.
2. In severe cases, the upper tarsal conjunctival epithelium near the fornix may break down, leaving a layer of fibrin called a 'pseudomembrane'.

In adults, epidemic keratoconjunctivitis is confined to the eye, but young children may also have a slight fever and a sore throat. The acute disease usually lasts for about 2 – 3 weeks. However, the small superficial opacities in the cornea may persist for many months, and cause discomfort, photophobia and slight blurring of the vision.

There is no specific treatment for the virus, so any treatment is essentially symptomatic. Antibiotic drops or ointment may help to prevent secondary

infection. In severe cases, local steroid drops (e.g. Predsol (prednisolone) drops 0.1%, 2 or 3 times a day) may help the inflammation to subside quicker.
- Pharyngoconjunctival fever is more common in children than adults. The most obvious symptoms are a sore throat and fever. The symptoms in the eye are less severe than in epidemic keratoconjunctivitis. Usually there are follicles on the conjunctiva which resolve after 2 or 3 weeks.

Epidemic haemorrhagic conjunctivitis

Epidemic haemorrhagic conjunctivitis (*Plate* 3c) was first reported in West Africa in the late 1960s. Since then the disease has appeared in most parts of the world. Because the first epidemics were about the same time as the American Apollo space mission, it is often called 'Apollo disease' in West Africa. The causative organism is a picorna virus (pico = small RNA virus), usually enterovirus 70.

Epidemic haemorrhagic conjunctivitis is highly contagious, and has a very short incubation period of only 1 – 2 days. Multiple petechial haemorrhages then appear all over the surface of the conjunctiva. The disease is acute, but short-lived, so that the patient usually makes a rapid and complete recovery. Occasionally, after a severe infection, there may be some permanent corneal or conjunctival scars.

Measles

Measles is a generalized viral infection which also invades the conjunctival and corneal epithelium. For this reason all children with measles have some conjunctivitis and superficial keratitis. Normally, these eye changes are quite mild compared to the other symptoms of the disease. However, measles in malnourished children is often very severe. It can cause serious corneal ulceration, blindness and even death. For further details, *see* Chapter 9.

Molluscum contagiosum (*Plate* 4f)

Molluscum contagiosum is a viral wart which appears on the margins of the eyelids. Virus particles are discharged from the wart into the conjunctiva, and cause a typical follicular conjunctivitis. The treatment is to remove the wart either by excision, cautery or curettage. The conjunctivitis will then resolve spontaneously.

Herpes simplex virus

The herpes simplex virus may cause conjunctivitis. However, it is much more important as a cause of corneal ulcers (See page 95).

Granulomatous conjunctivitis

Granulomatous conjunctivitis is the name for any unilateral conjunctivitis with a local inflammatory granuloma in the conjunctiva. It is often associated with swelling of the regional lymph nodes, and there may also be slight general malaise. Granulomatous conjunctivitis is sometimes called 'Parinaud's syndrome'.

Granulomatous conjunctivitis usually means that the conjunctiva has become by chance the route of entry into the body for some micro-organism. It is quite rare but there are many possible causes: –
- tuberculosis (probably the most common cause in hot countries)
- syphilis
- tularaemia (a bacterial disease of rodents)
- actinomycosis (a fungal disease)
- sporotrichosis (a fungal disease)
- lymphogranuloma venereum (a viral disease)
- cat scratch fever (cause unknown)
- parasitic worms, the larvae of flies and conjunctival foreign bodies may also produce similar conjunctival granulomas.

A biopsy and culture are usually necessary to identify the causative organism, and the correct treatment can then be given.

Allergic conjunctivitis

Allergy is an important cause of conjunctivitis. It occurs in four forms:
- vernal conjunctivitis (the most important)
- hay fever conjunctivitis
- phlyctenular conjunctivitis
- allergies to drugs or cosmetics

Vernal conjunctivitis (*Plates* 3f, 4a, b, *and* c)

Vernal conjunctivitis is the name for a chronic conjunctivitis which is especially common in children and which is probably due to allergy. It has not been possible to identify a specific allergen, but the most likely agent is some material in the atmosphere such as pollen. The disease is found all over the world, but is much more common and severe in hot countries.

Vernal conjunctivitis was originally called 'spring catarrh'. This is a poor name, because it is most common in climates where there is no spring. Also, the most important pathological changes are structural changes in the conjunctiva. Increased secretions (catarrh) are less important. The name vernal conjunctivitis is still not entirely suitable. 'Vernal' is only the Latin word for spring, and the disease occasionally involves the cornea as well as the conjunctiva.

Vernal conjunctivitis belongs to the same group of diseases as allergic rhinitis, asthma and eczema. These are called 'atopic' diseases, and are most common in children between the ages of 3 and 16. Occasionally, however, a younger child or a young adult may be susceptible. The characteristic of an atopic disease is a hypersensitivity reaction between the antigen in the air and the IgE antibody in the tissues. This reaction provokes the release of histamine and other toxins from the basophil and mast cells in the tissues. These toxins are then responsible for the symptoms of the disease. In temperate climates, most patients with vernal conjunctivitis have other evidence of atopic disease, such as asthma or eczema. However, in hot countries where vernal conjunctivitis is much more common, many patients have no other atopic disease.

The symptoms and signs of vernal conjunctivitis

The symptoms and signs may be seasonal, but they often persist throughout the year, and for many years. They are bilateral.

— Severe and persistent itching and irritation in both eyes is the characteristic symptom.
— There is often a sticky white discharge. It is caused by increased secretion of viscous mucus in the tears, so that the patients themselves often complain of 'string' or 'worms' in their eye. The sticky threads are the result of increased secretions of viscous mucus in the tears.
— Thickening of the conjunctiva with formation of papillae is a characteristic feature of vernal conjunctivitis. It occurs on the inside of the upper eyelid, or at the limbus, or at both sites.
— Changes on the upper eyelid conjunctiva
    The papillary hypertrophy on the inside of the upper eyelid is more common in older children. In the early stages the papillae give the surface of the conjunctiva a velvety appearance. They also obscure the underlying conjunctival blood vessels (*Plate* 3f). As the disease progresses, the papillae become larger and join together to produce giant papillae. These giant papillae fit together rather like cobble-stones (*Plate* 4a) The spaces between the papillae are filled with mucus, and it is possible to identify this mucus with special stains like Alcian blue.
— Changes on the limbal conjunctiva
    The changes at the limbus are more common in younger children. The limbal conjunctiva appears thick and swollen, and the underlying blood vessels may be dilated. (This vasodilatation at the limbus is unusual for a conjunctival disease. Dilated blood vessels at the limbus are nearly always the result of corneal or intraocular disease.)
    Also at the limbus, small pin-point white spots may appear on the corneal epithelium. These are necrotic areas of the epithelium, and stain with fluorescein. They are called 'Trantas' spots'.
    Increased pigmentation also occurs at the limbus in dark-skinned races. It often spreads to affect all the exposed conjunctiva between the eyelids. These pigmentary changes are fine and diffuse, and often very noticeable (*Plate* 4b *and* c).
    (One surprising feature of vernal conjunctivitis is that the severity of the symptoms often does not match the severity of the signs. Some patients may have very large papillae in their upper eyelids, but very few symptoms. Other patients may have severe itching but much less obvious changes in the conjunctiva.)
— Changes in the cornea
    Occasionally, vernal conjunctivitis may affect the cornea. This is probably because the thick mucus pulls off the corneal epithelial cells and the tarsal papillae rub against the cornea. Complications may also occur if the inflammation at the limbus spreads to the marginal cornea.
    The first sign of any complication in the cornea is a superficial punctate keratitis (*see* page 102).
    Just occasionally, the epithelial cells are stripped away to form a shallow oval ulcer, usually just above the centre of the cornea (*Plate* 4a). There is a lot

of mucus in the base of the ulcer. Sometimes, this mucus forms a thick sticky plaque which adheres firmly to the cornea and so prevents the ulcer from healing. Eventually, the ulcer will heal to become a vascularized scar. These ulcers are often bilateral.

Vernal conjunctivitis appears to die out in adult life. There is only a risk of permanent damage to the eye if corneal ulcers have developed. The very obvious inflammation and hypertrophy of the conjunctiva subsides and leaves little or no scarring. The changes at the limbus fade away much more quickly that those on the upper tarsal conjunctiva.

The treatment of vernal conjunctivitis

The most effective treatment is local steroid drops. In a typical case, prednisolone drops about 4 times a day for 1 − 2 weeks will relieve most of the symptoms. After that, drops perhaps twice daily will maintain the relief. Because the irritation and itching is so persistent, and because steroid treatment is so effective, many patients (or their parents) obtain further supplies from the local chemist or market pharmacy. They may then treat themselves excessively for many months or even years. Unfortunately, local steroid treatment can cause serious complications (see page 40). It is therefore essential to explain the dangers, and to make sure that the patient only has local steroid treatment under medical supervision.

Antihistamines, either locally or systemically, are not usually very effective, but they are worth a try.

Cromoglycate (Opticrom) prevents the release of histamine and other toxins from the mast cells. If it is used regularly, it will prevent the symptoms becoming so severe. However, the response is not as sudden or as complete as with steroids. Many patients find that by using cromoglycate, they can either reduce or completely stop any local steroid treatment. Cromoglycate also has the great advantage of having few, if any, side effects. The recommended dose is 1 drop to each eye, 4 times a day.

In advanced cases the response to medical treatment is sometimes disappointing, or it cannot be given because of side effects. In the past various surgical treatments have been used to destroy the papillae on the upper tarsal conjunctiva. If medical treatment fails to relieve the symptoms, there may still be a place for these surgical treatments: −
- Cryotherapy is least likely to cause permanent damage to the conjunctiva. The recommended treatment is to freeze the tarsal conjunctiva for about 30 seconds, thaw briefly, then freeze again for 30 seconds.
- Diathermy and cautery are both effective ways to destroy the papillae. However, they are both very painful and produce more long term scarring. They are not much used nowadays.
- Beta radiation is a very effective way to shrink the papillae. It is also easy and painless. However, there is always a risk that serious delayed side effects may occur many years after the treatment.

In desperation, people with severe vernal conjunctivitis have been told to wear occlusive goggles, or even emigrate to a cooler country if they can afford it.

Hay fever conjunctivitis

Hay fever conjunctivitis is an acute allergic reaction to pollen in the air, and it is usually associated with acute rhinitis. There are none of the structural changes which vernal conjunctivitis causes in the conjunctiva. The symptoms of hay fever conjunctivitis usually subside with a short course of antihistamine drops. Cromoglycate, and in severe cases local corticosteroids, may also be helpful.

Phlyctenular conjunctivitis

'Phlycten' is the Greek word for a blister and it describes the clinical appearance of this disease (*Plate* 5a). Phlyctenular conjunctivitis is caused by a localized hypersensitivity reaction to bacterial proteins in the bloodstream. These bacterial proteins are usually tubercular, and the highest incidence of the disease is in poor communities where tuberculosis is common. Children and young adults are most at risk.

Not every patient with a phlycten has tuberculosis. Sometimes, the phlycten is a hypersensitivity reaction to another bacterial protein (e.g. staphylococcus) or even a fungal infection (e.g. candida). Even if the response is to a tubercular protein, it does not necessarily mean that there are living bacilli in the body. The phlyctenular reaction itself represents a high degree of antibody formation and resistance to the infection. However, every patient with a phlycten is a tuberculosis suspect, and so should have a general examination, a Mantoux test and a chest X-ray if possible. A significant number of these patients have, or will develop active tuberculosis, and need appropriate treatment.

Phlyctens may appear anywhere on the bulbar conjunctiva, but are especially common at or near the limbus. It is not known why they only occur here, and not in other parts of the body. A phlycten first appears as a raised pinkish nodule surrounded by an area of hyperaemia. It then develops a necrotic grey centre surrounded by reactive inflammation. Finally the necrotic centre sloughs out and the phlycten heals with little or no scarring. The whole process takes about 2 weeks.

Sometimes, limbal phlyctens 'migrate' towards the centre of the cornea. The edge which is advancing upon the cornea shows superficial ulceration and inflammation. The limbal edge heals with vascularization and scarring. If the ulcer is not treated, it may eventually reach the central area of the cornea. The final scar is characteristically superficial and forms a wedge pointing towards the centre of the cornea. Conjunctival phlyctens produce only mild symptoms. However, corneal phlyctens cause considerable photophobia, pain and discomfort, and may leave significant scars.

Phlyctens respond very well to local corticosteroids. The inflammation will rapidly resolve and the amount of final scarring and visual loss will be far less. Some patients may of course need systemic treatment for tuberculosis.

Allergies to drugs and cosmetics (*Plate* 5b)

Almost any eye medication, or the chemical preservative, or eye cosmetics can provoke an allergic reaction in the conjunctiva. The eyelids are usually affected also. If the particular medication or cosmetic is no longer used, the reaction will subside.

Endogenous conjunctivitis

Endogenous conjunctivitis is the name for any spontaneous conjunctival disease which does not follow an external infection or allergy. The basic cause is usually unknown. These are some of the more common types of endogenous conjunctivitis: –

Keratoconjunctivitis sicca (dry eyes)

Keratoconjunctivitis sicca is quite common in old people and is often associated with rheumatoid arthritis. The lacrimal gland and accessory conjunctival glands produce fewer tears. The eyes therefore feel sore and gritty, and are prone to recurrent bacterial conjunctivitis. The epithelial cells in the exposed conjunctiva and cornea become degenerate and dehydrated, to produce a superficial punctate keratoconjunctivitis. This can be detected in the usual way with magnification and fluorescein dye (*see* page 102 and *Plate* 10a *and* b).

To diagnose keratoconjunctivitis sicca, it is necessary to demonstrate the lack of tears. This is done with a small strip of filter paper, the end of which is left in the lower fornix. The tears are absorbed by the filter paper and can be measured. The test is called 'Schirmer's test'.

The treatment is to use tear substitutes such as methyl cellulose drops frequently. In severe cases, it may help to close the lacrimal puncta with cautery, and so preserve the small amount of tears that are present. Antibiotic drops and ointment will help to prevent secondary conjunctivitis.

Ocular pemphigoid (*Plate* 4d)

In this condition, there is gradual shrinkage and fibrosis of the conjunctiva at the same time as keratinization of the conjunctival epithelium. It can spread to produce severe scarring of the cornea. There is no effective treatment for ocular pemphigoid.

Rosacea

Rosacea is a form of chronic conjunctivitis, which may involve the cornea. It is associated with an acne rash on the face and dilatation of the blood vessels of the face. Rosacea often improves with antibiotic and corticosteroid drops.

Traumatic conjunctivitis

Many different physical and chemical irritants can cause traumatic conjunctivitis. Conjunctival foreign bodies are extremely common, and are easy to miss both in the history and the examination. Snake venom conjunctivitis is fairly common in areas where the spitting cobra is found.

Psychological causes of conjunctivitis

Tension, anxiety or depression can produce symptoms all over the body. The exact pattern of these symptoms varies with the cultural background and with the individual patient. It is very common for young students who have no significant refractive error or evidence of eye disease to complain of irritation and discomfort in their eyes and difficulty in reading. It is of course necessary to check that there is no underlying organic disease. Probably the best treatment then is to reassure the patient that nothing is wrong, and to give some placebo drops.

Very rarely, hysterical patients deliberately damage their own conjunctiva in order to gain sympathy or attention. This is called 'conjunctivitis artefacta'.

Neonatal conjunctivitis (Ophthalmia neonatorum)

Neonatal conjunctivitis is conjunctivitis in a newborn child. The infant eye is especially susceptible to conjunctivitis, and the disease is more serious, for a number of reasons: –
– Many organisms which are pathogenic to the genital tract are also pathogenic to the conjunctiva. If the mother has any vaginal infection when she gives birth, there is a high risk of conjunctivitis in the newborn child.
– A newborn child produces few tears and the immune responses are not developed. Therefore the child is less able to fight any infection.
– The infant cornea is comparatively soft. An attack of conjunctivitis is more likely to infect and damage the cornea.
  A number of organisms can cause neonatal conjunctivitis: –
– Gonococcus is the most serious cause. It produces an acute conjunctivitis within the first few days of birth, and may cause corneal ulceration, scarring and eventually blindness.
– The TRIC agent is an organism similar to trachoma, which may be present in the female genital tract. It produces a more mild conjunctivitis, called 'trachoma inclusion conjunctivitis', within the first 2 weeks of birth.
– Staphylococcus and other organisms of a non-genital origin may also infect the infant conjunctiva.
  The treatment for neonatal conjunctivitis is basically the same as for any infective conjunctivitis. However, the risk of permanent damage to the cornea is so great that intensive treatment and very close observation are essential. The gonococcus is usually sensitive to many antibiotics including penicillin, but penicillin resistance is becoming more common. The TRIC agent will need at least 3 weeks of treatment with local tetracycline.

The diagnosis of conjunctivitis

It is important to try to diagnose the cause of conjunctivitis in order to give the correct specific treatment. *Table* 6.2 lists the basic features of the common types of conjunctivitis.

Acute conjunctivitis

This is usually caused by a bacterial or viral infection. Mucopurulent secretions indicate a bacterial cause: watery secretions and follicles indicate a viral cause.

Table 6.2. A summary of the common causes of Conjunctivitis

	Age and background of patient	Secretions	Duration of illness	Typical clinical picture	Cytology of conjunctival cells	Treatment
Bacterial conjunctivitis	Any	Mucopurulent	1 – 2 weeks	Conjunctival vaso-dilatation, sticky eyes, eyelid oedema (If chronic or recurrent look for eyelid or lacrimal disease)	Neutrophils	Antibiotic drops
Viral conjunctivitis	Any	Watery	1 – 8 weeks	Follicles, super-ficial punctate keratitis, pseudo-membrane if severe	Lymphocytes and monocytes	Symptomatic only
Trachoma	Any age but especially young children. Associated with poverty, dirt and flies	Slightly mucopurulent	1 month — 1 year +	Follicles, papillae, corneal pannus	Mixed neutro-phils and lymphocytes. Inclusion bodies seen	Tetracycline drops and ointment
Vernal conjunctivitis	Children and adolescents from any background	Stringy mucus	Chronic inter-mittent	Itching, papillae often cobble-stone, limbal infiltrate and pigment-ation. Keratitis and corneal ulcers if severe	Eosinophils	Cortico-steroid and cromoglycate drops
Xerophthalmia	Poor and mal-nourished infants and young children. Especially rice eating communiites	Watery and foamy	Chronic	Bitot's spot. Non-wetting of conjunctiva and cornea. Corneal ulcers if severe. Limbal pigmentation	Mixed	Vitamin A by mouth

Chronic or recurrent conjunctivitis

This may be caused by any abnormality of the conjunctiva, eyelids or lacrimal apparatus. There is usually secondary bacterial infection. The most common causes are ingrowing eyelashes, lacrimal sac infections, and conjunctival foreign bodies. Insufficient tear production is a common cause in old people.

Chronic conjunctivitis in children

This is usually caused by trachoma, vernal conjunctivitis or xerophthalmia. All of these conditions are common, and all are bilateral, so it is often difficult to make the correct diagnosis. Sometimes two of these diseases may be present together in the same patient, especially vernal conjunctivitis and trachoma. Remember that trachoma is a disease of bad hygiene and flies, and xerophthalmia a disease of bad nutrition. However, it may help to try to answer these questions: –

– How severe are the symptoms? Vernal conjunctivitis produces the most obvious symptoms, with severe itching of the eyes. In trachoma, the symptoms are irritation and discharge from the eyes. Xerophthalmia produces very few symptoms in the early stages.
– Are there changes on the upper tarsal conjunctiva? Papillae indicate either trachoma or vernal conjunctivitis. Follicles indicate trachoma.
– Are there any corneal complications? Xerophthalmia may produce extremely destructive corneal ulcers. Trachoma causes superficial keratitis, vascularization and scars in the upper part of the cornea. In vernal conjunctivitis, corneal complications are less common, but there may be punctate keratitis or central corneal ulcers.
– Are there changes at the limbus? Both vernal conjunctivitis and xerophthalmia cause pigmentation at the limbus. Vernal conjunctivitis causes inflammatory hypertrophy at the limbus, and in xerophthalmia there may be a Bitot's spot at the limbus.

Table 6.2 lists the different features of each of these diseases. It may also help to look at the following illustrations: –
– For trachoma, see Plate 6a – e.
– For vernal conjunctivitis, see Plates 3f, 4a and b.
– For xerophthalmia, see Plates 11e and f and 12a – c.

If laboratory services are available, a conjunctival culture or scraping may help the diagnosis of doubtful cases.

Degenerative changes in the conjunctiva

Pinguecula

A pinguecula is a fatty degenerative deposit. It is found under the conjunctival epithelium in the exposed interpalpebral fissure (Plate 5c). Pingueculas are common in old weather-beaten patients. There are not usually any significant symptoms. However, because the pinguecula is slightly raised above the normal conjunctival surface, it sometimes becomes inflamed.

Pterygium

A pterygium is a wedge of conjunctival tissue which grows over the surface of the cornea. For a full description, see Chapter 8.

Concretions (Plate 5d)

Concretions are tiny, hard, yellow or white granules which are found on the inside of the eyelids. They are caused by an accumulation of epithelial cells, mucus and debris in the conjunctiva. They eventually erode to the surface, where they may scratch the cornea and give a gritty feeling to the eye. It is possible to remove these concretions with the point of a needle using local anaesthetic drops.

Conjunctival tumours

Conjunctival tumours are quite common, and usually occur at or near the limbus. Most of them produce symptoms fairly early, and only rarely spread. They can usually be treated by local excision. Neglected conjunctival tumours can become large fungating masses filling the whole orbit, and may need radical surgery (*see Fig.* 18.7).
- Squamous cell carcinoma is the most common form of tumour (*Plate* 5e *and* f). The incidence increases with excessive exposure to sunlight, and irritation from dust, sand and smoke.
- Congenital dermoid cysts are found at the limbus, and are usually easy to excise.
- Papillomas, haemangiomas and melanomas are other forms of conjunctival tumour.
- Pigmented naevi are common especially near the limbus, (*Plate* 5c) and no treatment is usually necessary. However, if there is evidence of growth or inflammation, they should be removed by local excision.

7. Trachoma

Trachoma is one of the most common diseases in the world, and about 500 million people suffer to some extent. At least 2 million of these people are blind from trachoma, and many more have a significant visual handicap.

The earliest descriptions of trachoma are in ancient Egyptian, Babylonian and Chinese texts, but the word 'trachoma' was first used in Graeco-Roman times. It comes from the Greek word for 'rough' which describes the surface appearance of the conjunctiva in chronic trachoma.

Trachoma first attracted interest in Europe in the Napoleonic wars, when the British and French armies returned from Egypt. Many of the soldiers had contracted trachoma, and the disease spread in the community. However, it was about 100 years before the characteristic inclusion organisms were demonstrated in 1907, and another 50 years before the organism was first isolated in 1957.

The discoveries of the last 25 years have been especially important for the control of trachoma. We now know that the causative organism is sensitive to broad spectrum antibiotics. We also understand much more clearly why trachoma is such a severe and blinding disease in some situations, but fairly mild in others. At present, the total eradication of trachoma is almost impossible. However, the knowledge and technology are now available to control trachoma fairly cheaply, and so prevent blindness. Many areas are making effective use of this.

Geographically, the highest incidence of trachoma is in the dry, hot, dusty climatic zone which stretches from North India, through the Middle East to North Africa and the Sahel regions of Central and West Africa. It is also common in the rest of Central and South Asia, Indonesia, Northern Australia, Africa and Central and Southern America. It is always associated with poverty and unhygienic living conditions.

The organism which causes trachoma is at present called *Chlamydia trachomatis*. It is one of the Chlamydia group which have characteristics half-way between bacteria and viruses. Like bacteria, they multiply by binary fission and have some sort of cellular organisation. They are also sensitive to certain antibiotics, especially the sulphonamides and the tetracyclines. Unfortunately, Chlamydia are protected from the full effects of these antibiotics because, like viruses, they live inside the body cells.

C. trachomatis is found in the conjunctival and corneal epithelium, and also the mucous membrane of the genital tract. It seems to be responsible for two rather different conditions. The more severe form is trachoma, and the milder form is inclusion conjunctivitis. For this reason, the organism is sometimes called the 'TRIC agent' (short for trachoma inclusion conjunctivitis). There are in fact many different strains of *C. trachomatis*. Recent immunofluorescent antibody studies have shown that all the strains are very similar. However, serotypes A, B and C are more common in the eye, while serotypes D — K are more common in the genital tract.

The symptoms and signs of trachoma

The clinical picture of trachoma varies from a very mild condition with hardly any symptoms at all, to a severe and blinding disease. The symptoms are typical of any conjunctivitis, with an irritable red eye and a discharge which is usually slightly mucopurulent. In severe cases, there may be eyelid oedema, or pain and photophobia because the cornea is involved. In areas where trachoma is very common, it is usually first contracted in early childhood.

Trachoma is a chronic disease which progresses through different stages. McCallan, who worked in Egypt over 50 years ago, was the first person to describe these different clinical stages. His classification is still often used to describe a case of trachoma. However, it does not indicate whether the infection is mild or severe.

In the early stages of the disease, there are no specific signs. There are only the non-specific signs of conjunctivitis, e.g. hyperaemia of the conjunctival vessels, and increased secretions. A slit lamp examination may also reveal the early formation of papillae (*see Plate* 3e). This is sometimes called 'doubtful trachoma' or 'trachoma dubium'.

Stages 1 and 2 — Active trachoma

After about 1 – 3 weeks, more specific signs develop. This is Stage 1 — early active trachoma. As the disease progresses, the signs become more obvious, and this is Stage 2 — florid trachoma. The only real difference between the two stages is that Stage 2 is more severe. For this reason, it is common to describe the two together as active trachoma. The following signs are seen: –

i. Conjunctival changes (*see Plates* 6a – d *and* 3d). There are two forms of inflammatory response in the conjunctiva which are specific in established, active trachoma. These are follicles and papillae (*see* Chapter 6, page 64). It is usual to see both follicles and papillae, but sometimes one form is more common than the other.

– Follicles are subepithelial lymphoid nodules, which are usually just visible to the naked eye. As the disease progresses, they become larger and develop pale, necrotic centres. Follicles are most numerous in the fornices, especially the upper fornix. They are also found on the inside of the upper eyelid, and this is a characteristic feature of trachoma. There may also be follicles at the limbus of the cornea.

– Papillae are found on the surface of the conjunctiva, especially on the inside of the upper eyelid. They cause the conjunctiva to look velvety to the naked eye, and obscure the underlying blood vessels. With a slit lamp, it is possible to see each individual papilla with its central blood vessel.

In mild cases, only a few follicles or papillae can be seen on the upper eyelid conjunctiva (*Plate* 6a). In severe cases, the follicles and papillae will completely

obscure the underlying tarsal conjunctival blood vessels (*Plate* 6d). These severe
cases are likely to develop blinding complications later.
ii. Corneal changes (*Plate* 6e). The trachoma organism also invades the corneal
epithelium, especially the upper part under the upper eyelid. This is probably
because the upper cornea is in close contact with the upper eyelid.
– A punctate or diffuse superficial keratitis is an early sign of corneal
   involvement, which is usually only visible with a slit lamp. However,
   fluorescein dye will stain the individual epithelial defects, so that a faint green
   haze may be visible to the naked eye.
– As the infection becomes more severe, the inflammation in the superficial
   cornea becomes more obvious. Blood vessels grow from the limbus into the
   cornea. These blood vessels and inflammatory changes are called a pannus. In
   severe cases, the corneal epithelium may break down to form a shallow ulcer.

Stage 3 — Healing with scar formation (Plate 6f)

The period of active inflammation may persist for a few weeks, but eventually
healing with scar formation begins. At this stage, the disease is still active because
follicles and papillae can still be seen. However, the presence of scar tissue shows
that some healing is also occurring.

Scar tissue (sometimes called 'fibrous tissue') consists of collagen fibres. These
collagen fibres are formed following any damage to the tissues. They show that
the disease is becoming inactive, and that healing is taking place. The collagen
fibres are found under the conjunctival epithelium, especially in the upper tarsus.
Here they appear as fine white streaks obscuring the underlying blood vessels. In
severe cases, the fibrous tissue may form such a dense sheet that none of the
underlying blood vessels can be seen.

In the cornea, the inflammatory keratitis will gradually heal. However, there
may be some slight scarring in the upper part of the cornea, and the blood vessels
which have invaded the cornea usually persist. The follicles which may occur at
the limbus become scarred and shrink to form little pits. These are called
'Herbert's pits', and are diagnostic of trachoma (*Plate* 7a).

Stage 4 — Inactive trachoma with scars

At this stage, the disease has finally burnt itself out, and is inactive. Only the
scars remain. In mild cases, there are only a few faint scars on the upper tarsal
plate, which are of no significance. At the other extreme, the eye may be grossly
damaged, with severe scarring of the eyelids, conjunctiva and cornea. The
collagen fibres in the scar slowly contract, and this causes deformities especially
in the eyelids. Also, the fibrous tissue may replace specialized conjunctival cells,
and so the function of the conjunctiva may be affected. The changes produced by
this scarring are as follows: –
i. The eyelids are most susceptible to damage, especially the upper eyelid.
– The fibrous tissue develops mainly under the conjunctiva and in the tarsal
   plate. As the fibrous tissue contracts, the margin of the eyelid turns inwards
   against the eyeball. This is called 'entropion' (*Plate* 7b). The eyelashes then
   rub against the cornea. This is called 'trichiasis'.
– Fibrosis around the hair follicles causes displacement of the individual

eyelashes. They therefore emerge irregularly from the eyelid, instead of in a row, and they may rub against the cornea. In this case, there is trichiasis without entropion (*Fig.* 7.1).
- The tarsal plate may become thickened and deformed.
- The Meibomian glands may be obstructed, or even destroyed.

ii. The fornices and bulbar conjunctiva are also at risk of damage from fibrosis.
- The subconjunctival fibrosis obliterates the fornices. The glands which secrete mucus are mainly in the fornices, so these are also lost.
- The conjunctival epithelium may become keratinized. This means that it loses its moist, wettable surface, and becomes like skin.

iii. The lacrimal apparatus
- Any obstruction in the lacrimal passages may cause watering of the eyes and recurrent lacrimal sac infections.
- Occasionally, there may be damage to the lacrimal gland. This will reduce the production of tears.

iv. The cornea
The trachoma infection itself may cause slight scarring in the upper part of the cornea. However, this scarring does not usually extend to the pupil, and so causes little or no damage to the vision. Unfortunately, damage to the eyelids, conjunctiva and lacrimal apparatus may have serious effects upon the cornea.
- The ingrowing eyelashes constantly rub against the corneal epithelium, causing irritation, inflammation and discomfort. They may also cause recurrent corneal ulceration and scarring (*Plate* 7c, 7d *and Fig.* 7.2).
- Damage to the conjunctiva and to the lacrimal apparatus also weakens the defences of the eye. The risk of secondary corneal infections and further corneal scarring therefore increases.

The epidemiology of trachoma

Trachoma can vary from a mild to a very severe disease in different situations.

It is possible to produce a mild form of trachoma by inoculating a blind volunteer (who has had no previous infection) with the organism from an active case. The volunteer patient soon develops active trachoma with a typical follicular and papillary conjunctivitis. After a few weeks, however, the infection heals spontaneously with only very slight subconjunctival scarring and no significant damage to the eye. Another mild form of trachoma is found if a newborn child is infected at birth with trachoma organisms from the mother's genital tract. This usually presents as a mild follicular conjunctivitis, and heals spontaneously leaving little or no scarring. The mild form of the disease is called 'inclusion conjunctivitis', 'inclusion blennorrhoea', or sometimes 'paratrachoma'.

The most severe form of trachoma is called 'hyperendemic trachoma'. It is seen in some rural village communities, where almost everyone has either active trachoma or scars from an earlier infection. In these communities, many people may develop trichiasis or entropion, and corneal scars.

Why does the same infection produce a mild disease in one situation, and a severe blinding disease in another situation? Recent research has shown that several different factors influence the pattern of the disease. It is necessary to understand these factors clearly in order to plan suitable methods to control and prevent blindness from trachoma. The most important of these factors are as

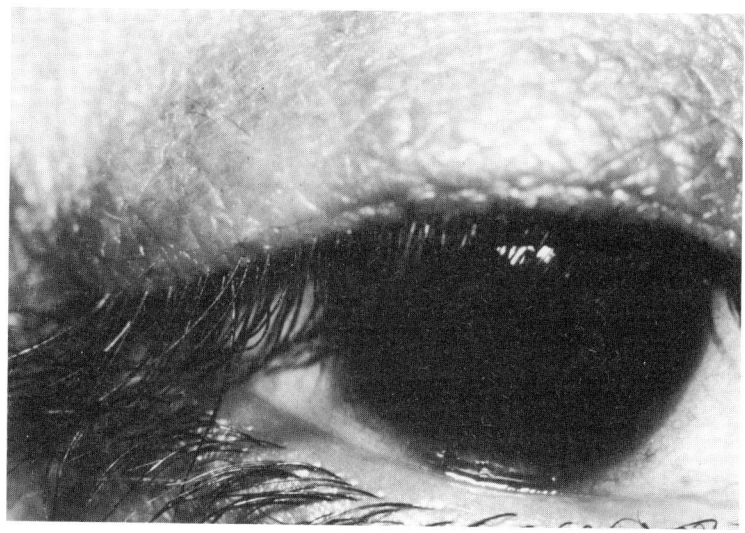

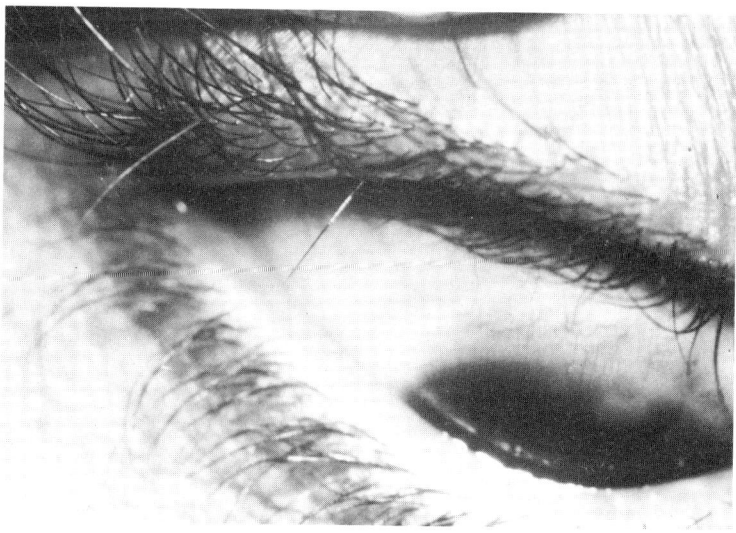

Fig. 7.1 Trichiasis. The ingrowing lashes are not seen until the eyelid is slightly everted.

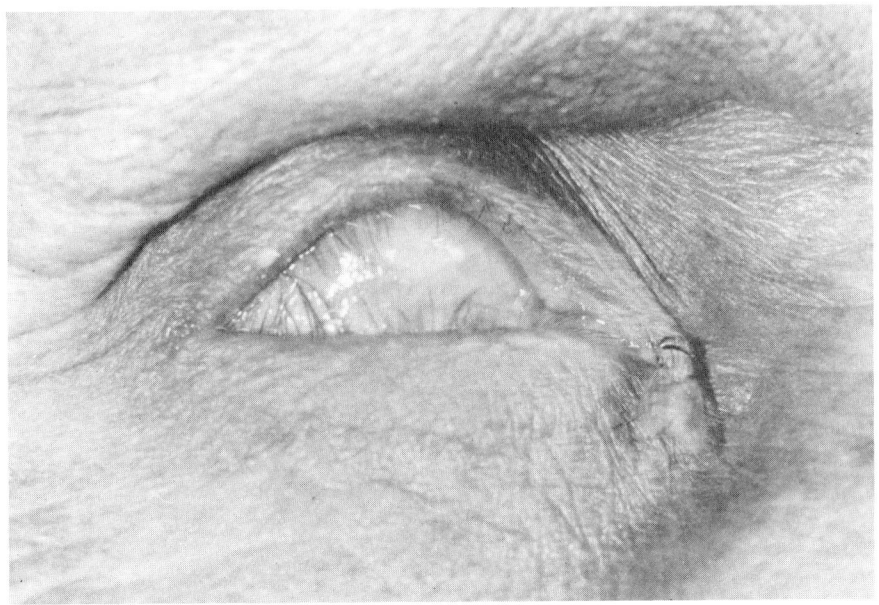

Fig. 7.2 Entropion with severe corneal scarring. Note the fly.

follows: −

1. Trachoma produces such poor and short-lived immunity that re-infection is very likely to occur. In an experimentally infected blind volunteer, there is only one cycle of the disease which heals with minimal scarring. However, in hyperendemic areas there are several cycles of the disease, one after the other. These re-infections produce a more severe form of the disease. It is also possible that continued re-infection with trachoma may cause a hypersensitivity reaction in the surrounding tissues. This would explain why the trachoma organism, which only seems to live in the epithelial conjunctival cells, can produce such deep scarring in the tarsal plate and the upper eyelid.

2. Trachoma is not a very infectious disease. It can only spread in poor, overcrowded communities where hygiene is bad and where conjunctival discharges frequently pass from eye to eye. This situation is sometimes called 'ocular promiscuity', just as sexual promiscuity describes close genital contact in a community. Most people who examine and treat trachoma patients every day do not themselves contract the disease. This is simply because they follow the basic rules of hygiene and personal cleanliness.

3. The main carriers of the infection are children below the age of 10, and especially pre-school children. The disease spreads from child to child by direct contact on the fingers of children and their mothers, and on clothes, handkerchiefs and pillows. Overcrowding, poor hygiene and, in particular, large numbers of flies all help the disease to spread. In areas where trachoma is a major problem, flies are often seen on the faces of young children. They feed on eye and nasal discharges, and therefore spread the infection from eye to eye (*Fig.* 7.3). In

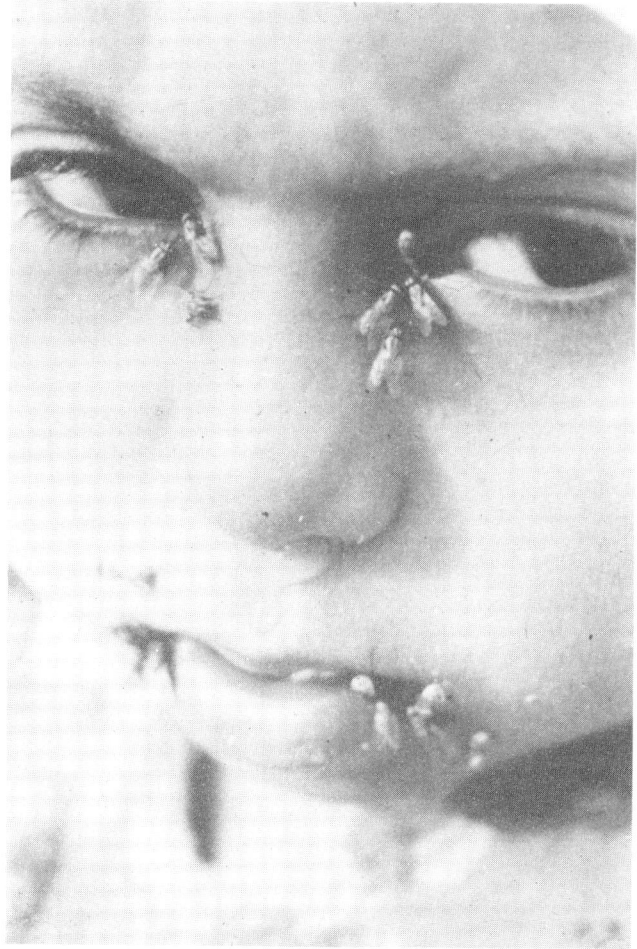

Fig. 7.3 A common sight where trachoma is a major problem.

hyperendemic areas, almost all young children have active trachoma. Most adults only have inactive trachoma scars, but some may still show active disease which is almost always a re-infection. Such re-infections are more common in adult women than in men. This is probably because women have closer contact with young children than men. It also explains why women are more susceptible to the late complications of trachoma.

4. The same conditions which help to spread trachoma also help to spread other types of infective conjunctivitis, especially bacterial conjunctivitis and adenovirus infections. These infections often come in seasonal epidemics, and usually occur when the greatest number of flies are found. Any secondary infection which occurs at the same time as active trachoma will produce a more severe clinical picture, and eventually lead to increased scarring (*Plate* 7d).

5. Trachoma is a much more severe and blinding disease in areas where heat and dust are a problem. There are probably several reasons for this: –
– Dust is a direct irritant to the eyes, and so increases the inflammatory reaction produced by the trachoma infection.
– Flies multiply rapidly in hot, dusty conditions.
– Dust provokes eye and nasal discharges. These discharges are the source of the infection, and are spread either directly or by flies.

A comparison of two areas in West Africa shows how important climatic factors are. Near the coast, the climate is very humid. Trachoma is common, but is not a very significant cause of blindness. Further north towards the Sahara desert, however, the climate becomes much drier, and blinding trachoma becomes increasingly more common. In all other ways the economic conditions and general way of life are almost identical.

6. Flies are very effective agents in transmitting trachoma. They lay their eggs on rotting rubbish or faeces, and so multiply more rapidly where there is poor public sanitation. One fly, Musca sorbens, lays its eggs in human faeces, and prefers to feed on eye and nasal discharges.

7. Whenever the standards of living improve, the incidence and severity of trachoma falls. Trachoma was a significant problem in Europe in the last century, but almost completely disappeared when living conditions improved. This was long before the discovery of any antibiotics, or even before there was any understanding of how trachoma is transmitted. Better living standards and personal hygiene prevent the spread of eye discharges from person to person, and also lessen the fly population.

8. In particular, trichiasis and entropion are the two complications of trachoma which cause blindness. The ingrowing eyelashes constantly irritate the cornea, and provoke further corneal ulceration, infection, vascularization and increased scarring. Almost all patients who are blind from trachoma have trichiasis or entropion.

Trachoma blindness in the community

The overall pattern of trachoma in the community varies very much from area to area: –
– In hyperendemic areas, most of the young children have active trachoma. The incidence of active infection then becomes less with increasing age. Nearly all adults show some degree of conjunctival scarring from trachoma. However, some adults, especially women, may still show active infection. Trichiasis and entropion become an increasing problem over the age of 15, and blindness from corneal scarring an increasing problem over the age of 30. The incidence of visual handicap from trachoma in a hyperendemic area can be as high as 10 per cent.
– In areas where the spread of the disease is less, either for climatic or hygienic reasons, many children may still have active trachoma. However, the scarring is less severe, and complications which can cause blindness, such as trichiasis and corneal scarring, are uncommon.
– In communities where hygiene is good, there is very little eye to eye spread of the disease, and so very few cases of trachoma. Trichiasis, entropion and blindness from trachoma do not occur. Where infections do occur, they often

originate in the genital tract, and cause secondary infection of the eyes, such as inclusion conjunctivitis in newborn children. It seems that a different strain of the organism is usually responsible for this genitally transmitted trachoma. It is probably just as virulent as the strain which is transmitted from eye to eye, but does not lead to blindness for all the reasons given above.

The diagnosis of trachoma

The characteristic signs of active trachoma are conjunctival follicles and papillae, especially on the upper tarsal conjunctiva. Inactive or burnt-out trachoma is usually indicated by any of the following signs: –
- Entropion or trichiasis of the upper eyelid.
- Scarring of the upper tarsal conjunctiva.
- Pannus blood vessels on the upper part of the cornea.
- Herbert's pits at the limbus.

These changes, both of active and inactive trachoma, can be identified with a simple magnifying lens, or even the naked eye.

The two diseases which are most often confused with trachoma are epidemic keratoconjunctivitis, caused by an adenovirus infection, and vernal conjunctivitis: –
- Adenovirus infection (*see* page 68) causes a more acute infection than trachoma. It produces superficial punctate keratitis over the whole cornea. By contrast, trachoma usually involves the upper cornea only. However, these fine corneal changes are very difficult to see with the naked eye.
- Vernal conjunctivitis (*see* page 70) is a chronic disease which is sometimes present as well as trachoma. The diagnosis of any type of conjunctivitis is also discussed on page 75 – 7.

The laboratory diagnosis of trachoma requires fairly specialized techniques and skills which are not usually available: –
- Giemsa stain or iodine can be used to demonstrate trachoma inclusion bodies in conjunctival scrapings. More recently, immunofluorescent staining techniques have been discovered which will demonstrate the organism more vividly. (The trachoma organism lives in the cells, and not in the conjunctival sac. To identify the organism, it is not enough just to take a conjunctival swab. It is necessary to obtain conjunctival epithelial cells by scraping the conjunctiva.)
- Trachoma can be cultured on certain living cells.
- It is now possible to identify antibody to the trachoma organism either in the patient's blood or in the tears.

The treatment of trachoma

The trachoma organism is sensitive to certain antibiotics, in particular the tetracyclines (tetracycline, chlortetracycline, doxycycline and oxytetracycline), the sulphonamides, and erythromycin. To a lesser extent it is also sensitive to penicillin and chloramphenicol. However, the trachoma organism lives inside the body cells, and so it is protected from the full effects of these antibiotics. The response to treatment is therefore much slower than when antibiotics are used in bacterial infections.

The antibiotic treatment may be given locally or systemically, but local treatment is usually best for the following reasons: –
– It is cheaper and most trachoma patients are poor.
– There is no risk of systemic side effects. Tetracycline can discolour and damage the teeth, and cause gastro-intestinal disturbances. Sulphonamides can cause severe hypersensitivity reactions.
– Local antibiotic treatment is also effective against bacterial conjunctivitis, which may be present as well as trachoma.

Tetracycline seems to be more effective than sulphonamides. It is also more effective against other bacteria. Both tetracycline ointment and oily suspensions are available. Two different dose schedules are recommended: –
1. Continuous treatment requires drops or ointment 4 times a day for 6 weeks. This is probably best for treatment of an individual patient.
2. Intermittent treatment requires drops or ointment 2 times a day for 1 week each month, for 6 months. This is probably best for treating the community.

If the infection is very severe, or if there is trachoma in the eye and the genital tract, local and systemic antibiotic treatment may be necessary. Even then, a week's course of systemic treatment is probably adequate. Longer periods of treatment increase the risks of side effects.

Patients with trachoma and vernal conjunctivitis need antibiotic and steroid mixtures, such as tetracycline and hydrocortisone. The same treatment has also been tried for patients who only have trachoma. It is possible that much of the tissue damage in trachoma is caused by an immunological reaction rather than by direct toxins from the organism. However, the results have been rather uncertain, and there are good reasons to be very cautious about steroid treatment. Local steroids should only be given under the direct supervision of a specialist.

The treatment of trichiasis and entropion

Trichiasis and entropion are by far the most common and important complication of trachoma. There is such a risk that the ingrowing eyelashes may cause corneal scarring and eventually blindness, that surgical treatment must be given as soon as possible. After surgery, the keratitis resolves, and some of the scarring gradually fades. This sometimes helps the cornea to gradually regain its transparency.

Unfortunately, there is not one, but very many different techniques for correcting trichiasis and entropion. In areas where there are few trained ophthalmic surgeons, it can be difficult for non-specialists or nurses to make the best choice. Then again, the tissues are deformed and scarred, and so the technique is often more difficult than the textbook illustration suggests. Most surgical methods for correcting trichiasis and entropion come under one of three headings: –
1. Removal of the ingrowing eyelashes is the simplest type of operation. It is especially suitable where there is no entropion, but only a few ingrowing eyelashes which irritate the cornea. It is no use pulling out the eyelashes (epilation), because they will only grow again. Cutting the eyelashes does more harm than good, because it makes them sharper and even more irritant. The following are all permanent methods of destroying the eyelashes: –
– Electrolysis. Inject with a local anaesthetic, and then insert the electrolysis

needle into the eyelash root along the line of the lash. Allow the current to flow for a few seconds. If the root has been successfully destroyed, it is possible to lift the eyelash out of the eyelid, rather than pull it out.

- Cryotherapy is a more recent technique. Apply the cryoprobe to the eyelid margin, and freeze the tissue for a few seconds at -25 °C. If possible, check the temperature with a needle thermocouple. Allow the tissue to thaw, and then freeze again. Unfortunately, cryotherapy very often causes depigmentation of the skin, which may be cosmetically unacceptable in dark-skinned patients. To avoid this complication, split the eyelid margin into two layers. The outer layer contains the skin and normal lashes, and the inner layer contains the ingrowing lashes. Only freeze the inner layer.
- Excision. If only a small area of eyelashes is misplaced, it is possible to excise these eyelashes together with their roots.

2. Splitting the eyelid margin (*Fig.* 7.4) is usually a simple operation, which can correct most cases of trichiasis or entropion. If any complications do develop, they do not leave the patient in a worse situation than before the operation.

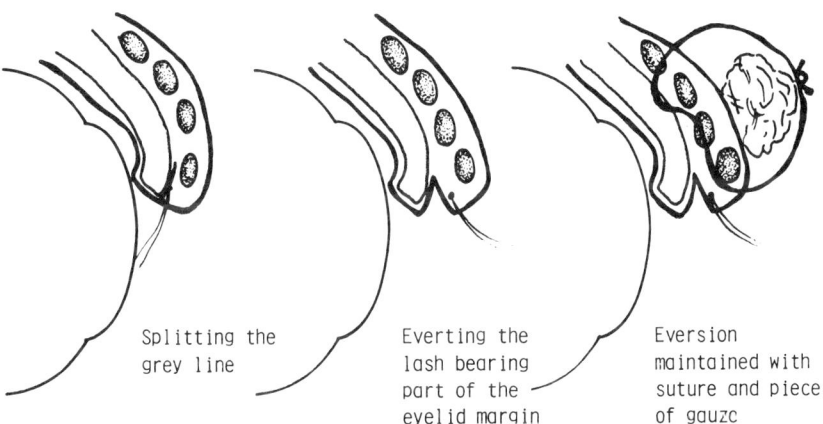

Splitting the grey line

Everting the lash bearing part of the eyelid margin

Eversion maintained with suture and piece of gauze

Fig. 7.4 Surgical correction of mild entropion.

Split the eyelid margin into two parts along the grey line. The inner part contains the conjunctiva and tarsal plate. The outer part contains the skin, orbicularis oculi muscle, the inverted eyelashes and their roots. The outer part is now free to rotate outwards. There are various ways to fix it in this new position, so that the eyelashes remain everted when the wound heals: –

- Put a small bandage over the eyelid margin. Use everting sutures to hold the eyelid in place while the defect fills up with granulation tissue (*Fig.* 7.4).
- Excise a small segment of eyelid skin and muscle from the eyelid margin. Everting sutures may also be used.
- A mucous membrane graft is a very effective but slightly more complex way of filling the gap at the lid margin. The easiest place from which to remove mucous membrane is the mouth.

3. Incision and rotation of the tarsal plate (*Fig.* 7.5) is an effective technique for severe entropion. However, if the operation is badly performed, or if complications develop, the eyelids may become very scarred or deformed. The technique is to divide the tarsal plate so that the eyelid margin containing the lashes is free to rotate outwards. Cutting through the tarsal plate inevitably means cutting through all the Meibomian glands, but significant complications

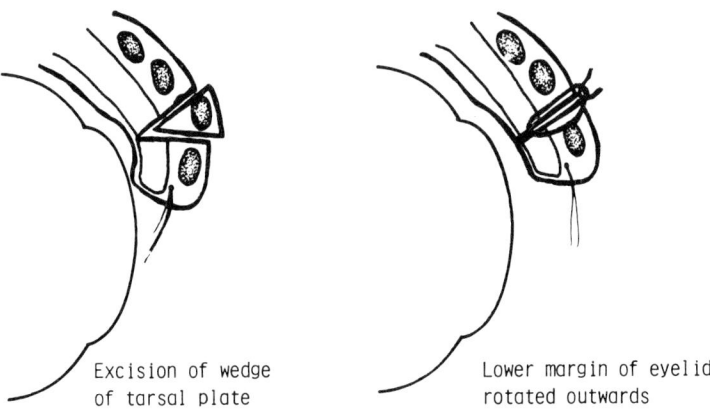

Excision of wedge
of tarsal plate

Lower margin of eyelid
rotated outwards

Fig. 7.5 Surgical correction of severe entropion.

do not seem to develop. It is possible to make an incision either from the skin or from the surface of the conjunctiva.

i. The skin approach is probably easier, and is called 'Snellen's operation'. This approach leaves the conjunctiva intact.
- Protect the eye with an eyelid guard.
- Remove a V-shaped wedge from the tarsal plate about 3 mm from the lid margin.
- Evert the lower fragment of the tarsal plate and the eyelashes. If it is necessary to increase the eversion of the eyelashes, make a small split along the eyelid margin.
- Use mattress sutures to fix the tarsal plate in its new position.

ii. The conjunctival approach effectively corrects any degree of entropion. However, it leaves rather a large open wound to fill with granulation tissue, and become covered with epithelium.
- Evert the eyelid.
- Divide the tarsal plate transversely about 3 mm from the eyelid margin and dissect free the front of the lower part.
- Rotate the lower strip of tarsal plate outwards, and fix it in its new position with mattress sutures.

Lacrimal and conjunctival complications

Lacrimal obstruction and conjunctival scarring may also require treatment. If the conjunctiva has become keratinized, and the fornices contracted, the cornea is likely to become scarred. It may help to use mucus and tear substitutes, such as methyl cellulose. Mucous membrane grafts from the mouth have also been tried to reconstruct the fornices in very severe cases, but the results have been very poor.

Corneal scarring and corneal blindness

This is the most significant complication of trachoma. Unfortunately, corneal grafting can only very occasionally restore the vision. Patients with severely scarred corneas from trachoma are often very poor risk cases for corneal grafting. This is because the conjunctiva is in a poor condition and because vascularization of the cornea may lead to graft rejection. Another difficulty is that corneal graft patients need careful supervision after the operation. This is often impossible for poor rural villagers.

It is essential to correct any trichiasis or entropion before performing a corneal graft. This is because an ingrowing eyelash will irritate the cornea, and destroy an otherwise successful corneal graft.

The prevention of trachoma

To prevent blinding trachoma, it is not necessary to eradicate the disease altogether. However, it is necessary to prevent the severe forms of trachoma which can so easily lead to blindness. There are several possible ways to do this: –
1. Improving personal and public hygiene is obviously the best way to eradicate blinding trachoma. However, for economic and cultural reasons, it is not usually possible to persuade people to change their traditional way of life. It is probably much better to aim for a few specific changes in a community which can significantly reduce the incidence of infection and re-infection with trachoma. Some examples are: –
– Supplying piped water, to encourage personal hygiene and the washing of clothes.
– Removing rubbish and faeces, to control the fly population.
– Teaching personal hygiene to primary school children and young mothers.
2. Antibiotics can be effective in three different ways: –
– By destroying the organisms in the individual patient, they help the infection to resolve earlier and reduce the risk of scarring.
– Most of the seasonal conjunctivitis which aggravates trachoma responds to antibiotic treatment.
– If the whole community is treated, there are fewer active carriers to spread trachoma.

In hyperendemic areas, all pre-school children and children in their first years at school are 'at risk'. It is possible either to treat them all, or preferably to examine them all and only treat those with active trachoma. It is much cheaper to pay for a drug prevention scheme now than to look after large numbers of blind people later.

3. The surgical correction of trichiasis and entropion is a valuable way to prevent blindness in the community. When patients first develop trichiasis or entropion, they have already suffered quite severe trachoma. However, the vision is usually still good, and the cornea fairly unscarred. If no treatment is given, progressive corneal scarring and blindness is likely to develop within 10 years.

In many areas, it is estimated that about 1% of the population needs corrective surgery for trichiasis and entropion. In a few areas it may be as high as 5% or even 10%. These figures show how urgent the need is to train some paramedical workers to perform trichiasis surgery.

4. Vaccination has been tried, but has not yet been successful.

For further reading

WHO, *Guide to Trachoma Control.* (1981) Geneva.

8.   The Cornea

The structure of the cornea is described in Chapter 2, and *Figs*. 2.1 and 2.2. The cornea has no blood supply. It obtains its metabolic needs from the blood vessels of the limbus and from the aqueous fluid in the anterior chamber. When the eyelids are open, oxygen from the atmosphere diffuses through the tear film into the cornea. When the eyelids are closed, the conjunctival blood vessels also nourish the cornea. The cornea has a very rich nerve supply, which makes it extremely sensitive to both touch and pain.

The cornea is the most important of the anterior structures in the eye. The only purpose of the eyelids, conjunctiva and lacrimal apparatus is to protect the cornea and keep it healthy and transparent. If they are diseased or damaged, inflammation or scarring in the cornea often follows. The cornea has an especially close relationship with the conjunctiva, and sometimes suffers from the same disorders. This is because the epithelium of the cornea is directly continuous with the epithelium of the conjunctiva.

Patterns of corneal disease

The cornea is exposed to the atmosphere, and so often suffers injury, inflammation or infection. Degenerative changes are also quite common.

The general word for any type of corneal inflammation is keratitis.
- If the inflammation is in the epithelium and Bowman's membrane, it is called 'superficial keratitis'.
- If the inflammation is superficial, but only occurs in certain, small discrete patches of the cornea, it is called 'superficial punctate keratitis (SPK)'.
- If the inflammation is in the stroma, it is called 'deep', 'stromal' or 'interstitial' keratitis.
- If there is inflammation and a significant loss of corneal epithelium, this is called a 'corneal ulcer'.

Because the cornea is such a specialized structure, any inflammation or injury is likely to cause some permanent damage or scar. The pattern of scarring will vary according to the nature of the original inflammation.

Many types of micro-organism can invade the cornea: viruses, bacteria, fungi or parasites. Most of these organisms come from outside, through the epithelium and into the cornea. However, a few may already be in the body, and migrate through the limbus.
- Viruses usually invade a healthy cornea through the epithelium. They often also infect the conjunctival epithelium, and so viral infection often presents as

superficial punctate keratoconjunctivitis. Viruses also cause corneal ulcers.
- Bacteria and fungi cannot normally penetrate the defences of a healthy cornea. They can only therefore enter if the defences are disturbed, or if there is a break in the epithelium. The bacteria often produce toxins, which cause necrosis and pus formation in the corneal tissue. This is called 'suppurative keratitis', or a 'suppurative corneal ulcer'.
  Leprosy, syphilis and onchocerciasis are all examples of organisms which enter the cornea from the body through the limbus. This is why they are mainly found in the stroma, and why any inflammatory reaction is usually a stromal keratitis.
  Sometimes the cornea is the site for a hypersensitivity reaction rather than a specific infection. These changes usually occur near the corneal margin, close to the limbal blood vessels.
The cornea is very sensitive to the outside environment.
- Hot dry air, dust or sand particles in the atmosphere, and smoke all irritate the corneal and conjunctival epithelium. In this way, any superficial infection is likely to get worse.
- Excessive exposure to ultra-violet light can harm the cornea and produce specific degenerative changes, such as solar keratopathy and pterygium.
- Poor hygiene obviously helps to spread eye-to-eye infections.
- Vitamin A deficiency specifically weakens the defences of the cornea.
  Indeed, the incidence of corneal scars in any community is a good indication of the general health, hygiene and nutrition of that community.
  The cornea is also prone to various degenerative changes called 'dystrophies'.

Corneal ulcers

There are many different types of corneal ulcer, but they all produce very much the same symptoms — pain, blurred vision, photophobia and watering.
- The pain is sharp, and fairly severe, because of the rich nerve supply to the cornea. Of course, in the occasional case of an anaesthetic cornea, there can be no feeling of pain.
- The vision is blurred because the ulcer makes the corneal surface irregular and may also make the cornea less transparent. Just how much vision is lost depends upon the size and position of the ulcer. Obviously, a central ulcer will affect the vision worse than a peripheral ulcer.
- Photophobia is very common, but it is not clear why. There is no proof that any of the corneal nerve fibres are sensitive to light.
- Watering and increased tears are a reflex response to the corneal damage.
  Examination of an eye with a corneal ulcer shows the following features:
- The ulcer itself is visible to the naked eye if it is large and deep, but superficial ulcers are not easy to see. It is therefore essential to instill fluorescein dye into the conjunctival sac, and so make these ulcers obvious (*Plate* 7e). There may also be inflammation in the corneal stroma around the ulcer.
- The anterior chamber may contain an inflammatory exudate in severe cases, and this may form a hypopyon (*Plate* 8c)
- The pupil is often slightly constricted.
- The ciliary vessels around the cornea are dilated (*Plate* 7e).
  It often helps the diagnosis to take a specimen of the ulcer for microscopy and

culture, if these facilities are available.
- Instill a drop of local anaesthetic to anaesthetize the cornea.
- Firmly scrape the edge of the ulcer with a small scalpel blade to collect any debris.
- Press some of this debris onto a slide for staining and microscopy, and inoculate some onto a culture plate.

Herpes simplex ulcers (Plate 7e and f)

Herpes simplex is a very wide-spread virus, and it is the commonest cause of corneal ulcers in an otherwise healthy eye. The virus is carried from person to person probably by direct contact. For this reason, herpes simplex usually enters the body through the face, especially around the eyes and mouth, and through the genital tract. Normally, the primary infection is so mild that there are no significant symptoms. Occasionally, however, there may be an attack of follicular conjunctivitis, or some vesicles on the eyelids or face associated with swelling of the regional lymph nodes. It is rare for the body to eliminate herpes simplex completely. The virus usually remains dormant until, months or even years later, secondary infection occurs. These secondary infections usually appear as localized epithelial ulcers, and recur at irregular intervals. Unfortunately, the cornea is one of the most common sites for these ulcers.

Herpetic ulcers often appear when the immune defences of the body are low, e.g. during an acute fever. Steroid drugs also specifically depress the cell-mediated immunity. It is therefore essential *not* to treat herpetic ulcers with mixtures of local antibiotics and steroids. The antibiotics will do nothing to the virus, and the steroids will only depress the immune defences of the body. The virus can then penetrate much deeper into the tissues, and the disease becomes much more serious. It is therefore very important to examine the cornea very carefully with fluorescein dye before using steroid drops.

Herpetic corneal ulcers may appear anywhere in the cornea. They are characteristically thin and branched, and are called 'dendritic' (which means tree-like) ulcers. Occasionally, the ulcer is larger and deeper, and is called an 'amoeboid' ulcer (*Plate* 7f). Herpetic corneal ulcers are usually only found in the epithelium and superficial layers of the stroma. This is why they are only visible with fluorescein dye. They heal spontaneously in about 2 − 4 weeks. An ulcer in the stroma will leave a residual scar, but the epithelium itself regenerates without scarring.

Unfortunately, herpetic infections can cause various complications: −
- Corneal anaesthesia often occurs after a herpetic ulcer, and may continue for months or even years.
- Recurrences are common. They occur at very irregular intervals, usually in the same eye as the first episode.
- Stromal keratitis (*Plate* 8a) may occur, especially in recurrent cases. The inflammation spreads to the deeper stromal layers of the cornea, and the whole of the cornea becomes oedematous and inflamed. Usually there is both stromal keratitis and ulceration of the corneal surface. Occasionally, however, there may be stromal inflammation without any epithelial ulceration. This condition is called 'disciform keratitis'.
- Iritis and secondary glaucoma are especially common when there is obvious

stromal keratitis.
- Indolent ulcers are chronic ulcers which follow a severe attack, and which will not heal. It seems likely that corneal anaesthesia and the destruction of the corneal stroma prevent the epithelial cells from growing over the irregular ulcer bed.

The treatment of herpetic corneal ulcers

Nowadays, antiviral drugs are the most effective method of treating herpetic ulcers. However, before these drugs were available, the treatment was to remove all of the diseased epithelium. Various techniques were used which are almost as effective as local antiviral drugs: –
- Débridement is a simple technique. Anaesthetize the cornea with local anaesthetic drops. Then gently wipe off the epithelium over and around the ulcer with a cottonwool bud. After débridement, it will be necessary to apply antibiotic and mydriatic drops or ointment (e.g. chloramphenicol and atropine) every day until the ulcer has healed. It will also be necessary to keep the eye padded. Padding the eye prevents the eyelids from moving over the cornea, and so helps the ulcer to heal.
- Chemical cauterization is another traditional technique. Phenol is probably the best agent, but alcohol and iodine can also be used. First anaesthetize and dry the cornea. Then moisten a wooden stick in 10% phenol and touch the edges of the ulcer with this stick. Phenol makes the epithelium turn white. After cauterization, the treatment is the same as for débridement (see above).

Antiviral agents inhibit the metabolism of viruses. However, viruses spend nearly all of their life cycle inside the host cells, and so are relatively resistant to any chemotherapy. For this reason, it is necessary to apply antiviral drugs frequently — once an hour for drops, and once every two hours for ointment. Iododesoxyuridine (IDU) has been available for some years now as drops or ointment. Acyclovir is a new antiviral agent which is available as ointment and can be given systemically. Prolonged treatment, especially with IDU, can sometimes produce toxic reactions.

Cycloplegic drops should also be given while the eye is painful. Because antiviral agents need such frequent application, it is not advisable to pad the eye.

Herpetic stromal keratitis is often very difficult to treat. Local corticosteroids are the best way to suppress the inflammation and to prevent corneal scarring, but they will also encourage the virus to proliferate. The usual treatment is therefore to give full doses of antiviral agents, and very small doses of local steroids. However, the use of steroids is best left to a specialist, and in cases such as these will need frequent and careful examination.

Indolent ulcers are difficult to treat and heal, but one of the following techniques may be helpful: –
- A tarsorrhaphy prevents lid movement over the ulcer, and so sometimes encourages the epithelium to heal.
- A flap of conjunctiva may be mobilized to cover the defect, and is occasionally effective.
- Corneal grafting can be used for a dense residual corneal scar, or to replace chronically diseased corneal tissue with healthy cornea.

Bacterial corneal ulcers (suppurative keratitis, *Plate* 8b *and* c)

The healthy cornea can resist invasion by pathogenic bacteria. However, if the natural corneal defences are weakened, these organisms can penetrate from outside and cause an acute infective corneal ulcer sometimes called 'suppurative keratitis'. Because the cornea has no blood supply, it is difficult for the body to mobilise its immune defences against the invading micro-organisms. If bacterial corneal ulcers are not treated, they often progress rapidly with serious complications. Certain factors increase the risk of bacterial corneal ulcers: –

– A foreign body, an abrasion or other injury, or an ingrowing eyelash which irritates the cornea — these all cause breaks in the corneal epithelium.
– Defective eyelid closure or proptosis which cause corneal exposure.
– Deficiency in the tear secretion or the tear film which cause the cornea to dry up.
– A loss of corneal sensation.
– Primary corneal diseases such as herpes simplex or vitamin A keratomalacia, which may become secondarily infected.
– Newborn infants are more susceptible to corneal infection than adults. This is because tear production is less, and the cornea itself is softer.

Bacterial corneal ulcers produce the same general symptoms as any corneal ulcer.The ulcer itself is usually in the centre or the lower part of the cornea because this is the most exposed part. It is also far from the blood supply and immune defences of the body.

The bacterial toxins provoke an acute inflammatory reaction in the surrounding tissues, which characterizes a bacterial corneal ulcer. All the constituents of pus are present — protein exudate, large numbers of neutrophils, dying cells and tissue debris. As a result, the surrounding cornea appears oedematous and infiltrated with white or yellow opaque material. The ulcer itself often appears shaggy and rough.

The anterior chamber often contains pus, which sinks to the bottom to form a hypopyon. The ciliary blood vessels are dilated.

Bacterial corneal ulcers can have many complications (*Plate* 9).

– Corneal scars usually remain where the bacterial ulcer has destroyed the corneal stroma. Even if the infection resolves in the early stages, either spontaneously or with treatment, some degree of corneal scarring is likely. Often these ulcers leave very dense scars.
– Some degree of iritis is always present. If this iritis is severe it may obstruct the flow of aqueous fluid, and so cause glaucoma.
– The ulcer may perforate into the anterior chamber. There is then a risk that the infection will spread into the eye. This is called 'endophthalmitis'. Eventually, the whole eye becomes shrunken and atrophic. This is called 'phthisis bulbi' (*see Plate* 9e).

If the perforation is only small it may help the infection to heal. This is because antibodies and cells from the vascular iris will come into contact with the infected cornea. In this case, the iris will stick to the back of the cornea, to form an anterior synechia.

Sometimes, after a large perforation, a thin fibrous scar forms across the cornea. If there is any obstruction to the flow of aqueous fluid, the pressure in the cornea will rise and the thin scar will then bulge forward. This condition is called 'staphyloma' (which means grape) (*see Plate* 9d).

Almost any pathogenic bacteria can cause corneal ulcers, but the most common are pseudomonas, staphylococcus and pneumococcus. To identify these organisms, it is necessary to use microscopy or bacteriological culture.

The treatment of bacterial corneal ulcers

Bacterial corneal ulcers are extremely destructive and may progress rapidly. Urgent and intensive treatment with antibiotics is therefore necessary. These antibiotics may be given locally as drops, ointment or subconjunctival injection, or they may be given systemically.

- Drops must be given every hour to provide effective drug levels in the cornea. It is possible to prepare one own's antibiotic solutions for this kind of intensive short term treatment. Simply add an ampoule of antibiotic powder to sterile saline or water to make a 1 or 2% solution. If methyl cellulose or a similar viscous substance is also added, the drops will adhere to the cornea longer.
- Ointments are useful at night, but they are not as effective as drops for intensive use. This is because it is uncertain how well the active ingredient comes out of the ointment base, and dissolves into the tears.
- Subconjunctival injections provide effective drug levels in the cornea (*see* page 37 for details and dosages). However, the injection is painful, and can only be given to children with an anaesthetic.
- Systemic antibiotic treatment is necessary if the ulcer has perforated, or if the infection has spread into the eye.

Organisms are usually more sensitive to one antibiotic than another. A bacteriological examination of the ulcer will help to identify the organism, and so indicate which antibiotic to choose. If it is not possible to identify the organism, it is best to give a mixture of antibiotics, and hope that at least one of them will be effective. In fact, even after a gram stain identification of the organism, it may still be advisable to give a mixture of antibiotics. This is because it is not always certain how the organism will respond to the antibiotics.

- Gentamicin and methicillin is a very useful combination of antibiotics for subconjunctival injection, especially if no bacteriological services are available. Gentamicin has a wide spectrum of activity against Gram-negative organisms, and methicillin is effective against most staphylococci.
- Gentamicin and carbenicillin is probably the best combination of subconjunctival drugs, if the gram stain shows gram-negative rods (presumably pseudomonas).
- Penicillin is usually recommended for Gram-negative cocci (presumably meningococci or gonococci).

A very wide range of antibiotics can be used as local drops. It is possible to buy some of these as commercial preparations. Others are antibiotic powders which dissolve in saline or water, and can be used in an emergency. It is accepted practice to use mixtures or combinations of antibiotics, especially when very little is known about the infecting organism. However, the antibiotics must be pharmacologically compatible. It may be necessary to modify or alter the treatment if there is no clinical improvement after 48 hours. Then again, the results of bacterial culture may indicate a more appropriate antibiotic. Mydriatic drops should also be given to keep the pupil well-dilated.

Fungal corneal ulcers

Fungal infections of the cornea are very rare in industrialized communities and temperate climates. However, a hot, humid climate helps the fungi to grow, and their spores to survive. Fungi usually live on vegetable matter. This is why any abrasions to the cornea from twigs, thorns, husks or seeds have a risk of fungal contamination. In rural communities, where the climate is hot and humid, superficial eye injuries with vegetable matter are frequent. In these communities, fungi may be almost as common as bacteria in causing corneal ulceration.

Fungi vary greatly in their virulence. Most fungi are not pathogenic at all, and some are only very weakly pathogenic. The infections they cause are therefore mild, and may recover spontaneously. On the other hand, a few fungi can produce quite virulent infections. In general, however, fungal infections are chronic and progress slowly for several weeks. Fungi cannot penetrate a healthy, uninjured cornea.

Fungal corneal ulcers have the same basic features as bacterial ulcers. However, fungal ulcers progress much more slowly. Therefore, the longer the ulcer has been present, the more likely it is to be a fungal ulcer. Fungal corneal ulcers often have a rough shaggy surface, and an irregular edge with localized extensions into the surrounding corneal stroma. These extensions are called 'satellite' lesions. There is often a lot of inflammation with anterior chamber exudate and hypopyon. There may also be a history of exacerbations and partial remissions. (*Plate* 8c has many of the features of a fungal ulcer.) Many fungal corneal ulcers have had weeks of intensive treatment for bacterial ulcers, without showing any clinical improvement.

If a fungal corneal ulcer is not treated, the cornea may eventually perforate, and the prognosis is poor. The eye is likely to become blind either from the complications of corneal perforation, or from corneal scarring. Occasionally the fungus and its inflammatory exudate grow in the anterior chamber. The pupil then adheres to the lens, the aqueous fluid cannot flow properly and secondary glaucoma develops.

It is possible to scrape the ulcer and demonstrate the fungi either by direct microscopy with Gram stain, or by fungal culture. Fungal cultures need incubation both at room temperature and at 37 °C. Unfortunately, fungi are difficult and slow to culture, so it may take several weeks to confirm the diagnosis. There is a wide range of possible pathogenic fungi, but the most common species to infect the cornea are Fusarium, Aspergillus and Candida.

The treatment of fungal corneal ulcers

The correct treatment can stop a fungal infection before it totally destroys the eye. Unfortunately, there are a number of reasons why the treatment of fungal corneal ulcers has very disappointing results: –
– Several fungicidal drugs are available, but many pharmacies and shops do not stock them. If they do have these drugs, they are usually made up as skin or

vaginal medicines, rather than for the eye.
- The particular fungus may not be sensitive to the particular drug which is being used.
- Treatment must be intensive and prolonged, and the response to treatment is slow.
- The patients are usually from poor, rural communities who often present late in the disease, and cannot afford long and uncertain treatment.
  The following drugs may all be useful for treating fungal corneal ulcers: –
- Natamycin can be used as a 5 — 10% suspension, or a 1% ointment. It has a wide range of antifungal activity, but poor penetration.
- Clotrimazole, miconazole and econazole are all antifungal agents with a good spectrum of activity and reasonable penetration. A 1% solution in arachis oil can be given as drops. These drugs also have some effect if given orally.
- Thiabendazole is an antihelminthic drug. It is also antifungal and is well absorbed by mouth. A dose of 25 mg per kg per day can be given by mouth, or it can be prepared as a 4% suspension, and given locally.
- Flucytosine is especially effective against candida. It is fairly non-toxic, and can be given orally in doses of 200 mg per kg per day.
- Nystatin and amphotericin B are both antifungal. However, nystatin is rather weak, and amphotericin B is rather toxic. It is therefore preferable to use other agents if they are available.

It is very important to apply any local antifungal drug every hour or every 2 hours, until there is no clinical evidence of infection.

Marginal corneal ulcers

Infective corneal ulcers usually occur near the centre of the cornea, where they are furthest away from the immune defences of the body. However, ulcers do sometimes occur at, or near the margin of the cornea. These ulcers may be infective, but they are usually caused by some sort of hypersensitivity or allergy.
- Phlyctens usually start in the conjunctiva, and are described in Chapter 6, page 73.
- Marginal infiltrates are small shallow ulcers with inflammation of the surrounding cornea (*Plate* 8d). These ulcers occur just inside the limbus, and are often multiple. Marginal infiltrates are probably caused by a hypersensitivity to staphylococcal toxins, and are often associated with chronic staphylococcal infections of the eyelids. The symptoms are not usually severe, and will heal spontaneously even without treatment. A small peripheral scar remains, but causes little or no loss of vision.
- Mooren's ulcers (ring ulcers) are severe and persistent ulcers which cover a large segment of the margin, and sometimes the whole limbus (*Plate* 8e). These ulcers may spread slowly towards the centre of the cornea. They then cause necrosis of the superficial layers of the cornea, and leave a vascularized and opaque scar. The symptoms of Mooren's ulcers are severe pain and photophobia. The cause is unknown, but is probably some kind of hypersensitivity reaction. Fortunately, Mooren's ulcers are fairly uncommon, but they are more frequent in the tropics.

The treatment for all these non-infective marginal ulcers is local steroid drops (e.g. Betnesol or Predsol drops, 4 times daily). However, steroids must be used with great care. If there is any danger that the ulcer might be an infective ulcer, steroids must not be given. Even if the diagnosis is certain, and steroids are given, it is essential to observe the patient at regular and frequent intervals. Sometimes, Mooren's ulcers do not respond well to steroid treatment. Surgical treatment, in particular excising the conjunctiva around the ulcer and cryotherapy to the conjunctiva, has been tried in severe Mooren's ulcers. The results unfortunately are often poor.

Exposure corneal ulcers

Exposure corneal ulcers develop when the eyelids or tear film do not cover the cornea adequately. For this reason these ulcers are associated with defects of the eyelids, facial palsies, proptosis or unconsciousness. Exposure corneal ulcers often have a well-defined upper border which marks the line of the upper lid across the cornea (*Plate* 11a). Secondary infection by bacteria is also very common. It is very important to try to restore adequate eyelid cover for the cornea, and to keep the cornea well lubricated with tear substitutes. It is also important to treat the secondary infection with local antibiotics.

Neuroparalytic keratitis is similar to exposure corneal ulceration, and it is caused when the cornea loses its sensation and therefore its protective reflexes. Neuroparalytic keratitis is common in leprosy, and after any severe virus infection of the cornea, such as herpes simplex or herpes zoster.

Vitamin A deficiency and measles are very important causes of severe corneal ulceration in young children. *See* Chapter 9.

Vernal eye disease may cause corneal ulceration in children and adolescents. *See* Chapter 6.

Diagnosis of corneal ulcers

It is usually easy to diagnose a corneal ulcer if fluorescein drops are available. However, to give the correct treatment, it is necessary to identify the cause of the ulcer, and this is much more difficult. Table 8.1 lists the common causes of corneal ulcers and their main features.

Even if the exact cause of the ulcer is unknown, it is essential to try to answer three questions: −
− Is this a bacterial infection? Bacterial ulcers need urgent and intensive treatment to prevent blindness. Other ulcers may become secondarily infected with bacteria. It is therefore wise to give prophylactic antibiotics locally to any corneal ulcer.
− Is this a herpetic ulcer? Herpetic ulcers are very common. They vary greatly in appearance and in their response to treatment. Even without treatment, they eventually heal, but steroid treatment makes the ulcer very much worse.
− Is it safe to use steroids? Steroids should not normally be used because of the problems with herpetic ulcers. Unfortunately, many patients have had their sight destroyed by using local steroids for corneal ulcers. However, some marginal ulcers and vernal ulcers respond specifically to steroids.

Table 8.1. Common causes and main features of corneal ulcers

Cause of ulcer	Predisposing factors	Clinical appearance	Treatment
Herpes simplex (common)	Any patient. Recurrences common	Irregular. Usually only superficial. 'Dendritic'	Débridement or antiviral agents NOT steroids
Bacterial infection (common)	Following injury or in an unhealthy cornea	Central or lower cornea. Often slough around ulcer and hypopyon	Intensive local and subconjunctival and possibly systemic antibiotics NOT steroids
Fungal infection (uncommon)	Only in warm humid conditions. After injury with vegetable matter	Same as bacterial infection. Chronic	Antifungal agents NOT steroids
Nutritional corneal ulcers	Malnourished children especially with vitamin A deficiency or following measles	Xerosis of conjunctiva and cornea. Usually central and lower half of cornea. Ulcers may occur in both eyes	Vitamin A orally. General treatment. Local antibiotics. and possibly antiviral agents NOT steroids
Marginal ulcers (Mooren's ulcer, phlyctenular ulcer, marginal infiltrates)	Any patient	At or near limbus	Local steroids
Vernal ulcer	Children and adolescents	Central oval ulcer. Signs of vernal conjunctivitis (papillary hypertrophy in both eyes). Itching	Local steroids. Débridement may help

Superficial punctate keratitis (*Plates* 4e, 10a *and* b)

Superficial punctate keratitis is the general name for any corneal condition which produces localized punctate lesions on the epithelial surface of the cornea. The eyes feel gritty and uncomfortable, and there may be a reflex increase in tear production. There may also be some very slight blurring of the vision. The individual lesions are not usually visible to the naked eye. However, with fluorescein stain, a faint green haze appears on the surface of the cornea. If a slit lamp is used, each individual epithelial lesion can be seen. It is necessary to observe carefully the distribution and character of the lesions, and also the conjunctiva. This often helps to determine the specific cause. There are many different causes of superficial punctate keratitis, but the following is a list of the more common causes: −

1. *Adenovirus infection* (epidemic keratoconjunctivitis, *See Plate* 4e) The lesions are in the epithelial and subepithelial layers, and are usually all over the cornea. Characteristic changes also occur in the conjunctiva.
2. *Trachoma*. The lesions are mainly in the subepithelial layers, and are near the upper limbus. There are also characteristic conjunctival changes.
3. *Vernal conjunctivitis*. The lesions are superficial and are especially noticeable near the limbus. Again, there are characteristic conjunctival changes.
4. *Onchocerciasis* (*Plate* 21c) The lesions are mainly beneath the epithelium, but are all over the cornea.
5. *Leprosy*. Punctate keratitis may occur in lepromatous leprosy. There will usually be other signs of leprosy in the skin.
6. *Dry eyes* (keratoconjunctivitis sicca) is caused by diminished tear production and is quite a common disease in old people. The lesions are superficial and only occur on the lower, exposed parts of the cornea. The treatment is to use methyl cellulose, or some other type of artificial tear drop, at frequent intervals. In severe cases, it may be helpful to destroy the lacrimal punctum. The small amount of tears which are present will then be unable to drain away.

If the cause of superficial punctate keratitis is known, it is possible to give specific treatment. If the cause is uncertain, it is best to treat the disease symptomatically. Artificial tear substitutes will be necessary during the day, and antibiotic ointment at night.

Stromal keratitis (interstitial keratitis, *Plate* 8a)

Stromal keratitis can be caused in two different ways. Sometimes micro-organisms enter directly from the body tissues, through the limbus and into the stroma of the cornea. Onchocerciasis, leprosy and syphilis are the most common organisms to infect the cornea in this way. However, stromal keratitis may also result from the extension of a superficial infection. An example of this is the stromal keratitis which can occur following a herpes simplex infection.

In the early stages of stromal keratitis, there is oedema and cellular infiltration of the corneal stroma. As the disease progresses, vascularization and scarring also appear. The cornea is hazy, and so patients complain of blurred vision. It is important to treat the specific cause of the keratitis. If the epithelium of the cornea is intact, and does not stain with fluorescein dye, then steroid drops can also be given. Local steroid drops normally suppress the inflammation in the corneal stroma. Unfortunately, any scarring is usually permanent.

Corneal dystrophies

Corneal dystrophies are degenerative diseases of the cornea, and are nearly always bilateral. Some of these dystrophies are basically ageing changes and a few of them are hereditary. Fortunately, most corneal dystrophies which seriously affect the vision are rare.
- Arcus senilis appears as a white ring just inside the limbus (*see Plate* 16b). It is very common in old people, but is not pathological.
- Keratoconus changes the shape of the cornea from spherical to cone-shaped, and will cause significant loss of vision.
- Fuchs' dystrophy can also cause significant loss of vision. The endothelial

cells degenerate, and the cornea becomes oedematous.

There are several other rare corneal dystrophies. The only effective treatment for advanced corneal dystrophies is corneal grafting.

Corneal oedema

In a normal cornea, the endothelial cells transfer fluid out of the stroma into the anterior chamber, and so keep the cornea dehydrated. If the endothelial cells cannot function properly for any reason, the cornea thickens and becomes oedematous. Special instruments are necessary to detect this increased thickness, but the oedema gives the cornea a hazy appearance which is visible to the naked eye (*see Plates* 8a, 20f *and* 21b). There are three basic causes of corneal oedema: –

– Stromal keratitis, which causes inflammation of the cornea (*see above*, page 103).
– Damage to the corneal endothelial cells, either by disease (a corneal dystrophy) or after an operation such as a cataract operation.
– A severe rise in the intraocular pressure, so that the corneal endothelial cells cannot transfer fluid from the cornea into the anterior chamber (*see* Chapter 14).

The earliest symptoms of corneal oedema are blurred vision, and seeing coloured rings (or haloes) around white lights. Small drops of fluid in the oedematous cornea split white light into the colours of the spectrum, and so a rainbow halo is seen. If the corneal epithelium is also oedematous, superficial blisters will develop in the epithelium. These blisters are usually very painful.

Corneal oedema can be a symptom of angle closure glaucoma. For this reason, it is very important to check the intraocular pressure of any patient with corneal oedema.

Pterygium (*Plate* 10c *and* d)

A pterygium consists of hypertrophic conjunctival epithelium. It grows from the limbus towards the centre of the cornea in the shape of a wedge ('pterygium' means wing). A pterygium only occurs in the exposed, part of the cornea between the eyelids. It usually starts nasally, but occasionally temporally, in the 3 o'clock or 9 o'clock position. The main part of the pterygium (nearer the limbus) is more vascular than the surrounding conjunctiva, and has blood vessels which run radially towards the tip of the pterygium. At the tip of the pterygium there is degeneration and opacification of the superficial cornea. The whole of the pterygium is raised above the corneal surface.

The stimulus which causes a pterygium to grow is excessive exposure to ultra-violet sunlight. Less important factors may be dry, hot and dusty conditions. This is why pterygia are most common in people who live outdoors in sunny areas. Pterygia usually grow slowly throughout life. However, they are normally more active, vascular and fleshy in young people, and become thin and atrophic in old people. Pterygia are possibly more common in blacks, because they are more likely to form scar tissue.

Normally, the only significant symptom of a pterygium is a slight cosmetic blemish. However, because pterygia are raised above the corneal surface, they are prone to recurrent episodes of mild inflammation. The patient may complain of irritation to the eye, and dilated blood vessels may be visible on the pterygium. A large pterygium may even reach the pupil, and partially blurr the vision.

The attacks of intermittent inflammation may be treated with vasoconstrictor drops (e.g. zinc and adrenaline), or with short courses of local steroids. It is possible to excise the pterygium surgically. Many patients ask for this surgery for cosmetic reasons, but it is best to try to persuade them against excision. The reason for this is the very high rate of recurrence after surgery, especially in young people with active, fleshy pterygia. The only real indication for excision is if the pterygium is covering the pupil and there is a risk of visual loss. There are reports of pterygium excisions which claim to reduce the incidence of recurrence after surgery. However, it is more probable that recurrences are due to the natural reaction of the conjunctival and corneal epithelium, which surgery cannot alter. The most effective way to prevent regrowth of the pterygium after excision is to use local anti-inflammatory or immunosuppressive drops, or irradiation.

To excise a pterygium: –
– Apply local anaesthetic drops to the conjunctiva, and inject the base of the pterygium with local anaesthetic containing dilute adrenaline.
– Grasp the main part of the pterygium with fine-toothed forceps. Use a scalpel blade to dissect the pterygium off the cornea. Only minimal excision is necessary.
– Dissect the conjunctiva and the pterygium away from the limbus, and excise it about 3 – 5 mm. from the limbus. This will leave an area of bare sclera.

The treatment after a pterygium excision is most important. Steroid drops or ointment must be applied regularly until all signs of inflammation have resolved. This may take 4 – 6 weeks. If it is available, surface irradiation with beta rays from a Strontium 90 applicator reduces the recurrence rate. The treatment can be given either immediately after the operation, or a few days later. The usual technique is to place the applicator over the bare area of the sclera and the limbus, and give a dose of up to 3000 rad. Higher doses may cause delayed lens opacification. There is some evidence that drops containing cytotoxic drugs (e.g. methotrexate, cyclophosphamide etc.) may reduce the recurrence rate.

It is just possible that tinted sun glasses may give the cornea some protection against ultra-violet light, and so reduce the incidence of pterygia.

Solar keratopathy (*Plate* 10e)

Excessive exposure to ultra-violet sunlight sometimes causes changes in the cornea called 'solar keratopathy' or 'climatic droplet keratopathy'. This condition occurs as a horizontal band just below the centre in the most exposed part of the cornea. In the early stages, there are fine subepithelial droplets and a fine frosting at the level of Bowman's membrane, but there is no significant visual loss. In the advanced stages, however, yellow nodules and cysts are visible to the naked eye, and the vision may deteriorate. Solar keratopathy is especially common in people who live by the sea in desert climates.

It is important not to confuse solar keratopathy with band degeneration of the cornea (*Plate* 10f). Both conditions occur at the level of Bowman's membrane and appear as horizontal bands in the exposed part of the cornea. However, band degeneration of the cornea is a fine calcific deposit. It is sometimes associated with chronic uveitis, but may develop for no obvious cause. It is fairly easy to treat band degeneration. First give local anaesthetic and scrape away the corneal epithelium. It is then possible to remove the calcific deposit. Apply drops of a chelating agent such as sodium versenate which dissolves calcium, and at the same time gently scrape the cornea. There is no specific treatment for solar keratopathy, but severe cases may benefit from corneal grafting.

Corneal scars (*Plates* 9 and 11a)

The only part of the cornea which can regenerate easily is the epithelium. Damage which is confined to the epithelium will therefore heal without scarring. Any deeper damage or inflammation to the cornea is likely to leave a scar. In hot countries where there is a high incidence of corneal diseases, such scars are very common. A corneal scar has two basic clinical features: vascularization and opacification.
- Vascularization is the growth of blood vessels into the cornea, as a response to inflammation. When the inflammation subsides, the vessels slowly regress and eventually empty altogether. It is sometimes still possible to see these 'ghost vessels' with a slit lamp. However, obvious vascularization of the cornea usually indicates that the original inflammatory process is still active.
- Opacification occurs because the collagen fibres are arranged irregularly in the fibrous tissue scar, and are therefore opaque. Faint scars may very gradually fade over many years, but otherwise corneal scars are permanent. In severe scars, lipid, calcium or amyloid deposits may occasionally develop. A nebula (which means 'cloud') is a name for a faint corneal scar, and a leucoma (which means white spot) is a name for a more dense localized scar.

Corneal scarring is the result of many different corneal diseases. These diseases include three of the major blinding tropical eye diseases — trachoma, nutritional corneal ulcers, and onchocerciasis. The pattern of scarring varies, however, and can sometimes help to determine the original disease, if this is not obvious from the history and other ocular signs.
- Trachoma produces scars which are often at the upper limbus, and spread downwards from there (*Plate* 7c). The scars are nearly always bilateral, superficial and associated with corneal vascularization. Conjunctival scars are also present, and there is trichiasis of the eyelashes.
- Nutritional corneal ulcers produce dense scars in the central and lower cornea, but not often in the upper cornea. The scars are often bilateral, especially in xerophthalmia, but do not spread to the conjunctiva.
- Onchocerciasis causes deep and diffuse scars which start at the 4 and 8 o'clock positions on the limbus, and spread inwards (*Plate* 21d *and* e). The scars are usually bilateral.
- Herpes simplex produces a unilateral and irregular corneal scar.
- Suppurative keratitis produces a large and dense unilateral scar.

The treatment of corneal scars

The aim of treatment is to improve first the vision and second the cosmetic appearance of the patient. However, it is important to assess many different factors before deciding what treatment, if any, to give.

1. Is the original disease active? For example, if trachoma is still active, or if there is irritation to the cornea from trichiasis, it is necessary to treat these conditions first. When the inflammation and vascularization in the cornea subside, the opacity may gradually become much less dense.

2. Where is the scar and how large is it? The scar may cover the pupil totally, partly or not at all. The iris may adhere to the back of the cornea, and so distort the pupil. It is also important to note how dense, deep and vascular the scar is.

3. At what age did the scarring occur? Corneal scarring in early childhood is likely to make the damaged eye lazy, or amblyopic (see p. 201). The earlier the age when the scarring occurred, the more amblyopic the eye will be.

4. How healthy is the other eye? If the other eye is normal, it is more likely that the scarred eye will be amblyopic. A patient who already has good vision out of one eye has less to gain from treatment.

5. Is there also a squint, nystagmus, poor fixation of the eye or poor projection of light? All these signs indicate that the retina and optic nerve have either never developed normal function, or have lost it through amblyopia or disease. It is therefore very unlikely that surgical treatment will significantly improve the vision. Without accurate projection of light, it is not worth even considering surgery.

There are several possible ways to improve the vision of patients with corneal scars. If the scar does not totally cover the pupil, spectacles may help. The cornea at the edge of a scar looks transparent, but is often distorted. This distortion produces a significant refractive error, and especially astigmatism. This astigmatism can sometimes be corrected with spectacles.

There are two methods of improving the vision by allowing the patient to 'see round' the opacity. The first method is to use mydriatic drops, which dilate the pupil. The second is a better and permanent method, and is called an 'optical iridectomy'. The iridectomy alters the position of the pupil aperture, so that it is in line with the clear cornea (Plate 11a). An iridectomy is usually a fairly straightforward operation, and the iris of a normal eye very easily prolapses through a limbal incision. However, the iris of a diseased eye may adhere both to the lens and to the back of the cornea. This means the operation may be difficult to perform without causing further intraocular damage. After a successful optical iridectomy, patients usually have considerable astigmatism. This is because they are not looking through the centre of the cornea.

The most sophisticated treatment for corneal scars is corneal grafting, sometimes called 'keratoplasty' (Plate 11b). The technique is to excise the central part of the diseased cornea, usually about 7 mm in diameter, and suture healthy cornea from a donor eye in its place. The usual source of the donor cornea is from the eye of a recently dead person. Occasionally, it is necessary to remove an eye with a healthy cornea from a living patient. Very occasionally, a patient may be blind in one eye but still have a healthy cornea. He can then have a graft of his own corneal tissue from one eye to the other. It is normal to transplant the full thickness of the cornea. If the corneal scar goes no deeper than the anterior corneal layers, however, a partial thickness (or lamellar) corneal graft may be all that is necessary. It is usual to hold the graft in place with a single continuous monofilament 10/0 nylon or perlon suture. This does not irritate the eye or cause blood vessels to grow into the graft. Unfortunately, areas where corneal scars are very common usually have very little specialist eye care. These are also the areas where people are usually least willing to donate eyes for grafting after death.

A corneal graft operation requires great technical skill. It also requires close supervision of the patient for many months after the operation to prevent graft rejection. Graft rejection means that the graft is invaded by blood vessels and lymphocytes from the patient because it is foreign tissue. This causes inflammation and oedema of the graft which finally goes opaque. To prevent rejection, it is usual to give immunosuppressive drugs for some months. Steroid drops are used locally in nearly all cases, and steroids and other drugs are sometimes used systemically.

Other complications may also occur as well as rejection.

Unfortunately, the patients who most need corneal grafts are often most likely to reject them. Severely scarred corneas usually have extensive vascularization also. Blood vessels from the patient's cornea will therefore invade the graft, and lymphocytes will attack. There is no purpose in performing a corneal graft operation on an eye with extensive conjunctival disease or an eyelid abnormality. Normal eyelids, conjunctiva and tear film are essential for a corneal graft to stay clear.

Very many people who are blind from corneal disease could see again if they received treatment. Unfortunately, the medical services in many hot countries are not sophisticated enough to give these people the treatment they need. However, most of this corneal blindness is preventable. Efforts to prevent corneal scarring in the whole community are probably more worthwhile than the treatment of a few individuals.

It is possible to improve the cosmetic appearance of an eye with a corneal scar by tattooing the cornea. The method is to shave off the superficial cornea and then scratch pigment into the corneal stroma. The pigment should be the same colour as the iris or pupil. Tattooing the cornea is only recommended when the vision is very poor in the damaged eye, and the other eye is normal. Corneal grafting will also improve the cosmetic appearance of the eye. However, corneal graft material is too precious to be used for cosmetic reasons alone. If a corneal scar is so large that the eye has no vision, and if it is ugly or painful, then it is better to enucleate the eye and replace it with an artificial eye (*Fig.* 8.1).

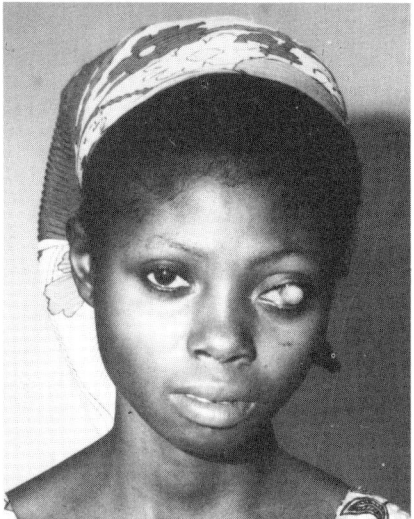 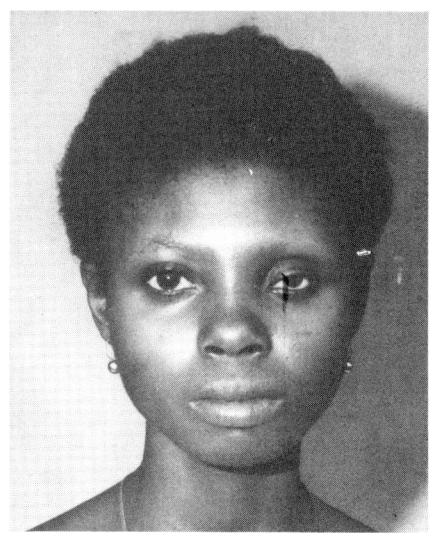

Fig. 8.1 A staphyloma scar. The eye was removed, and even a cheap mass-produced artificial eye greatly improved the appearance.

9. Nutritional Corneal Ulceration and Xerophthalmia

Nutritional corneal ulceration is a disease which only young children get. It is also completely preventable. Every child with this disease therefore means that someone has failed. The parents have failed to feed their child properly. The local community has failed to help one of its poorest and weakest members. Doctors and politicians have failed to give basic health care where the need is most urgent.

For fifty years now, we have known the basic facts about nutritional corneal ulceration, and every year, new research brings new understanding. We have the knowledge and the technology to eradicate this disease, and yet the incidence has not even begun to fall. WHO estimates that every year 100 000 – 200 000 children suffer from nutritional corneal ulceration. Only about a quarter of these children recover with reasonable eyesight. Another quarter go either partially or completely blind, while the remaining half die in the acute stage of the illness.

Many different factors cause nutritional corneal ulceration. These factors all exist in conditions of poverty, but the most important factor is dietary deficiency of vitamin A. Vitamin A deficiency produces a clinical condition called 'xerophthalmia'. Xerophthalmia means 'dry eyes', but the name is misleading. In xerophthalmia, tears are produced as normal, but the conjunctiva and the cornea resist wetting by these tears. There are many causes of 'dry eyes' in adults, but the only important cause in young children is vitamin A deficiency.

It is possible to study specific vitamin deficiencies in laboratory animals. In real life, however, children do not suffer from single dietary deficiencies, and they nearly always have protein energy malnutrition as well. To make it worse, most of these children suffer from recurrent infections, especially gastroenteritis, and may also have intestinal parasites. One very important infection, especially in Africa, is measles. In fact, in some African communities, measles may cause more cases of corneal ulceration than vitamin A deficiency itself.

Fig. 9.1 shows the metabolism of vitamin A, and the factors which cause vitamin A deficiency. *Fig.* 9.2 shows some of the factors which cause corneal ulcers in malnourished children. The causes of nutritional corneal ulceration are clearly very complex, but the remedy is simple. A proper diet of cheap, nutritional foods, which even the poorest families could buy, would greatly reduce the incidence of this disease. Furthermore, a basic child welfare scheme with immunisation against measles could probably eradicate corneal blindness. Programmes to eradicate vitamin A deficiency have a high priority in WHO, and for two good reasons. Vitamin A deficiency causes extreme personal suffering

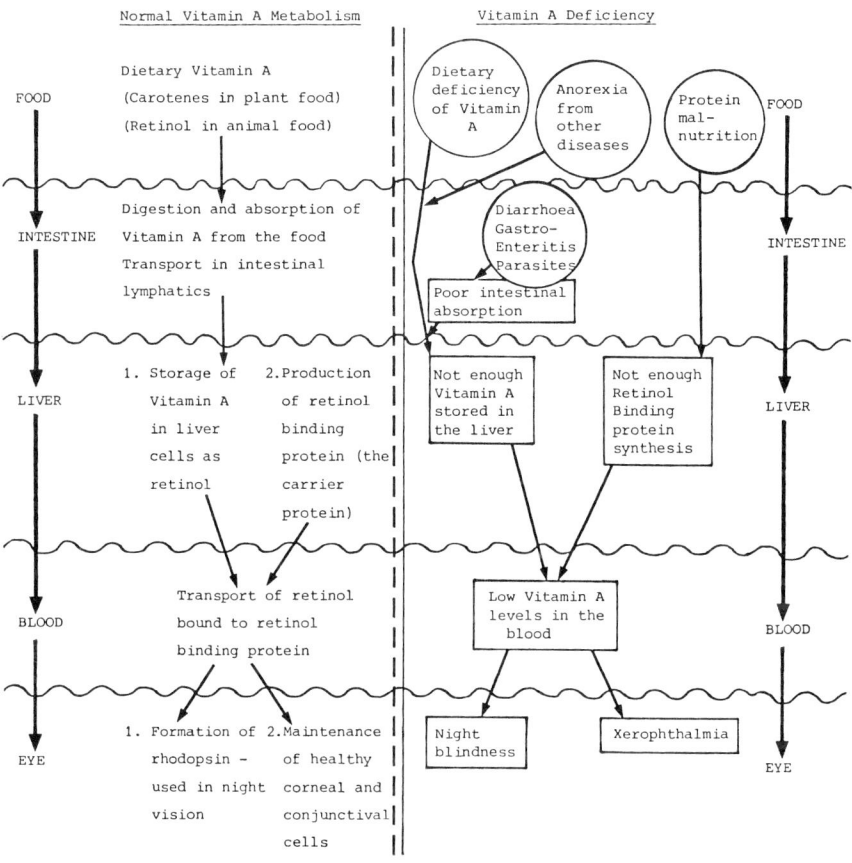

Fig. 9.1 The left side of this diagram shows how vitamin A passes from the food to the eye in a healthy person. The right side of the diagram shows the main causes of vitamin A deficiency. These are indicated by circles: ○

and economic loss all over the world. It is also completely preventable.

The rest of this chapter is divided into six sections: –
– The biochemistry and physiology of vitamin A
– The signs and symptoms of vitamin A deficiency in the eye
– Protein energy malnutrition, intercurrent infections and measles
– The treatment of nutritional corneal ulcers
– The epidemiology of nutritional corneal ulcers
– The prevention of blindness from nutritional corneal ulceration

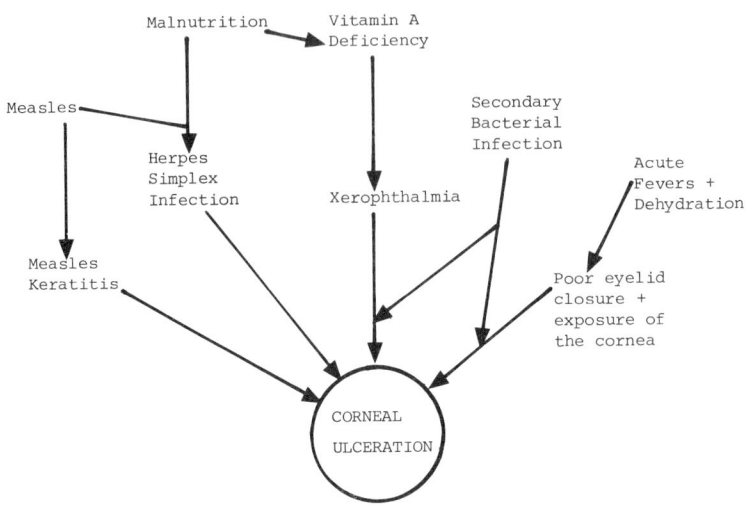

Fig. 9.2 Nutritional corneal ulcers in children are usually caused by several different factors working together to damage the cornea. Some of the more important causes are shown in the following diagram.

The biochemistry and physiology of vitamin A

The earliest records of xerophthalmia and resulting corneal ulceration are in ancient Egyptian and Chinese texts. However, the cause remained unclear until recently. An experiment early this century showed that animals develop a condition similar to xerophthalmia if they eat a diet deficient in fat. Then, in 1921, doctors diagnosed xerophthalmia in Danish orphanage children whose diets were deficient in milk. During the last fifty years, our knowledge of the biochemistry and physiology of vitamin A has greatly increased. Vitamin A (or retinol) is a fat-soluble unsaturated alcohol, and it seems to be an essential vitamin for most animals.

1. Dietary sources of retinol

There are two sources of dietary retinol for humans: animal foods and plant foods. Table 9.1 lists the concentration of vitamin A in some of these foods.
- Animal foods contain the active vitamin retinol, but some foods are much richer in retinol than others. The liver, which stores retinol, is the best source. Milk products are also very rich in retinol.
- Plant foods contain carotene pigment, which is chemically related to retinol. There are in fact many different carotene pigments. They are all converted

Table 9.1. The concentration of vitamin A in different foods

Animal Foods	in iu of Retinol per 100 g or 100 ml	Plant Foods	in iu of Carotene per 100 g or 100 ml
Fish liver oil	100 000 +	Red palm oil	50 – 100 000
Animal liver	10 000	Carrots	10 000
Butter	3 000	Spinach	10 000
Cheese	1 500	Sweet potatoes	5 000
Kidney	1 000	Apricots, mangoes	2 000 +
Eggs	1 000	Tomatoes	1 000
Fish	200	Green beans	1 000
Fresh milk	150	Yellow maize	350
Meat (mutton, beef etc.)	20	Wheat	slight
Lard	negligible	Rice	
		Potatoes	} negligible
		White maize	
		Cassava	

Adapted from *Vitamin A,* T. Moore, Elsevier, Amsterdam, 1957

into retinol in the wall of the intestine, but some are converted more effectively than others. The pigment which gives the highest yield of retinol is beta-carotene.
— Some plant foods are much richer in carotene than others. The best source of carotene is red palm oil. Green leafy vegetables (e.g. spinach) and orange coloured fruit and vegetables (e.g. carrots, mangoes, papayas) are also very good sources (*Plate* 11c). Starchy white cereals and root crops (e.g. rice, cassava), which are often the staple diet of poor people, contain little or no vitamin A (*Plate* 11d).
— The International Unit (iu) is officially discouraged, but is still widely used to express vitamin A activity in foods.

1 iu is equivalent to
$$\begin{cases} 0.3\ \mu g \text{ of retinol} \\ 0.6\ \mu g \text{ of beta-carotene} \\ 1.2\ \mu g \text{ of other carotenes} \end{cases}$$

1 μg or microgram = 1/1 000 000 of a gram)

2. *Absorption and storage* (*see Fig* 9.1)

Retinol and the carotenes are fat-soluble. During digestion in the intestine, they are emulsified and absorbed. Retinol is more effectively emulsified and absorbed than the carotenes. In ideal conditions, about 90% of ingested retinol, and about 70% of ingested carotene is absorbed. However, if the intestine is diseased or has a heavy load of parasites, absorption may be much less.

Cooking improves the absorption of carotenes. The best way to prepare vegetables to get the maximum absorption of carotenes is to fry them. Frying both breaks up the cells and provides fat in which the carotene dissolves. If plants are eaten raw, not ground up enough, or not cooked enough, the carotene pigments may not be released from the plant cells. These carotenes may then pass

Table 9.2

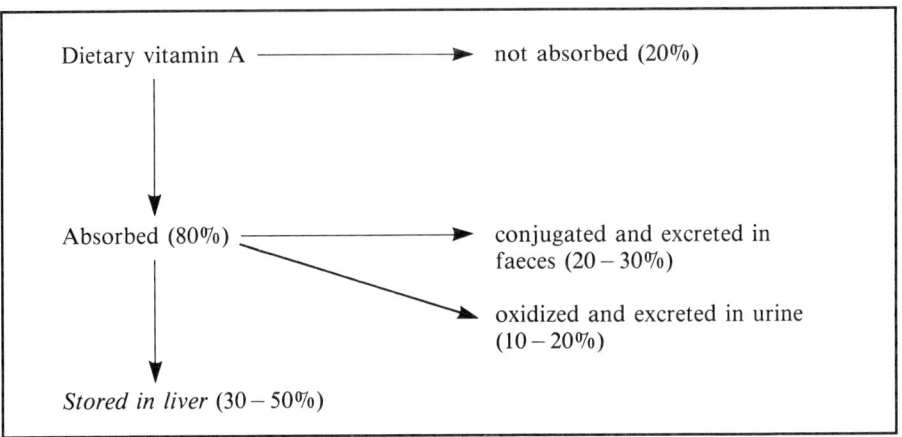

undigested through the alimentary tract.

Carotenes are slowly converted to retinol in the wall of the intestine. All the absorbed retinol is then transported in the intestinal lymphatics to the bloodstream. Most of this retinol is taken up and stored in the liver. The rest of the retinol is either conjugated with glucuronic acid and excreted in the bile, or metabolized and excreted as degradation products in the urine. Table 9.2 shows what happens to a single dose of vitamin A.

The liver stores retinol very effectively, and it can maintain adequate serum levels for up to six months. This is why vitamin A deficiency needs only intermittent doses of retinol.

3. Transport from the liver to the tissues

Two conditions are necessary for this: –
– First, there must be some retinol stored in the liver.
– Second, the carrier protein, retinol binding protein (RBP) must be synthesized in the liver. Retinol must be bound to RBP before it can be released into the plasma.

In a healthy individual, retinol and RBP are both present in the liver. Retinol bound to RBP can therefore enter the circulation and be utilized.

In vitamin A deficiency, however, there is not enough retinol stored in the liver. The RBP therefore remains in the liver, and does not enter the circulation.

In protein deficiency, the opposite is true. There is not enough RBP synthesized in the liver. The retinol therefore remains stored, and does not enter the circulation.

4. Functions of vitamin A

The maintenance of healthy epithelial tissues is the most important function of vitamin A, but it is not clearly understood. Normally, special epithelial cells called 'goblet cells' secrete mucus. This mucus is an effective wetting

agent, and so epithelial surfaces are normally mucous membranes. In vitamin A deficiency, however, two changes occur which cause the epithelial tissues to dry up: –
– First, there is a loss of goblet cells, and so less mucus is produced.
– Second, the epithelial surfaces become skin-like (keratinized). Keratinized epithelium resists wetting more easily than normal epithelium.

In theory, these changes occur in mucous membranes all over the body, but in practice they are only apparent in the conjunctiva and the cornea of the eye.

A skin condition called 'perifollicular hyperkeratosis' seems to result from vitamin A deficiency. In this condition, keratin tissue builds up around the hair follicles.

The formation of visual purple is the only function of vitamin A which has been defined biochemically. The aldehyde form of vitamin A is called 'retinal'. Retinal combines with opsin (a protein found in the photosensitive part of the rods in the retina) to form visual purple. When the retinal molecule is exposed to light, it changes from one chemical form (isomer) to another. Further chemical changes then produce the electrical impulse which the brain eventually interprets as light. Vitamin A deficiency produces a condition called 'night blindness'. In night blindness dark adaptation and the ability to see in the dark are specifically diminished.

Vitamin A deficiency depresses the appetite and also the immune reponses in experimental animals. These changes may also occur in man.

5. Vitamin A deficiency in young children

Young growing children are much more at risk from vitamin A deficiency than adults. There are two reasons for this: –
– First, the vitamin A requirement per unit of body weight is much greater for a child than an adult. The recommended daily intake of vitamin A per kg body weight is 65 μg (125 iu) for an infant, but only 12 μg (36 iu) for an adult. (The total requirements for infants and adults are therefore very similar.)
– Second, a child cannot store vitamin A in the liver as well as an adult.

Clinical vitamin A deficiency is common in children with inadequate vitamin A in their diets, but extremely rare in adults. Even if adults are deprived of vitamin A in experimental conditions, it is many months before any signs of vitamin A deficiency appear.

The signs and symptoms of vitamin A deficiency in the eye

Table 9.3 shows the fairly generally accepted classification of the signs of vitamin A deficiency in the eye. These signs are divided into two: primary signs and secondary signs.
– The primary signs are specific for xerophthalmia. They start with the least severe and end with the most severe.
– The secondary signs are not specific for xerophthalmia, but they are likely to indicate vitamin A deficiency.

Everyone who is concerned either with child welfare or eye disease in areas where malnutrition is common should be familiar with these basic signs of xerophthalmia.

Table 9.3. Classification of xerophthalmia

Primary signs	
X1A	Conjunctival xerosis
X1B	Bitot's spot with conjunctival xerosis
X2	Corneal xerosis
X3A	Corneal ulceration with xerosis
X3B	Keratomalacia
Secondary signs	
XN	Night blindness
XF	Xerophthalmia fundus
XS	Xerophthalmia scars

X1A — Conjunctival xerosis (Plate 11e *and* f)

Changes occur on the bulbar conjunctiva, especially the exposed parts. Look for the following features, which may be widespread, or localized to small patches of the conjunctiva: –

– Dryness causes the conjunctiva to lose its normal, shiny lustre and look like wax or paint instead. It also becomes 'unwettable', so that the tear film breaks up and leaves dry patches. As the conjunctiva thickens and loses its transparency, the underlying blood vessels are more difficult to see. When the eye moves, it is sometimes possible to see wrinkles and folds in the thickened conjunctiva.

– Increased pigmentation gives the conjunctiva a fine, diffuse, smoky grey-brown appearance, especially near the limbus in the interpalpebral fissure. This pigmentation is common in xerophthalmia, but it is also a feature of vernal conjunctivitis.

– A creamy white debris is sometimes found, especially in the canthi, the lower fornix, or the lid margins around the openings of the Meibomian glands. This debris is a feature of advanced conjunctival xerosis.

All these changes can be difficult to detect in the early stages. For this reason, it is better not to diagnose vitamin A deficiency on the basis of conjunctival xerosis alone.

Conjunctival xerosis is fully reversible with vitamin A treatment, and this must be given.

X1B — Bitot's spot with conjunctival xerosis (Plate 11f)

A Bitot's spot is a small plaque of material on the surface of the bulbar conjunctiva, and nearly always in the interpalpebral fissure. The material is usually foamy, but may look waxy or greasy, and may contain pigment from eye make-up. If the material is wiped away, it leaves a dry conjunctival bed with a rough surface. A Bitot's spot usually occurs temporal to the limbus, but it is occasionally nasal. It is either oval in shape, or forms a triangle pointing away from the limbus. There is often increased pigmentation of the conjunctiva around the Bitot's spot.

It seems probable that a Bitot's spot forms because the eyelids do not wipe the bulbar conjunctiva properly. Sometimes a structural defect (e.g. a squint or an eyelid abnormality), exposes part of the conjunctiva. A Bitot's spot is likely to form on this exposed area.

A Bitot's spot is a very obvious sign, and if other conjunctival signs are also present, then vitamin A deficiency is very likely. Bitot's spots do not always indicate vitamin A deficiency, however, and are sometimes seen in older children and adults who are obviously well-nourished. Other disorders at the limbus which may be confused with Bitot's spot are discussed on page 229.

X2 — Corneal xerosis (Plate 12a)

Corneal xerosis is an extension of the conjunctival signs onto the cornea. It is much less common than conjunctival xerosis, but it is a highly specific sign. The surface of the cornea looks rough, dull and irregular. The break up time of the pre-corneal tear film shortens to less than 10 seconds. To measure the break up time: –
– Instill a fluorescein drop into the eye.
– Wait until the patient blinks.
– Measure how many seconds the fine tear film remains on the surface of the cornea before it breaks up.

Corneal xerosis indicates an eye which is at great risk of developing serious corneal damage. However, with early treatment at this stage, it is still fully reversible.

X3A — Corneal ulceration with xerosis (Plate 12b and c)

There are many causes of corneal ulceration (see page 102), but the following features are characteristic of corneal ulceration from xerophthalmia: –
– Both conjunctival and corneal xerosis are present.
– Both eyes are diseased to some extent.
– The ulcers are in the central and lower part of the cornea.

Often there is very little pain, tissue reaction or inflammation. However, if there are any signs at all of corneal ulceration, urgent treatment is necessary. Corneal ulceration is not fully reversible. There will always be some corneal scarring, and severe cases will almost destroy the eye. Even so, it is surprising how vigorous treatment can reduce quite extensive corneal destruction to much smaller corneal scars.

X3B — Keratomalacia (Plate 12d)

Keratomalacia is the last and most severe sign of xerophthalmia. Part, or the whole of the cornea very quickly degenerates and 'melts away'. A mass of white or yellow gelatinous, necrotic matter replaces the normal cornea. Keratomalacia has two striking features: –
– The onset is very rapid.
– There is no significant tissue reaction or inflammation.

Very often the intraocular contents extrude. Many of these eyes then progress either to phthisis bulbi, or to staphyloma formation (see page 97 and Plate 9).

The sudden 'melting' of the cornea is not really understood. It is possible that collagenase enzymes are formed in the cornea. These enzymes then dissolve the collagen and cause rapid tissue destruction. Secondary infection of the ulcer does not seem to be necessary to start the ulceration, but it is bound to occur and cause complications.

XN — Night blindness

Vitamin A is necessary for the light sensitive rods in the retina to function properly. Vitamin A deficiency therefore produces poor dark adaptation and poor night vision (nyctalopia). It is possible to detect night blindness either by electroretinography or dark adaptation tests. However, because both these methods require sophisticated equipment and a co-operative patient, they can only really be used in research. In practice, it is usually necessary to question the parents carefully about the child's behaviour, and to explain what night blindness is. Parents can often then recognize and describe night blindness, and a diagnosis is possible.

There are other possible causes of night blindness, especially retinitis pigmentosa (*see* page 148).

XF — Xerophthalmia fundus

Vitamin A deficiency seems to produce a characteristic change in the retina. Pale yellow spots appear, especially near the course of the retinal vessels, and also in the retinal periphery (*Plate* 12e).

XS — Xerophthalmic scars

There are many causes of corneal scarring. Therefore it is impossible to be sure if a corneal scar is from a previous episode of xerophthalmia or not. Xerophthalmic scars vary from a very faint scar to total destruction of the eye. Corneal scars from xerophthalmia are usually in the lower part of the cornea, and they are usually bilateral. One eye may, however, be much more scarred than the other. Corneal scars in a malnourished child with no history of trauma or other eye infections strongly indicate xerophthalmia.

Protein energy malnutrition, intercurrent infections and measles (*see* Fig. 9.2)

Protein energy malnutrition

Protein energy malnutrition (PEM) obviously causes widespread and complex changes in the body. In general, PEM retards growth and development, and weakens a child's resistance to infection. More specifically, it upsets the metabolism of vitamin A. In protein deficiency, there is not enough RBP synthesized in the liver. Less retinol can enter the bloodstream, and so the body tissues are deprived of vitamin A. This is why children with both vitamin A deficiency *and* PEM have more severe eye lesions than children with vitamin A deficiency alone.

A child who receives treatment for PEM often has a sudden 'growth spurt' as growth returns to normal. This sudden growth increases the utilization of any vitamin A stores. Appropriate action will then be necessary to replace these

PLATE 1

Chapter 3

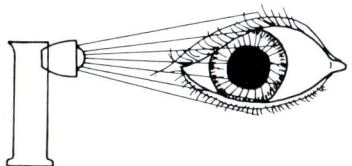 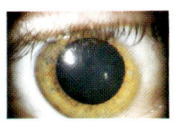

a. A normal eye seen with diffuse illumination.

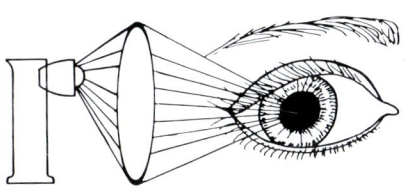 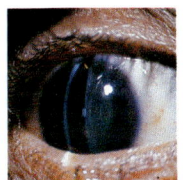

b. A normal eye seen with focal illumination.

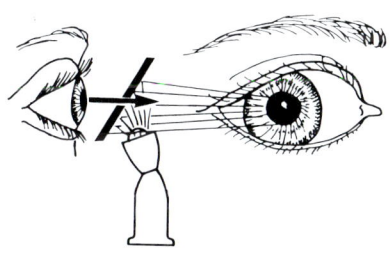 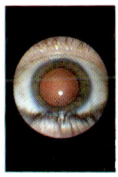

c. A normal eye seen with coaxial illumination.

PLATE 2

Chapter 5

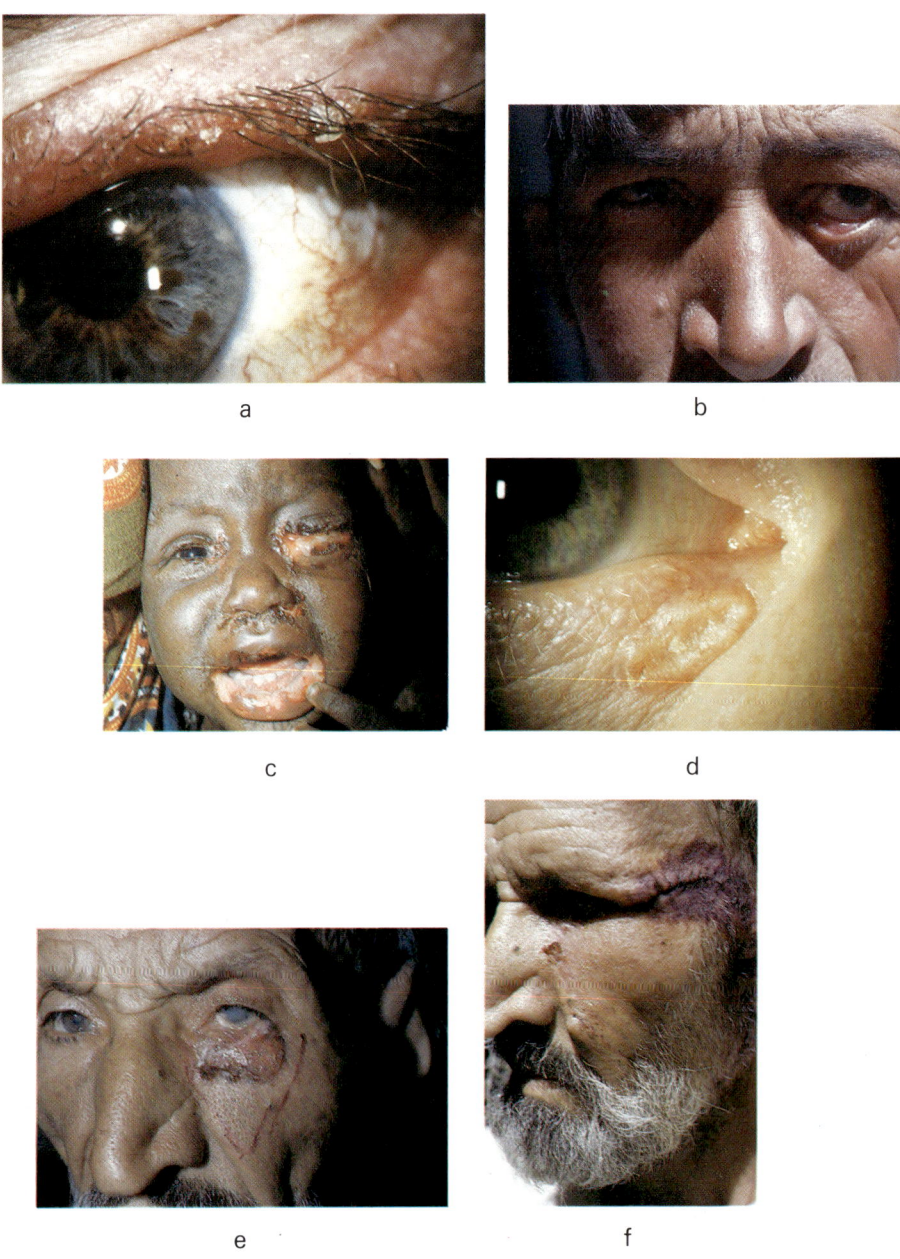

a

b

c

d

e

f

a, Seborrhoeic blepharitis. Note the scales adhering to the eyelashes.

b, Contracture and ectropion of the lower eyelid following cutaneous leishmaniasis.

c, Early cancrum ulcers in the mouth and eyelid. The child recently had measles.

d, Early rodent ulcer.

e *and* 2f, A large rodent ulcer. A wide margin of healthy tissue should also be removed. A large flap of skin has been rotated in from the lateral part of the cheek to fill in the defect.

PLATE 3

Chapter 6

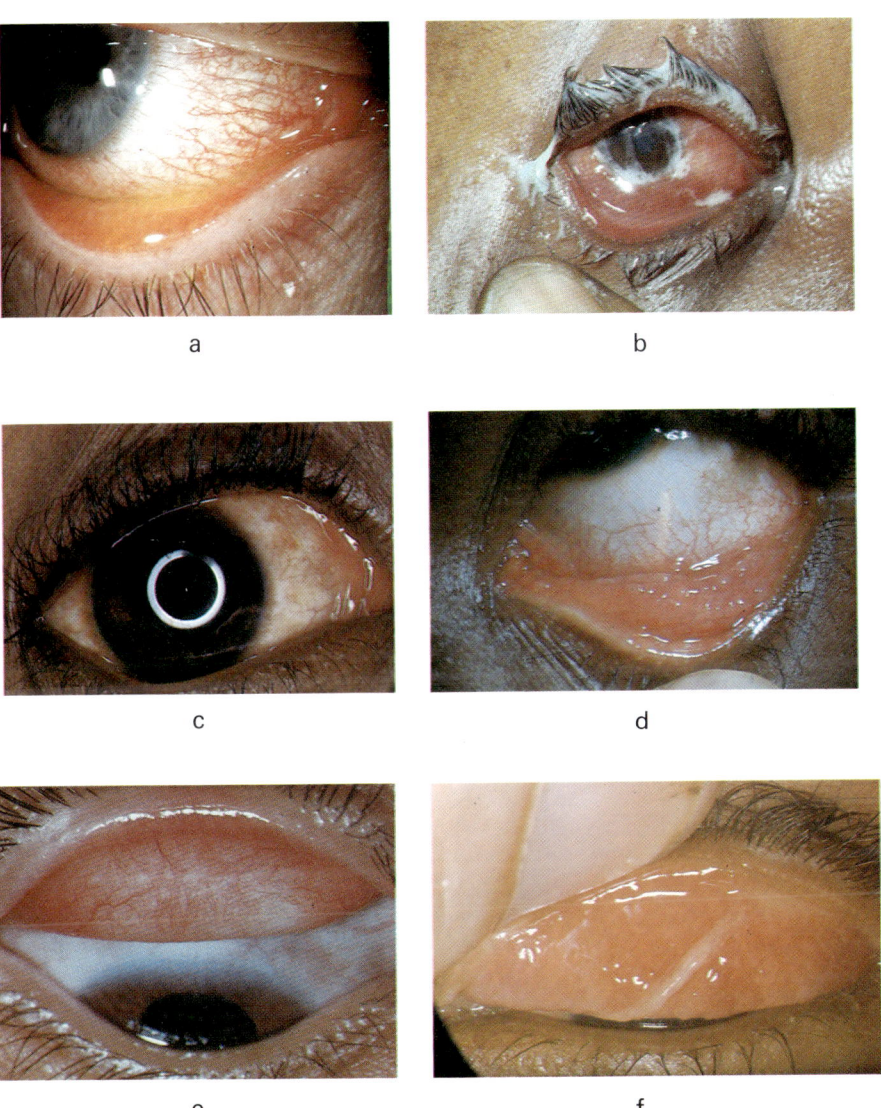

a

b

c

d

e

f

a Acute viral conjunctivitis. Note the dilated blood vessels towards the fornix. Also the increased watery tear secretion, which is coloured by the fluorescein dye.

b Acute bacterial conjunctivitis. Note the dilated blood vessels, the oedematous conjunctiva, and purulent discharge.

c Acute haemorrhagic conjunctivitis. Note the petechial haemorrhages.

d Follicles in the lower fornix. The patient has trachoma.

e Dilated blood vessels in the upper tarsal conjunctiva. The patient has early trachoma.

f Vernal conjunctivitis. Note how papillary hypertrophy obscures the normal conjunctival blood vessels. A thick mucus thread is present.

PLATE 4

Chapter 6

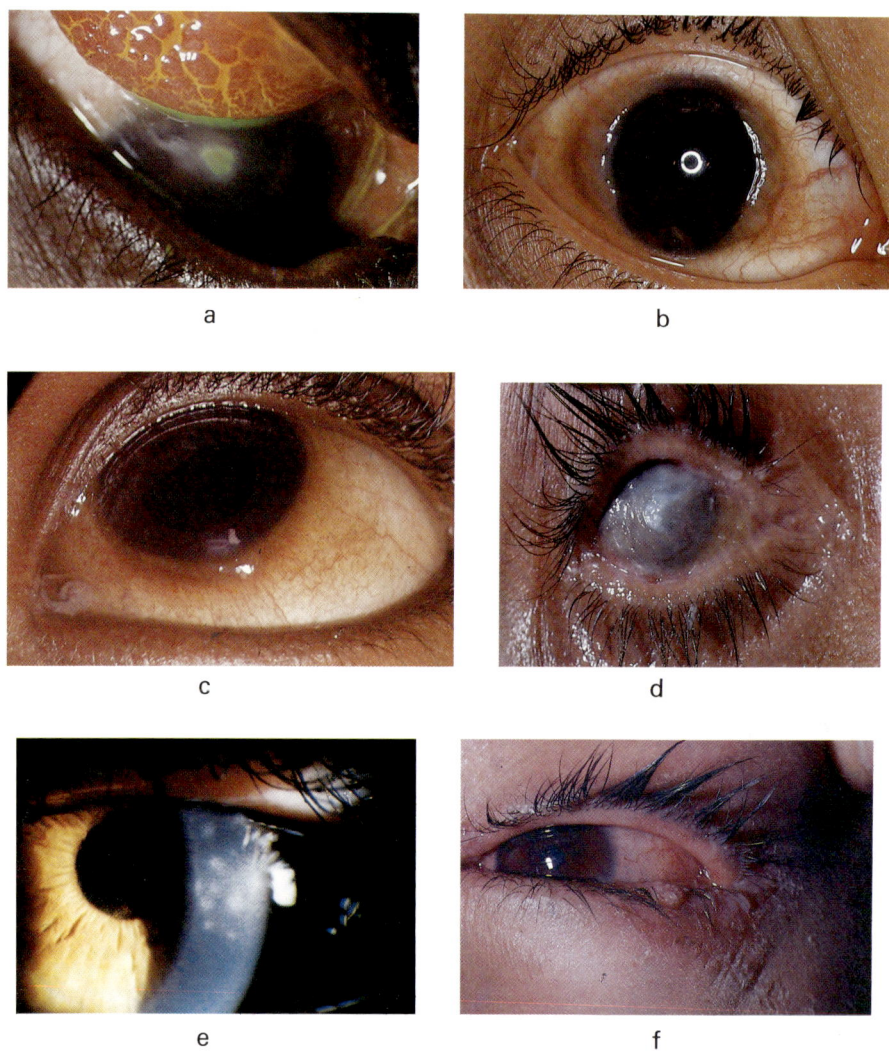

a Vernal conjunctivitis. The upper eyelid has been everted to show the cobblestone papillae on the upper tarsal conjunctiva. Note also the ulcer on the cornea.

b Vernal conjunctivitis. Note the fleshy hypertrophy at the limbus, and the increased pigmentation.

c Vernal conjunctivitis. Note the strand of mucus, the pigmentation only in the exposed conjunctiva, and the tiny white Trantas spots at the limbus.

d Benign mucous membrane pemphigoid. The conjunctiva and cornea are keratinized, and the fornices are obliterated.

e Adenovirus keratoconjunctivitis. Note the punctate opacities in the cornea. These opacities are only visible where the focal beam of the slit lamp passes through the cornea.

f Molluscum contagiosum. The patient presented with chronic conjunctivitis which persisted until the wart was removed.

PLATE 5

Chapter 6

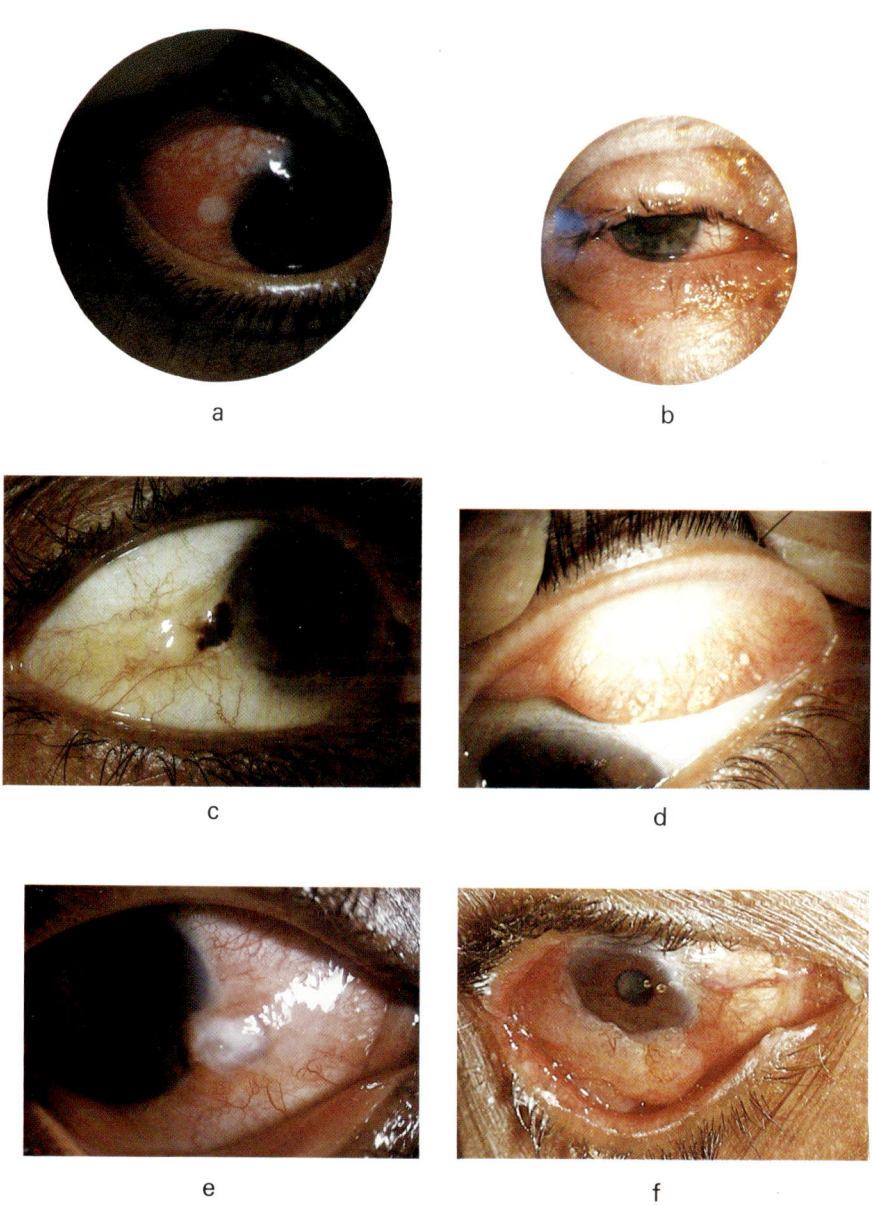

a

b

c

d

e

f

a Phlyctenular conjunctivitis.
b A severe allergic reaction to eye drops. Note the conjunctival vasodilatation, and the eczema of the eyelids.
c A pigmented naevus and a pinguecula lying side by side at the limbus.
d Concretions and scars following chronic conjunctivitis.
e A very early carcinoma at the limbus. This can very easily be excised.
f A more advanced conjunctival carcinoma. It is still possible to excise it locally.

PLATE 6

Chapter 7

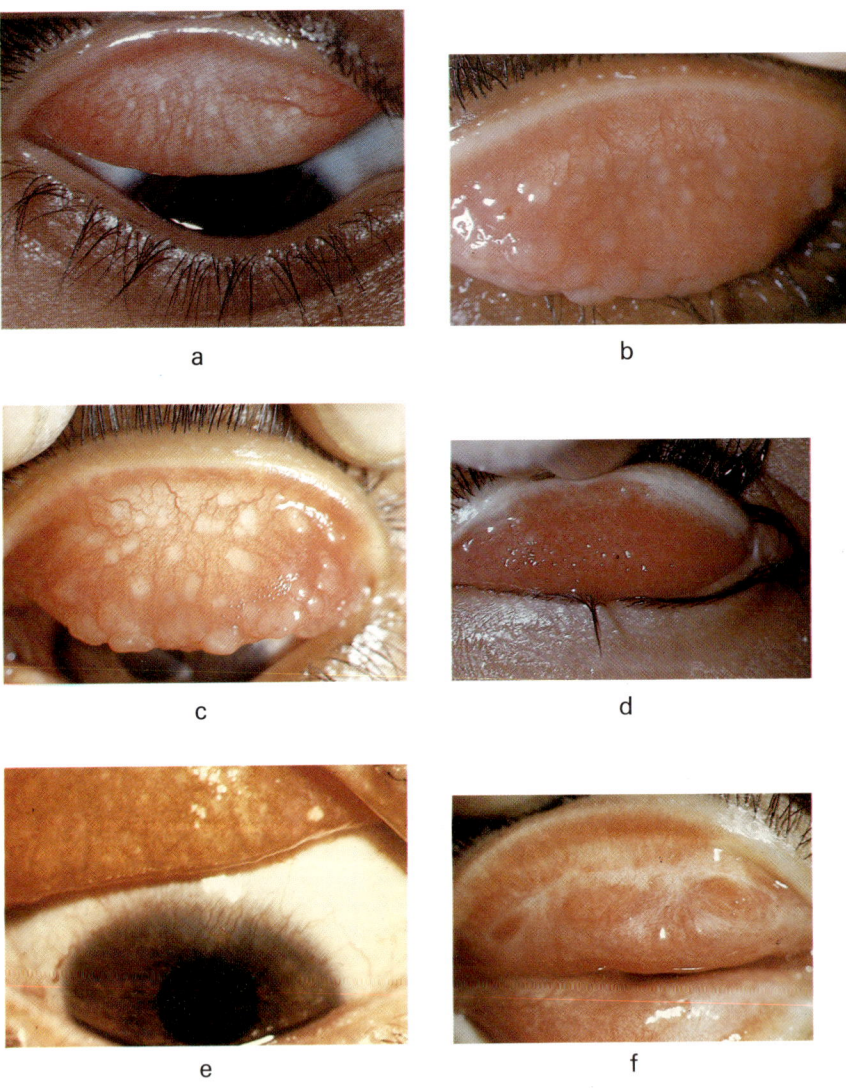

a

b

c

d

e

f

Plate 6a-d The upper tarsal conjunctiva in active trachoma. Note how the inflammatory changes progressively obscure the underlying blood vessels.
a Mild active trachoma with scattered follicles and a mild papillary hypertrophy. The conjunctival blood vessels can easily be seen.
b Moderate active trachoma with many large follicles and some papillary hypertrophy. The conjunctival blood vessels can just be seen.
c Moderate active trachoma. The follicles are exceptionally large in this case.
d Severe active trachoma with many follicles and obvious papillary hypertrophy. The conjunctival blood vessels cannot be seen at all.

e Corneal pannus. The lower half of the cornea is normal. Note the blood vessels growing down from the upper limbus, and the papillae on the upper tarsal conjunctiva.
f Scar formation and papillary hypertrophy on the upper tarsal conjunctiva.

PLATE 7

Chapter 7

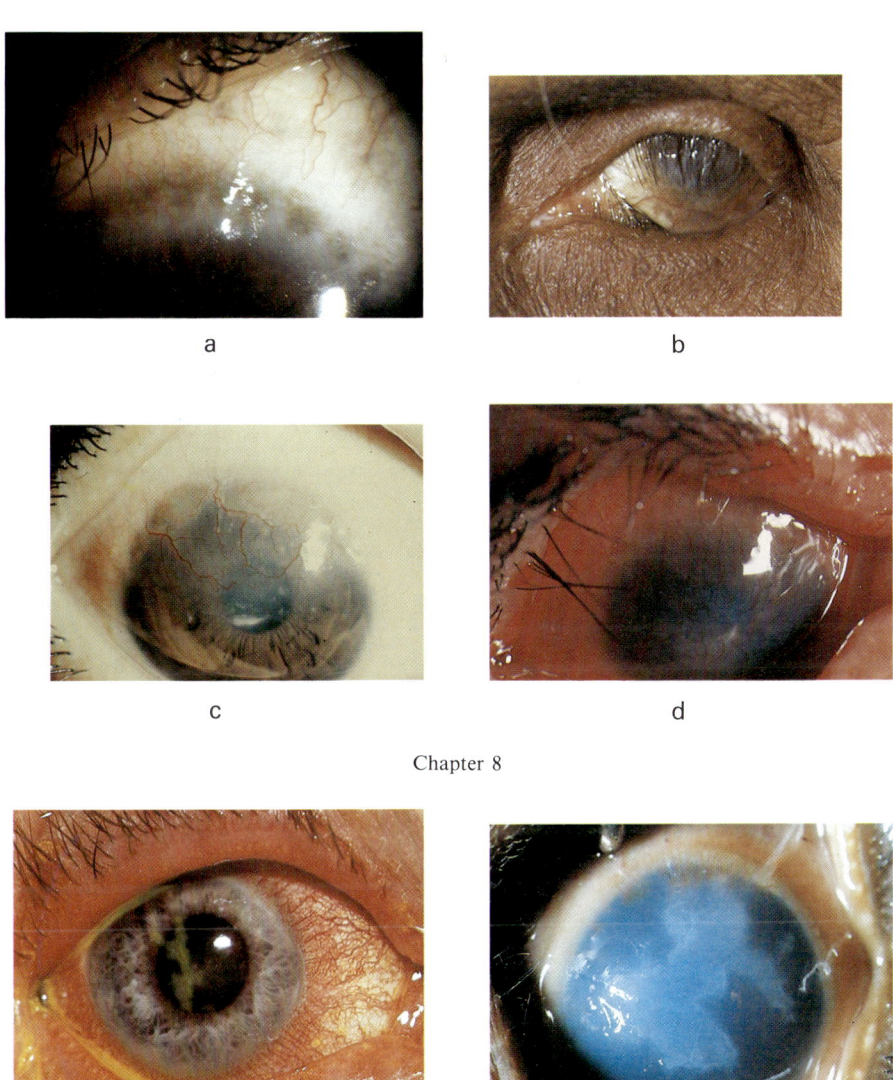

a

b

c

d

Chapter 8

e

f

a Herbert's pits.

b Entropion. In this patient, both the upper and lower eyelid are turned in. Most of the lower eyelid lashes have rolled right in and cannot be seen.

c Quite marked corneal vascularization and scarring. Note how the upper cornea is affected.

d Acute secondary bacterial conjunctivitis in an eye with chronic trachoma. Note the trichiasis and corneal scarring.

e A dendritic herpes simplex corneal ulcer with fluorescein stain. The cornea looked normal to the naked eye before adding fluorescein.

f A severe 'amoeboid' herpes simplex ulcer. The ulcer is visible even without fluorescein. The patient was a young child recovering from measles.

PLATE 8

Chapter 8

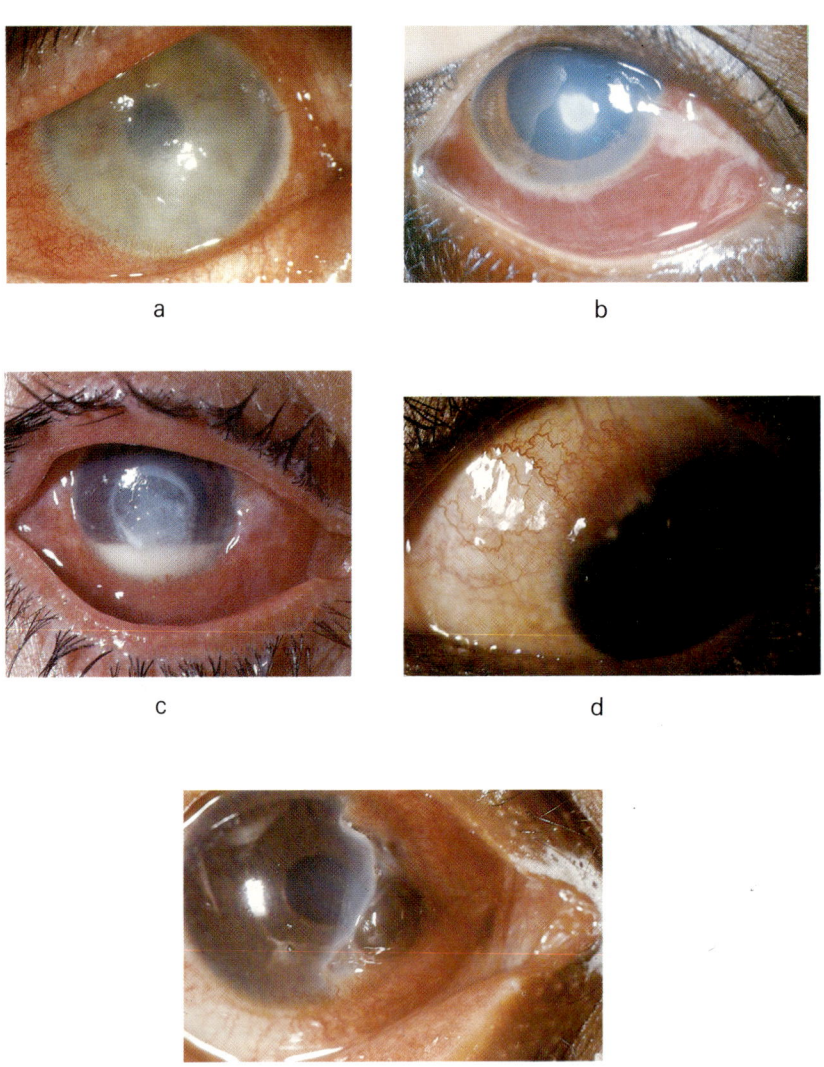

a

b

c

d

e

a Stromal keratitis. Note the generalised corneal oedema, and the dilatation of the ciliary blood vessels.

b Bacterial corneal ulcer (suppurative keratitis). Note the slough in the ulcer bed. The patient had a subconjunctival haemorrhage following a subconjunctival antibiotic injection.

c Suppurative keratitis. Note the large hypopyon and the ragged edge of the ulcer.

d Marginal corneal infiltration. Note the position of the lesions just inside the limbus.

e A severe Mooren's ulcer. The cornea has perforated and the iris has prolapsed through the hole. Any severe corneal ulcer may perforate in this way.

PLATE 9

Chapter 8

The Complications of Corneal Ulcers

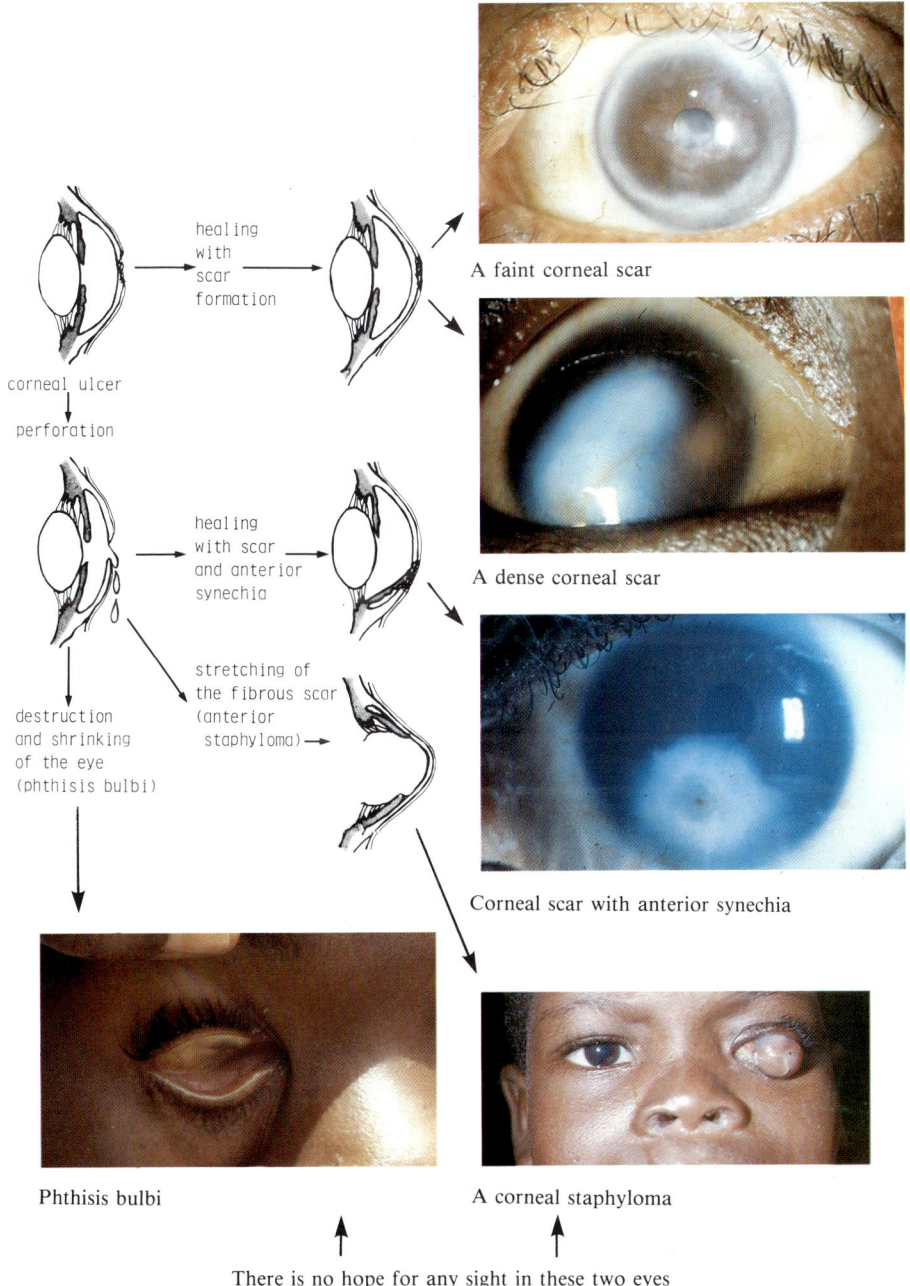

healing
with
scar
formation

A faint corneal scar

corneal ulcer

perforation

healing
with scar
and anterior
synechia

A dense corneal scar

destruction
and shrinking
of the eye
(phthisis bulbi)

stretching of
the fibrous scar
(anterior
staphyloma) →

Corneal scar with anterior synechia

Phthisis bulbi

A corneal staphyloma

There is no hope for any sight in these two eyes

PLATE 10

Chapter 8

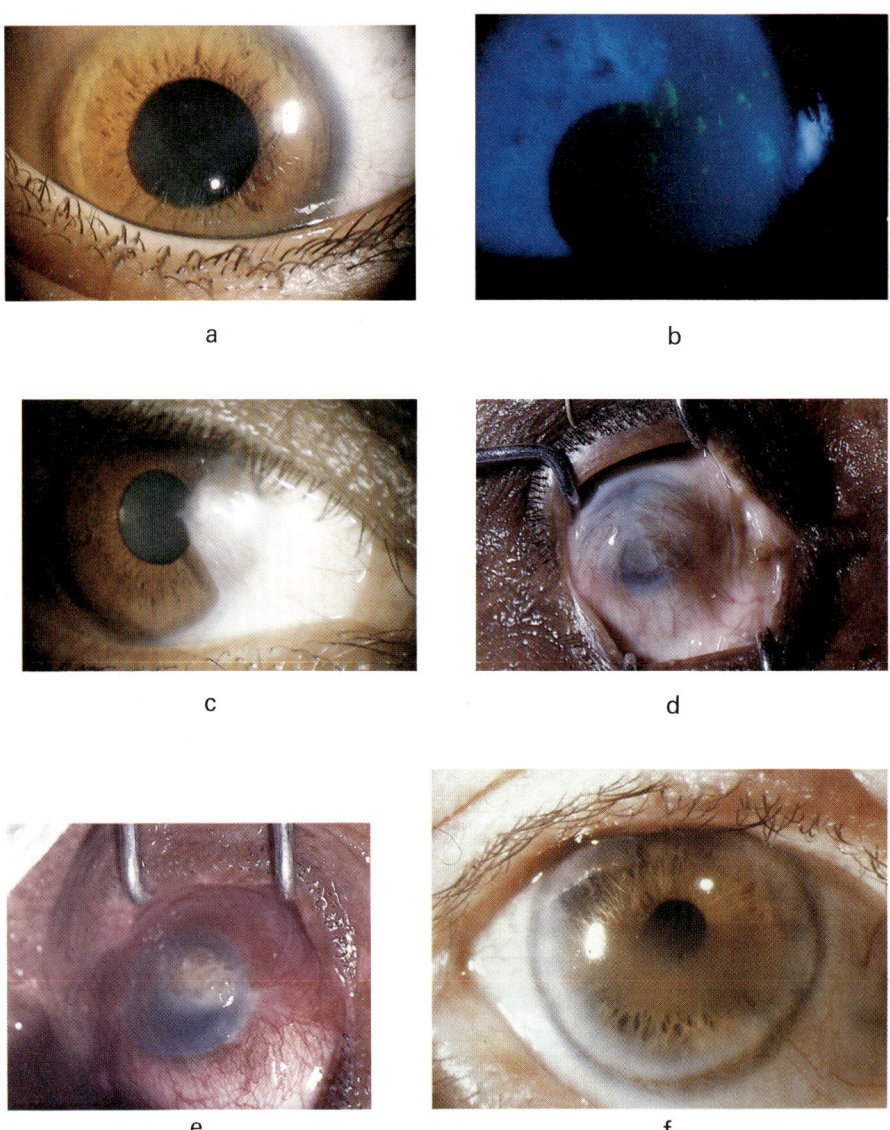

a

b

c

d

e

f

a – b Superficial punctate keratitis. The cornea looked normal until fluorescein drops were instilled. *a*. With white light just a faint green haze can be seen. *b*. With blue light the stain is more obvious.
c A pterygium. In this case, the lesion has reached the pupil margin, but the vision is still normal.
d Pterygium. In this case a pterygium is growing over the pupil from both the nasal and temporal side. There is also a mature cataract, and the pupil has been dilated.
e Solar keratopathy. Note the yellow vesicles in the exposed cornea.
f Band corneal degeneration.

PLATE 11

Chapter 8

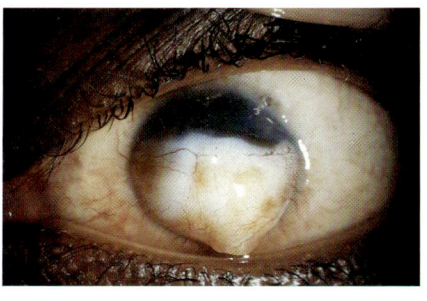

a

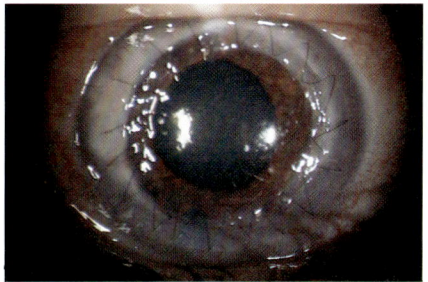

b

Chapter 9

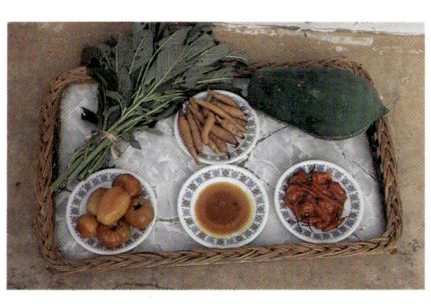

c

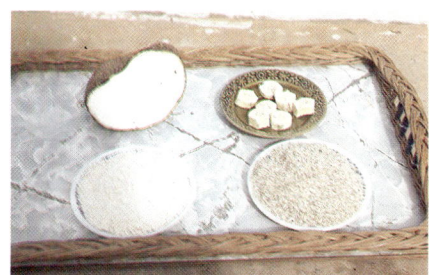

d

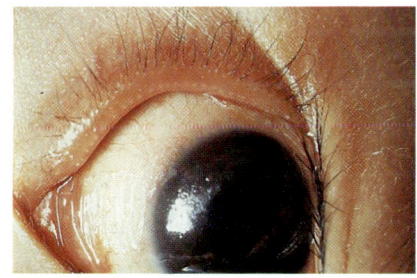

e

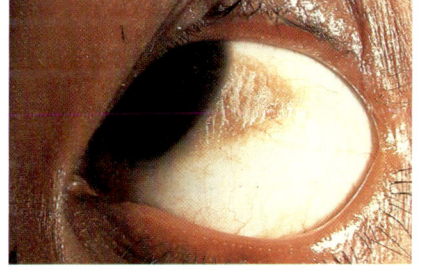

f

a A very dense corneal scar from exposure keratitis. Note the fatty deposits in the cornea, and the flat top to the scar. The patient had an optical iridectomy, and can now see well enough to walk around without help.

b A successful corneal graft.

c These vegetable foods are pigmented, and are rich in Vitamin A: − red palm oil, carrots, spinach, papayas, tomatoes, peppers.

d These vegetable foods are pale, and are very low in Vitamin A: − plantain, cassava, yam, rice.

e Conjunctival xerosis. These early changes are very difficult to detect. Note the creamy white debris which is lying on the surface of the cornea.

f Bitot's spot. The increased ·conjunctival pigmentation is often, but not always, present.

PLATE 12

Chapter 9

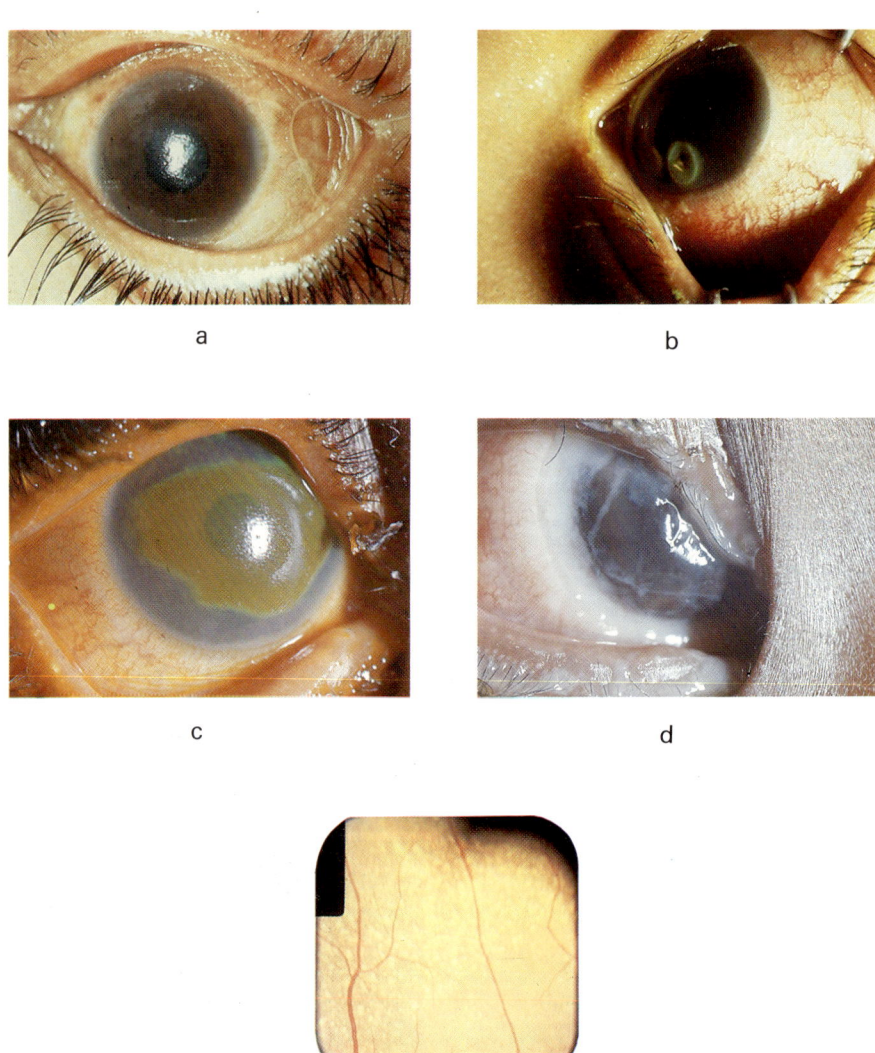

a Corneal and conjunctival xerosis. The light reflection from the cornea is altered, and the conjunctiva is dry, thickened and slightly pigmented.

b Corneal xerosis with ulceration. The ulcer is only in the lower part of the cornea, and is stained with fluorescein.

c A large superficial ulcer stained with fluorescein. The child had measles.

d Keratomalacia. The cornea has completely dissolved away, and a thin sheet of fibrin covers the iris. The child had measles.

e Xerophthalmia fundus.

PLATE 13

Chapter 10

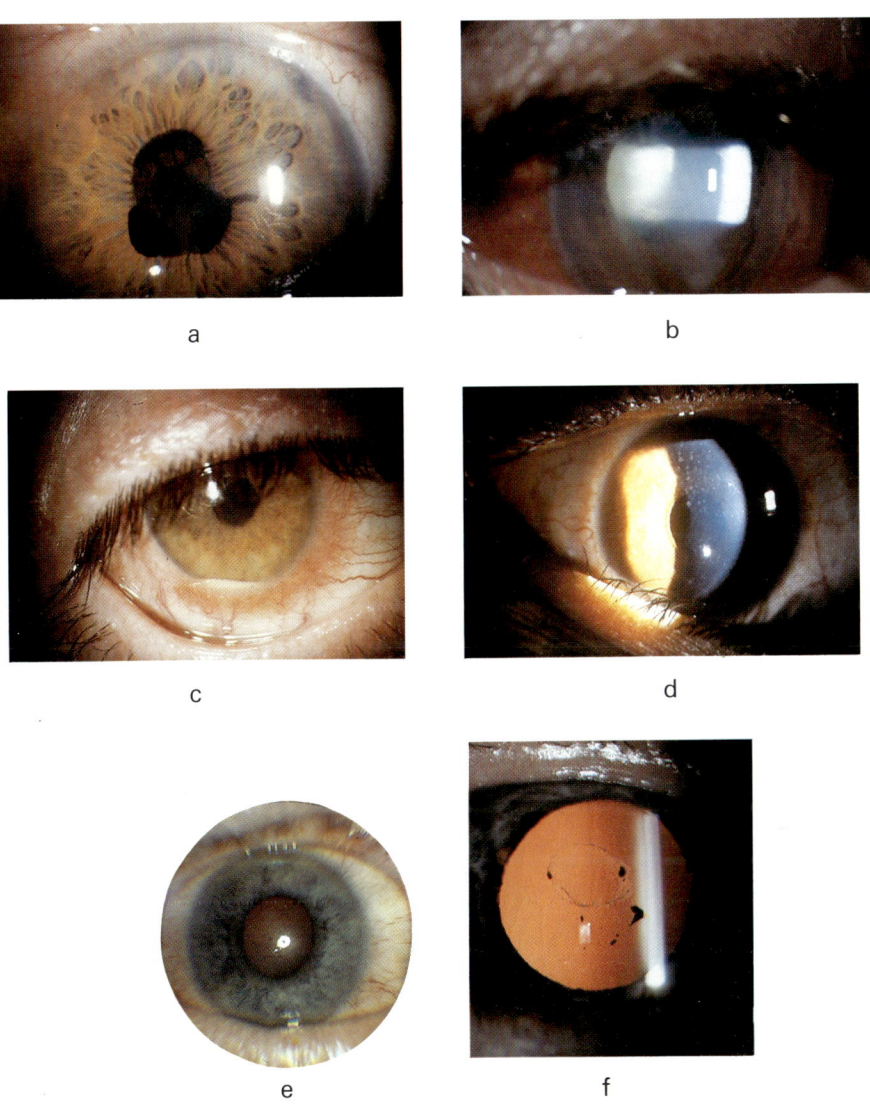

a

b

c

d

e

f

a Old iridocyclitis. The pupil has been dilated, but the iris has stuck to the lens in places. There are also deposits of iris pigment on the lens surface.

b Acute iridocyclitis: aqueous flare. Note the reflection of the beam of light from a slit lamp as it passes through the anterior chamber.

c Acute iridocyclitis. Note the dilatation of the ciliary blood vessels and the small hypopyon.

d Acute iridocyclitis. The tiny keratic precipitates on the back of the cornea are just visible in the slit lamp beam, but nowhere else.

e Iridocyclitis seen with an ophthalmoscope. Note how the shadows of the keratic precipitates are just visible against the red reflex.

f Old iridocyclitis seen with an ophthalmoscope. Note how the pigment deposits on the surface of the lens are only visible when the pupil has been dilated.

PLATE 14

Chapter 10

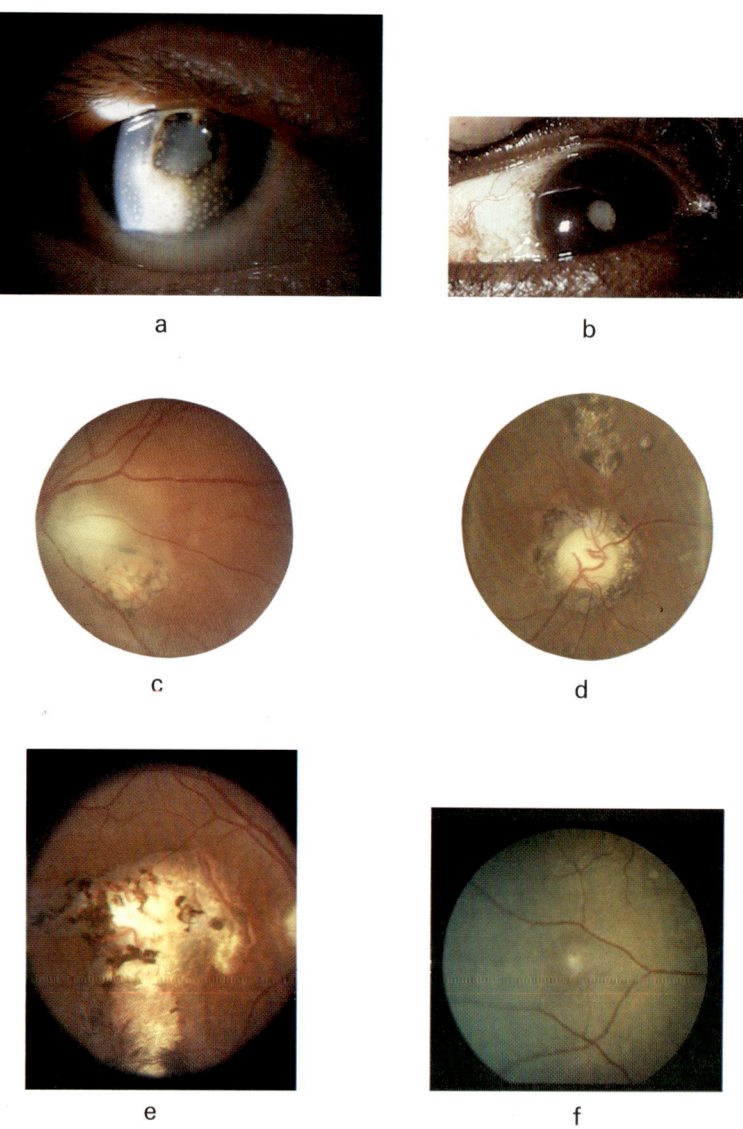

a

b

c

d

e

f

a Chronic iridocyclitis. Note the very large 'mutton fat' keratic precipitates and the irregular pupil.
b Old iritis with secondary lens opacity. Note the constricted pupil and specks of iris pigment on the lens surface.
c Acute choroiditis. Note the white oedematous retina next to an area of old choroiditis.
d Old choroiditis from syphilis.
e Old choroiditis, probably from toxoplasmosis. There is both hypertrophy and atrophy of the choroidal pigment, and atrophy of the choroidal blood vessels. The lesion has a distinct edge.
f A small choroidal tubercule in miliary tuberculosis.

PLATE 15

Chapter 11

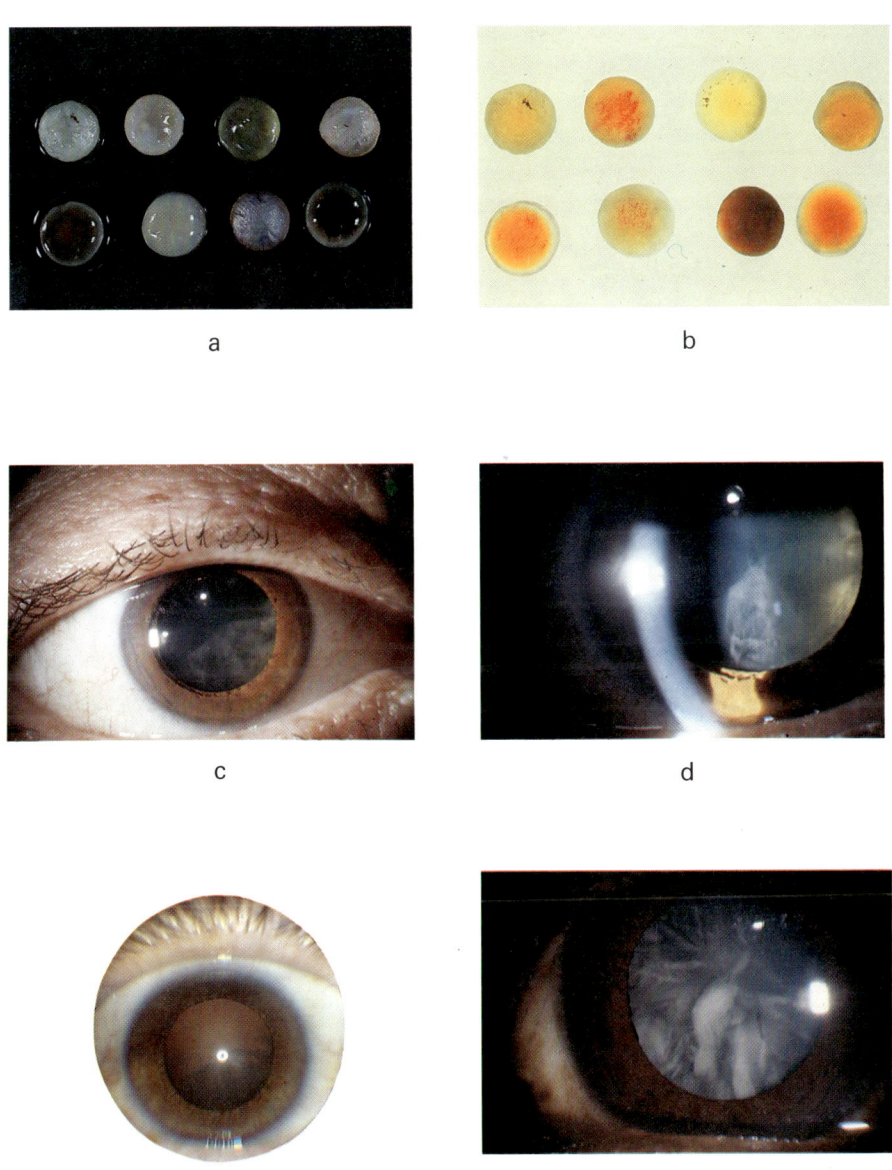

a

b

c

d

e

f

a *and* b Eight cataractous lenses. In *Plate* 15a the light is coming from in front, and in *Plate* 15b from behind.

c An early cortical lens opacity seen with diffuse illumination.

d The same eye seen with focal illumination from a slit lamp.

e The same eye seen with coaxial illumination from an ophthalmoscope.

f A more dense cortical lens opacity seen with diffuse illumination.

PLATE 16

Chapter 11

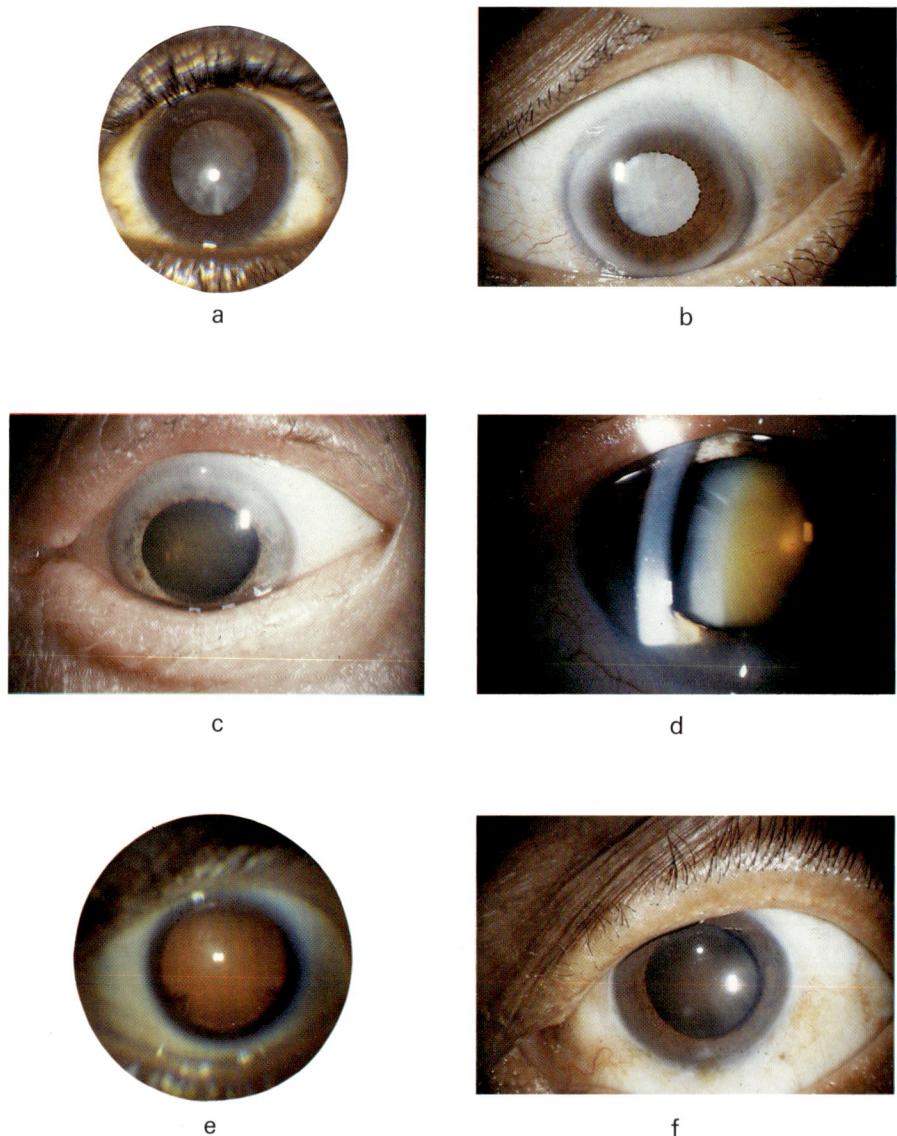

a The same eye as *Plate* 15f seen with coaxial illumination from an ophthalmoscope.
b A mature white cataract. There is also arcus senilis in the cornea.
c Early nuclear sclerosis seen with diffuse illumination.
d The same eye seen with focal illumination from a slit lamp.
e The same eye seen with coaxial illumination from an ophthalmoscope.
f A 'black' cataract. This is a totally opaque lens, but it looks very similar to a normal eye (*Plate* 1a).

PLATE 17

Chapter 11

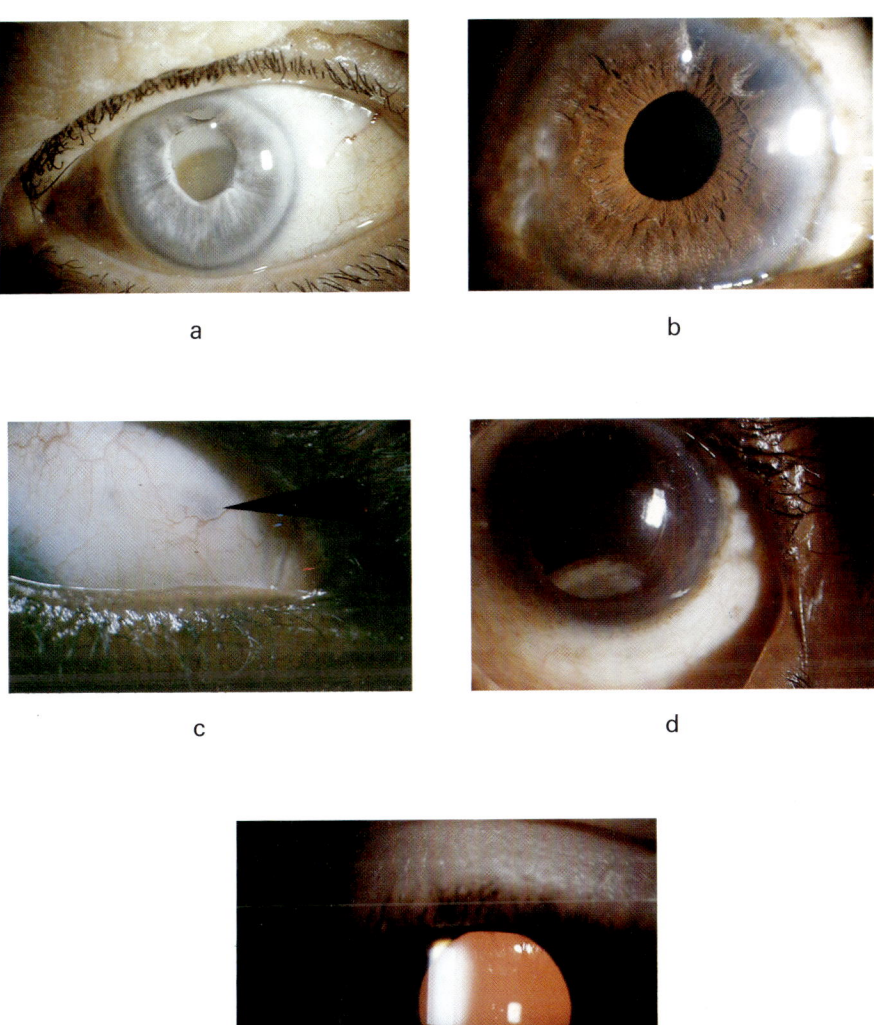

a

b

c

d

e

a A hypermature cataract. The yellow nucleus can be seen inside the milky-white cortex.
b An aphakic eye. (Compare this with the normal eye, *Plate* 1a).
c An eye after couching. The dark spot in the sclera at the tip of the pointer is the entry point into the eye.
d An eye after couching. The dislocated lens in the lower vitreous is just visible through the dilated pupil.
e A transparent but subluxated lens. The edge of the lens can be seen when the red reflex is observed through a dilated pupil.

PLATE 18

Chapter 12

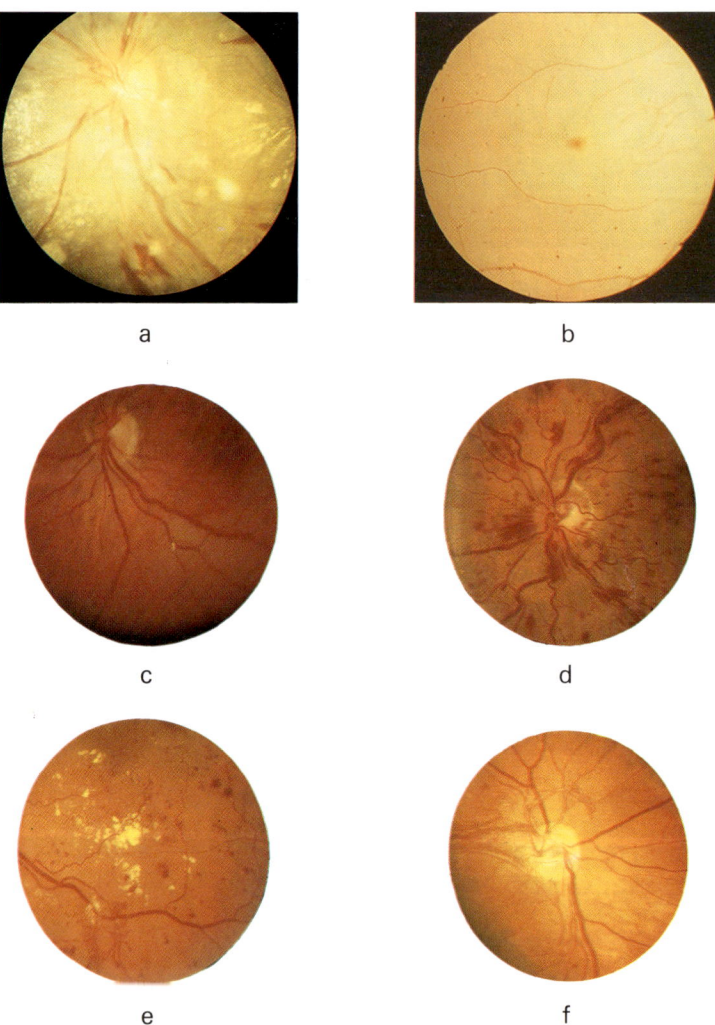

a

b

c

d

e

f

a Advanced hypertensive retinopathy. Note the 'cottonwool' exudates and flame-shaped haemorrhages. At the extreme right, the hard exudates can be seen radiating from the macula. Papilloedema is also present.

b Total central retinal artery occlusion. The retina is white and oedematous, and the blood vessels are hardly visible. The macula is a pink spot.

c Branch retinal artery occlusion. Note the yellow embolus in the lower temporal artery. That segment of the retina is pale and oedematous and obscures the choroidal outline.

d Central retinal vein occlusion. Note the extensive haemorrhages and dilated blood vessels.

e Diabetic retinopathy. Note the 'dot and blot' haemorrhages and the hard exudates. There is an area of new vessel formation at the bottom of the picture, and arterio-venous nipping where the artery and vein cross on the left. The patient also had mild hypertension.

f Proliferative diabetic retinopathy. Note the new vessels growing from and around the optic disc.

PLATE 19

Chapter 12

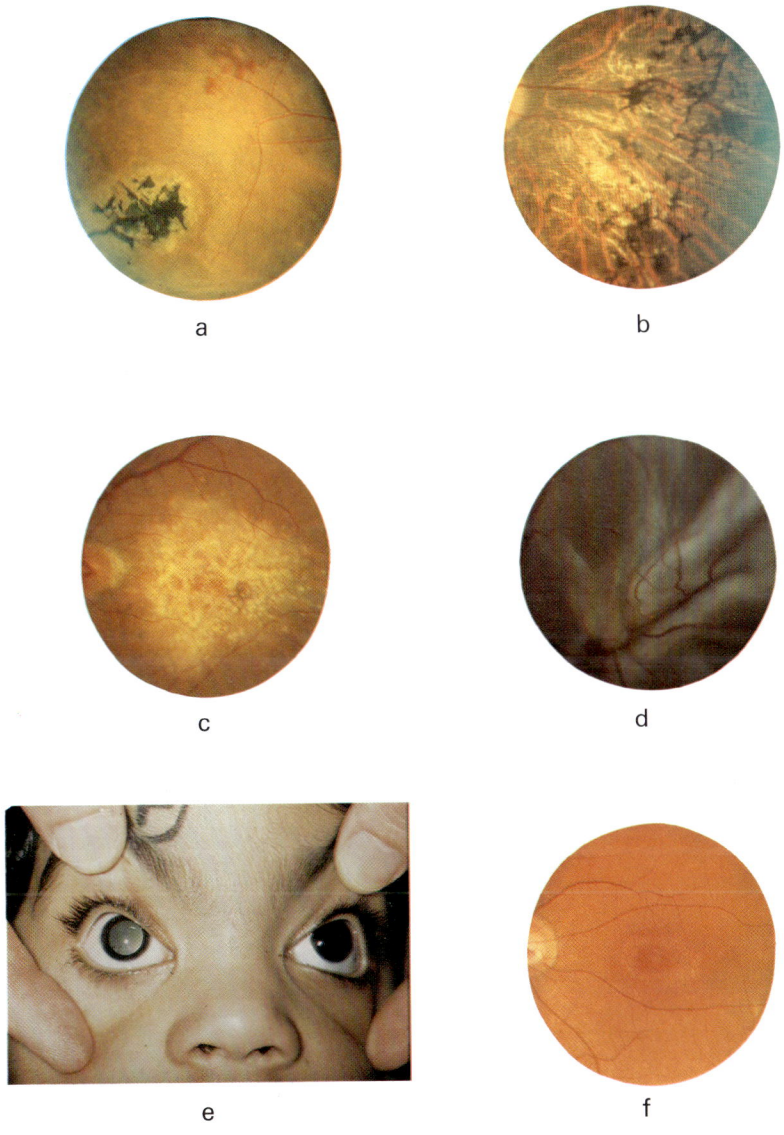

a Sickle-cell retinopathy. Note the 'fan' of new vessels at the top of the picture, and the patch of pigmentation at the bottom.

b Retinitis pigmentosa. Note the pattern of the pigment, and the thin retinal arteries.

c Senile macular degeneration.

d A detached retina. Note the folds and dark appearance of the retina. Note also the choroidal pattern of pigmentation cannot be seen.

e An early retinoblastoma. Note how this looks very like a cataract.

f A severe case of chloroquine retinopathy. Early cases are very difficult to detect.

PLATE 20

Chapter 13

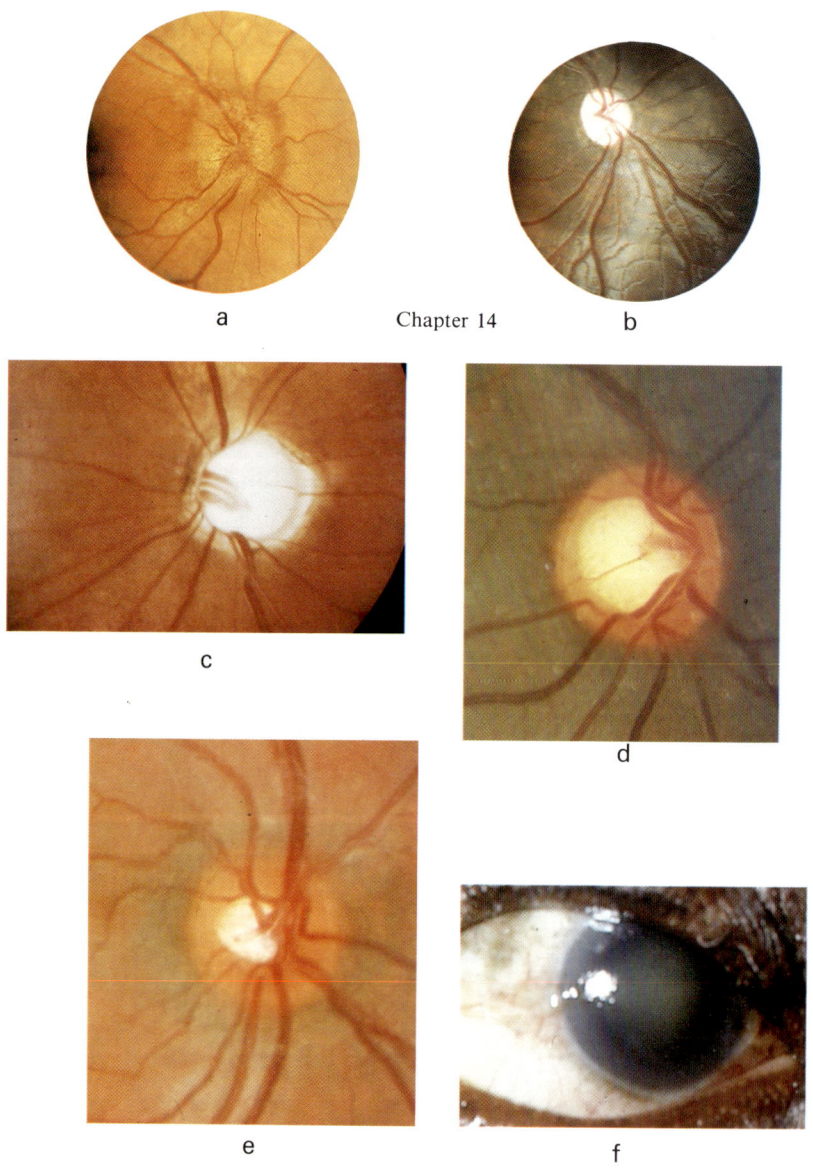

a   Chapter 14   b

c

d

e   f

a Papilloedema. Note the swollen disc with new blood vessels. The surrounding retina and retinal vessels are normal.

b Primary optic atrophy. Note the pale optic disc.

c Advanced glaucomatous optic atrophy. The entire optic disc is very pale. The retinal blood vessels disappear at the edge of the disc, and can be seen out of focus in the centre of the disc.

d Early glaucomatous optic atrophy. Just over half the total disc area is pale and cupped.

e A normal optic disc showing physiological cupping. Only a very small portion of the disc is cupped in the centre or on the temporal side.

f Very advanced glaucoma. Note the dilated pupil and the hazy, oedematous cornea.

PLATE 21

Chapter 14

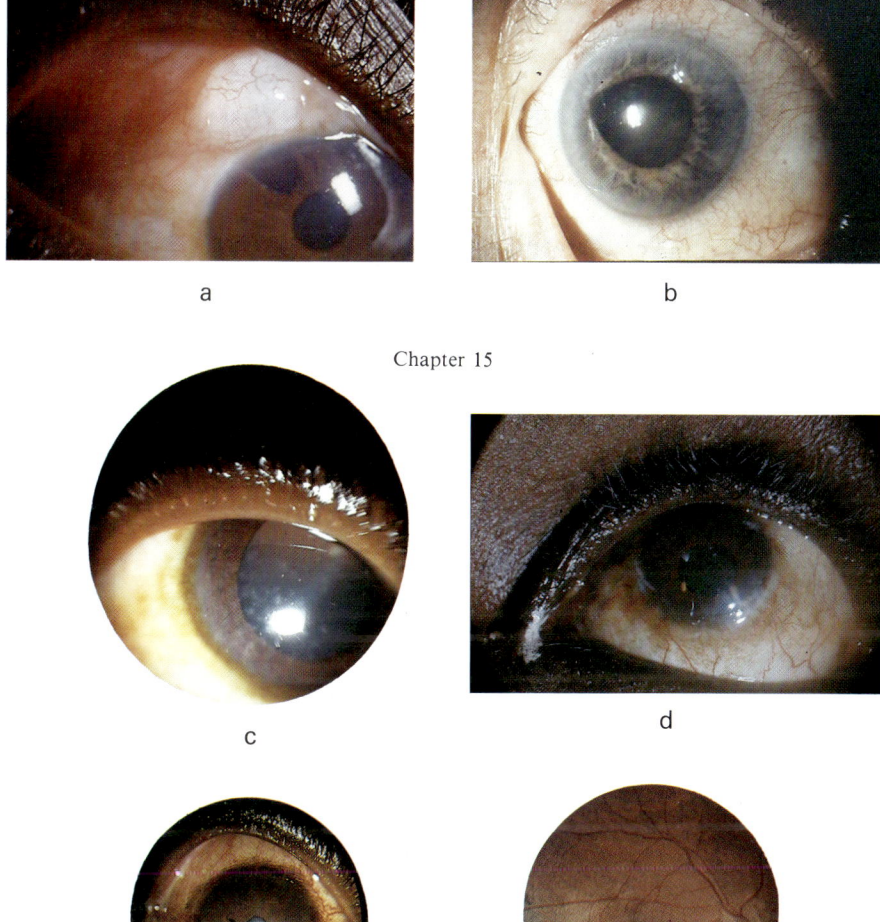

a

b

Chapter 15

c

d

e

f

a The eye after a trabeculectomy operation.

b Acute angle closure glaucoma. Note the ciliary injection, corneal oedema and half-dilated, slightly irregular pupil.

c 'Snowflake' corneal opacities. The opacities in this picture are much larger and more obvious than usual.

d Early sclerosing keratitis. The white opacity starts at the limbus in the interpalpebral fissure. Note the irregular, distorted pupil.

e More advanced sclerosing keratitis. Note the irregular pigmentation at the limbus.

f 'Mottling' and some atrophy of the pigment epithelium temporal to the macula. There are also some pigmentary changes around the optic disc.

PLATE 22

Chapter 15

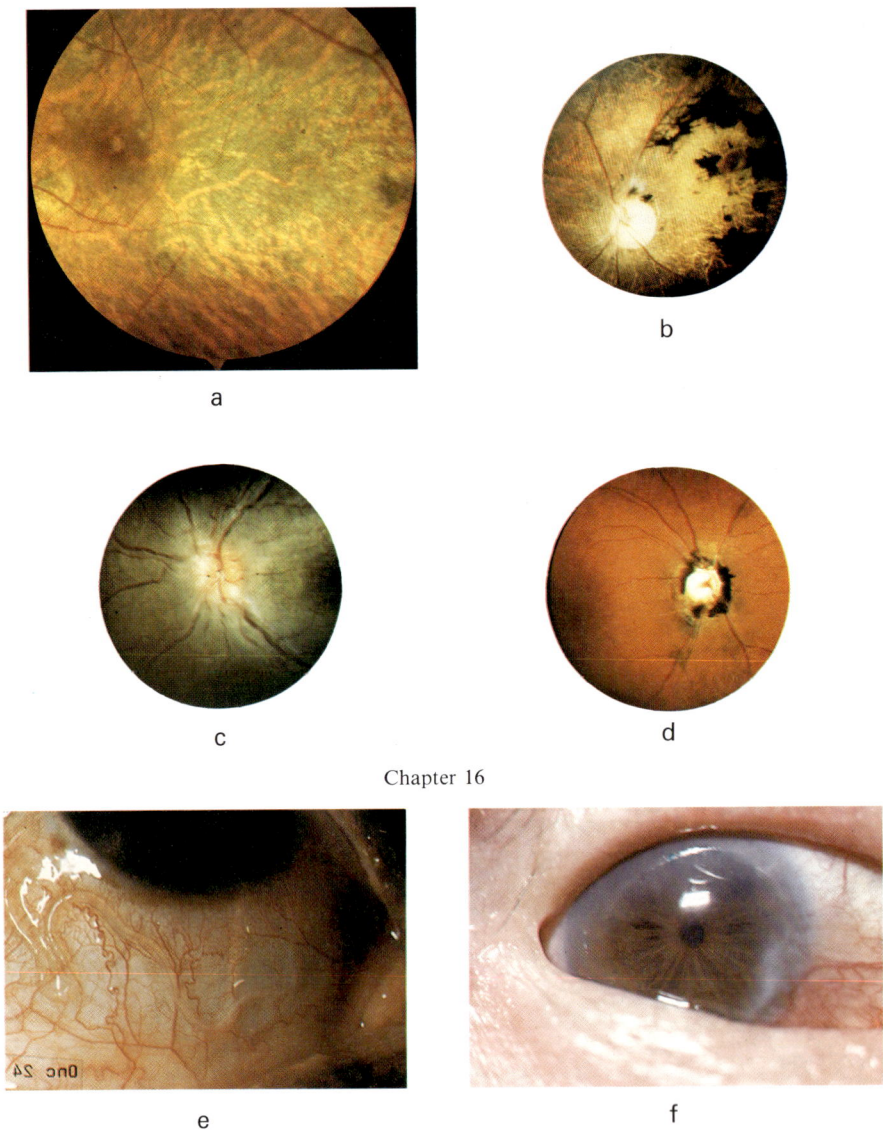

Chapter 16

a Atrophy of the pigment epithelium and the choriocapillaries temporal to the macula.

b Advanced chorioretinal atrophy and excess pigmentation. Note too the optic atrophy.

c Optic neuritis in onchocerciasis.

d Onchocercal optic atrophy. Note the increased pigmentation and fibrous tissue on and around the optic disc.

e A Loa loa worm under the conjunctiva.

f Lepromatous leprosy. There is interstitial keratitis shown by the white appearance of the margin of the cornea. There is episcleritis shown by the dilated episcleral vessels. There is chronic iritis with constriction of the pupil. Note also the loss of eyelashes.

PLATE 23

Chapter 19

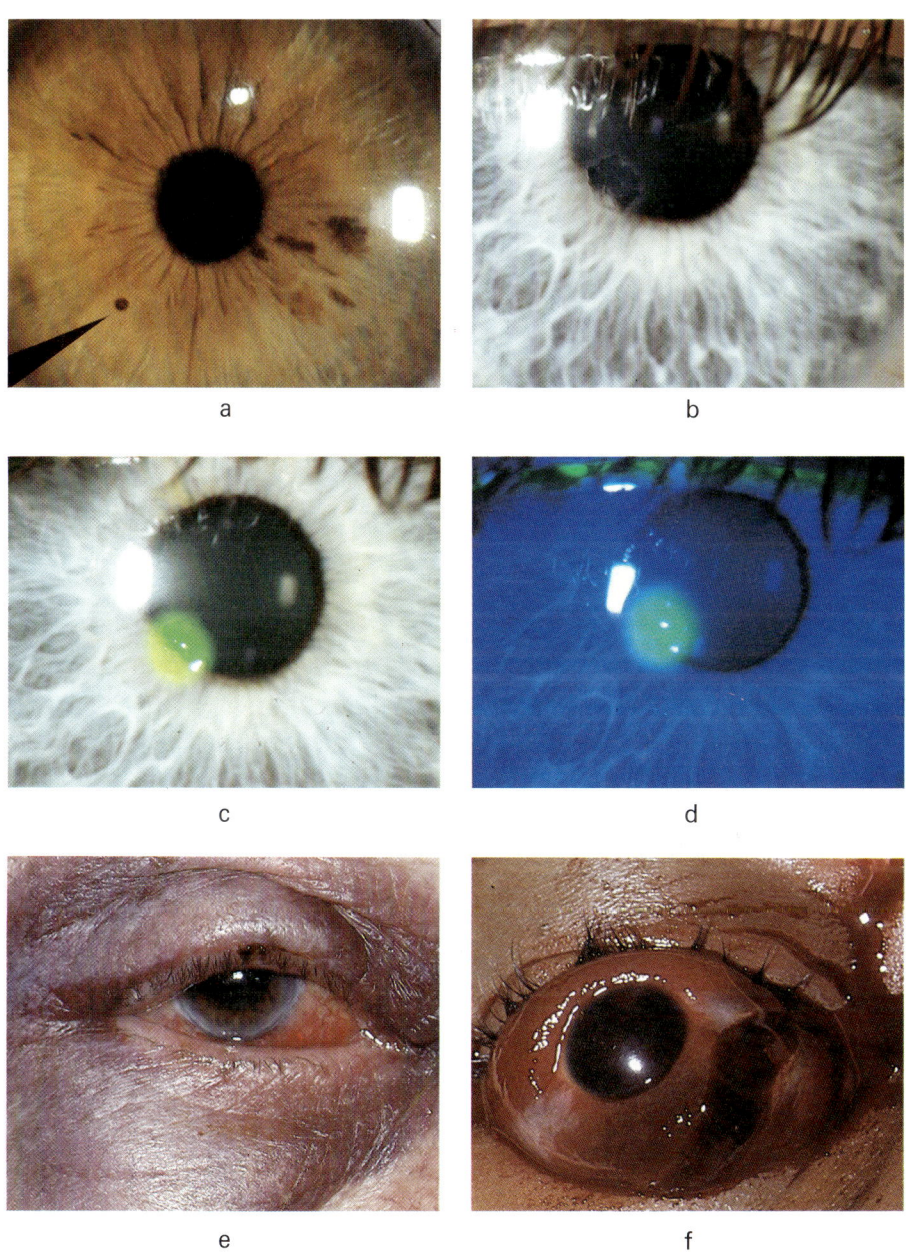

a

b

c

d

e

f

a A small corneal foreign body (shown with an arrow).
b A small corneal abrasion which is almost invisible.
c The same corneal abrasion with fluorescein stain.
d The fluorescein stain is more obvious in blue light.
e Bruised and swollen eyelids and a conjunctival haemorrhage following a blunt injury to the eye.
f A penetrating scleral laceration, a 'blackball' hyphaema and an eyelid laceration.

stores, so that there is no danger of vitamin A deficiency.

There are many ways to assess PEM in young children. It is usual to measure either the arm circumference or the child's weight for age, and to look for any signs of oedema.

Generalized infections

Generalized infections (e.g. measles, gastroenteritis or malaria) often precipitate acute xerophthalmia and corneal ulceration. Such infections lower vitamin A levels in the body in two ways: –
– They increase the metabolic needs of the body.
– They depress the appetite, and so reduce food intake.

Malnourished children are especially prone to infections. During the acute illness, they often lie exhausted and dehydrated, sometimes with poor closure of the eyelids and a diminished blink reflex. In hot, dry climates especially, there is a great risk that the exposed part of the cornea may become ulcerated. This explains why malnourished children develop corneal ulcers mainly in the lower parts of the cornea.

Measles (Plate 12c and d, Plate 7f)

Measles is a much more important cause of corneal ulceration than any other infection. Measles seems to be more severe in blacks, and this susceptibility may be racial. Indeed, in many parts of Africa, more than half of all cases of child blindness are from corneal ulceration following measles. There is some doubt whether these ulcers can be from vitamin A deficiency, because the children often seem to have adequate dietary vitamin A. It is certain, however, that nearly all of these children are malnourished.

Measles is not like most other childhood infections, because the measles virus actually invades the conjunctival and corneal epithelium. During an attack of measles, even healthy and well-nourished children develop superficial keratoconjunctivitis. Normally, this resolves completely, but in malnourished children it may progress to severe corneal ulceration.

We now know that secondary herpes simplex infections of the cornea are common after measles. The herpes simplex virus often lies dormant in the tissues. Malnutrition and measles together depress cellular immunity, so that the herpes virus becomes active and causes a severe infection. In a normal person, herpes simplex causes a localized superficial ulcer in the cornea, or a 'cold sore' on the lip. However, after measles in malnourished children severe necrotic ulcers may develop, especially in the eye and in the mouth (see Fig. 9.3).

Intestinal parasites

Intestinal parasites do not seem to upset the metabolism of vitamin A, but they may lower the absorption of carotenes and retinol from the intestine.

Nutritional corneal ulceration in children is a very complex disease indeed. Clearly the three most important factors are vitamin A deficiency, protein energy malnutrition and measles. However, there are many more factors, and not all of

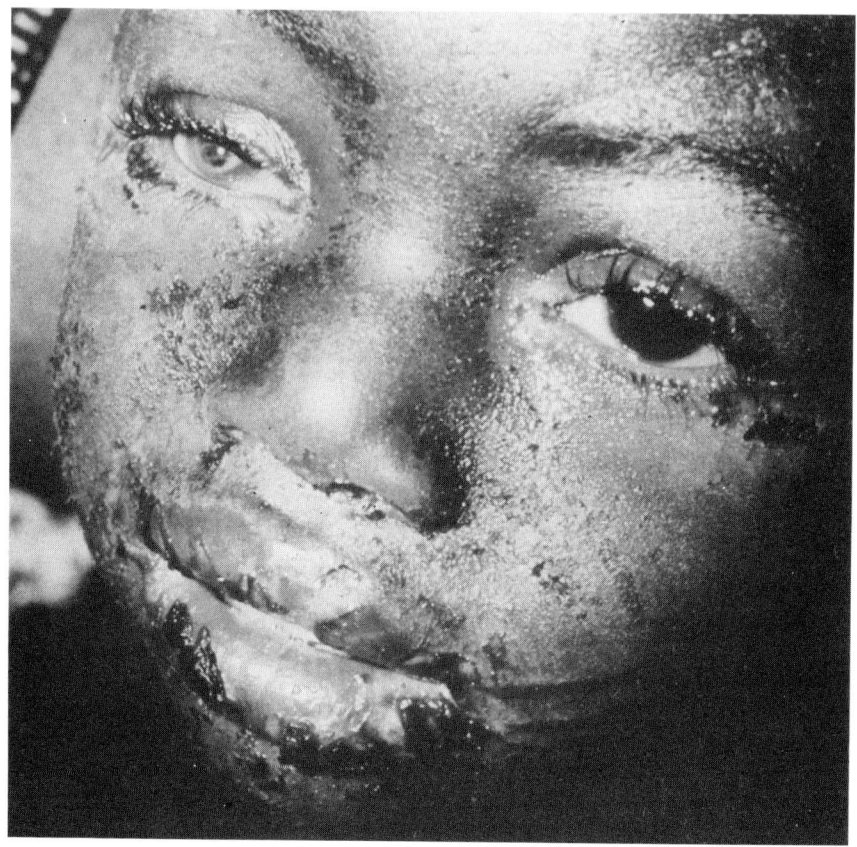

Fig. 9.3 A perforating ulcer in the right eye and mouth ulcers. The child had measles.

them are fully understood. Further research may of course improve our understanding. On the other hand, effective action could prevent this disease and make further research unnecessary. Surely this is not too much to hope?

The treatment of nutritional corneal ulcers

It is necessary to correct any underlying nutritional deficiency or general illness, and to give local treatment to the eyes. However, it is not enough just to dispense injections, tablets and eye ointment. It is also important to recognize the social, economic and family problems which have caused the disease. In other words, it is necessary to 'treat' nutritional corneal ulceration in the widest sense of the word.

Nutritional and general treatment

Massive doses of vitamin A are necessary for: –
– all children with active corneal ulceration,

Table 9.4. The recommended doses of vitamin A

		Dose by mouth		
		mg	iu	
Emergency treatment of	Day 1	110	200 000	(For children less
children with	Day 2	110	200 000	than 1 year old,
xerophthalmia or	2 weeks	110	200 000	half this dose should
corneal ulcers	later			be given)

(If the child is severely ill with gastro-enteritis or unable to swallow, the first dose should be an intramuscular injection of water-soluble vitamin A)

Preventative treatment in the community.			
Children under 1 year old	55	100 000	Repeat every 4 – 6 months
Children over 1 year old	110	200 000	Repeat every 4 – 6 months
Children at birth	27.5	50 000	
Mothers just after giving birth	165	300 000	
Pregnant and lactating mothers	11	20 000	Weekly

— all children with any of the signs of xerophthalmia,
— all severely ill or malnourished children from areas where xerophthalmia occurs, even if there is no clinical evidence of xerophthalmia.

Table 9.4 shows the doses of vitamin A which WHO recommends. Most preparations of vitamin A also contain small doses of vitamin E (tocopherol). Vitamin E seems to improve the absorption and utilization of vitamin A.

If vitamin A capsules are not available, the child must eat foods which are rich in vitamin A. It is also important to correct any protein energy malnutrition.

Many malnourished children also need treatment for dehydration, pyrexia, bronchopneumonia, gastroenteritis, measles or intestinal parasites.

Local treatment to the eye

All eyes with evidence of corneal ulceration need local treatment. Even eyes without ulcers may need treatment to prevent ulcers forming. It is necessary to handle eyes with advanced ulceration very gently, so that the ulcer does not perforate. It may also be necessary to restrain the child, to prevent him from rubbing his eye.

— Antibiotics. Bacterial infection is probably not a primary cause of these corneal ulcers. However, bacteria are certainly very common secondary invaders. Ulcers with clinical evidence of established bacterial infection (hypopyon, or infiltration of the cornea around the ulcer) need broad-spectrum antibiotic drops or ointment every hour. Subconjunctival and systemic antibiotics may also be helpful in severe cases. Antibiotic ointment 3 or 4 times a day can also help to prevent corneal infection in more mild cases.
— Antiviral agents. Herpes simplex infection may cause some of these ulcers, especially after measles. The treatment for herpes simplex is local antiviral agents every 1 or 2 hours (*see* page 96).
— Padding an eye often increases the local bacterial content. On the other hand, it prevents dehydration and exposure of the cornea. Padding also helps the

epithelium to heal, and reduces pain and photophobia. It is probably helpful to pad eyes with active acute corneal ulcers.
- Make sure the eyes are properly closed.
- Apply the pad very carefully, especially if the child is young.

If the eyes are not properly closed, the pad will rub against the cornea and cause further damage.

Some sick children have not developed ulcers, but cannot close their eyes properly. The mothers of these children will need to learn how to close the eyelids, and to apply plenty of antibiotic ointment. This ointment will lubricate and protect the cornea. Any severely ill young child who has poor eyelid closure is at risk of developing corneal ulceration. It is very important to prevent this.
- Mydriatics are necessary for all cases of active corneal ulceration. The most common treatment is atropine 1% drops or ointment once a day.

Surgery

Some surgeons have tried to save eyes with severe keratomalacia either by emergency corneal grafting, or by using conjunctival flaps. However, there is usually no indication for emergency surgical treatment. Most of these children are too ill to tolerate a general anaesthetic, and the necrotic and diseased tissues are unsuitable for surgery. Recovery is often considerable with medical treatment alone.

The epidemiology of nutritional corneal ulcers

Nutritional corneal ulceration is very closely associated with poverty and malnutrition. The reasons are obvious: –
- Poor people generally eat vegetable foods because they are cheap. However, the best sources of dietary retinol (e.g. liver, butter, cheese, kidney, eggs and milk) are all expensive animal foods.
- Fats help the absorption of retinol and the carotenes, but poor people usually eat very little fat of any kind.
- Some vegetable foods are excellent sources of carotene (*Plate* 11c). However, most starchy white foods, which are the staple diet of many poor communities, contain very little carotene (*Plate* 11d). The highest incidence of xerophthalmia is in areas of South India, Bangladesh and Indonesia, where rice is the staple food.

In some areas, the basic food is rich in vitamin A (e.g. red palm oil on the West African coast, or cow's milk among some nomadic tribes). In these areas, vitamin A deficiency is very uncommon. On the other hand, some local languages have special words for night blindness or Bitot's spot. These words indicate that the community is traditionally prone to vitamin A deficiency.

Vitamin A deficiency sometimes occurs even when foods rich in vitamin A are cheap and easily available. There may be taboos, religious customs or cultural reasons why children do not eat these foods, or the child may simply not have acquired the taste. In some communities, it is the custom to wean small children with mainly starchy cereals and root crops.

In some areas, nutritional corneal ulceration is especially common at certain times of the year. These are the times when fruits and green vegetables rich in vitamin A are not available, or when there are seasonal epidemics of intercurrent infection.

The clinical pattern of xerophthalmia is very variable. In Africa, the early signs of xerophthalmia are uncommon, but measles is a very important factor. In India and Indonesia, conjunctival and corneal xerosis is much more common, but measles is less important.

Young children between 6 months and 3 years are more at risk from acute destructive corneal lesions. Children over 3 years old, however, are more likely to have milder conjunctival changes without corneal destruction. It is possible that younger children are more susceptible to protein energy malnutrition and intercurrent infections.

Breast feeding generally protects against xerophthalmia. However, in communities where xerophthalmia is common, the mother's diet may be so poor in vitamin A, that her milk is deficient in it. In this way, the weaning child cannot build up adequate stores of vitamin A in the liver.

There are many reasons why an unsophisticated mother should not wean her child too early. The risk is especially great if she then gives her child artificial milk which is deficient in vitamin A (e.g. dried skimmed milk, or sweetened condensed milk). Most countries now insist that such milk is fortified with vitamin A before it is sold.

Poor people from city slums are in some ways worse off than poor people from villages. They are less likely to eat fresh vegetables and milk products, and more likely to wean their children earlier. On the other hand, preventative measures from governments and health authorities are more likely to reach them.

Measuring Vitamin A levels.

There are many ways to measure vitamin A levels in a community or an individual: –
– Dietary analysis is an important way to study the community, but it is not a useful way to study an individual patient.
– Biochemical tests give a good indication of vitamin A levels. Some examples are: –
   – spectrophotometry or fluorometry, used to assay vitamin A,
   – immunodiffusion, used to assay the serum retinol binding protein.
   However, both these methods are much too complex for ordinary use.
– Clinical assessment of the eye is the best and easiest way to diagnose vitamin A deficiency in an individual. It is also very valuable in community surveys.
   There are problems in community surveys. For example: –
– Conjunctival xerosis and Bitot's spot are relatively common signs, but they do not always progress to blindness. On the other hand, the corneal signs are much less frequent, and therefore harder to assess in a survey. However, they are much more likely to indicate a severe risk of blindness.
– Xerophthalmia scars give a good indication of the incidence of blindness in a community. However, the scars may be the result of another disease, not always xerophthalmia.

Table 9.5. The diagnosis of xerophthalmia in the community

Criterion		*Minimum % of the population at risk*
Clinical		
X1B	Bitot's spot	2.0 %
X2 + X3	Corneal xerosis and corneal ulceration	0.01%
XS	Xerophthalmia scars	0.1 %
Biochemical		
Serum retinol (vitamin A) less than 10 μg/100 ml		5.0 %

WHO has established certain criteria, which indicate that xerophthalmia is a serious problem in the community (*Table* 9.5).

The prevention of blindness from nutritional corneal ulceration

'Prevention is better than cure.' This old saying is more true of nutritional corneal ulceration than any other eye disease. It is true that prompt, effective treatment saves either the sight or life of a few children. However, there are many more who are permanently blind when they first seek medical treatment — and even more who never receive any treatment at all.

Any programme of prevention must have two essential features: –
– It must be based in the community, rather than the hospital.
– It must have co-operation and co-ordination between different sciences such as ophthalmology, nutrition, agriculture, community medicine and education.

Measures for prevention are possible at different levels in the community. The government may intervene to improve the health of the nation as a whole. Or else individual mothers may receive nutritional advice and support. Nutritional corneal ulceration is a complex problem, and there is no simple remedy. A preventative measure which is appropriate in one community may not be appropriate in another. The following list describes some of the measures which different communities have taken.

1. Distribution of massive dose capsules (Table 9.4, p. 121)

Vitamin A capsules containing 55 mg (100 000 iu) are easy to obtain and very cheap. In fact, the biggest expense in this programme is the distribution, and not the cost of the capsules themselves. A single dose of 55 mg for children under 1, and 110 mg for children over 1, can protect against vitamin A deficiency for up to 6 months. It is important not to give more than one dose of vitamin A a month. Children who have had more than one dose a month sometimes show signs of vitamin A toxicity — headaches, vomiting and nausea.

Pregnant women and lactating mothers also need vitamin A. However it is advisable to give small doses more frequently. If the woman is pregnant, there is a risk that a single massive dose might damage the fetus.

Children at risk need vitamin A capsules for the first 5 years of life. The community must therefore be well-organized to make capsule distribution effective. The most common reason why capsule distribution programmes fail is that they do not reach the children most in need of protection.

2. Fortification of foods

It is necessary to identify one particular food which all the children in the community eat, and which is processed at one or two central factories. It is usually possible for these factories to fortify the food with vitamin A, without changing the taste or appearance.

3. Horticulture and agriculture

It is often difficult to persuade members of a community to change their diet and agricultural methods. However, in order to treat vitamin A deficiency at source, it is necessary to encourage people to grow and eat the right sorts of food. Green leafy vegetables (e.g. spinach) and orange coloured fruit and vegtables (e.g. carrots, mangoes, papayas) are very rich in carotene. They are also cheap and easy to grow.

Seed improvement may increase the Vitamin A content of fruit and vegetables. Improved methods of food preservation will make vitamin A rich foods available throughout the year.

4. Nutrition and health education

Nutrition and health education is possible in many ways and at many levels, e.g. radio, television, schools, adult education classes and hospital out-patient waiting areas. It is only young children who are at risk from xerophthalmia, and they are totally dependant on their mothers. For this reason, the aim of any programme must be to educate the mothers and future mothers of young children. These mothers will need advice about: −
− weaning in general,
− which weaning foods to choose,
− how to choose cheap, nutritional foods when money is a problem.

It is preferable if advice about weaning is part of a comprehensive programme of child care. Some hospitals have special nutritional rehabilitation centres for malnourished children *and* their mothers. The children receive treatment, and the mothers receive advice and guidance. The treatment of a malnourished child should always include some sort of nutritional advice.

5. Immunization

Immunization programmes can prevent many serious childhood illnesses, especially measles. The measles vaccine is a living, but attenuated virus, and it needs very careful storage. Unfortunately, many vaccine schemes for measles have failed because the vaccine has died. Recent clinical trials with a new vaccine have given very encouraging results. This new vaccine is a stable aerosol measles vaccine, which could possibly eradicate measles. The eradication of measles would, of course, be a benefit in itself. It would also be a major advance in the prevention of nutritional corneal blindness in children.

For further reading

1. World Health Organisation (1982), *Vitamin A Deficiency and Xerophthalmia.*, Technical Report Series 672. Geneva.

2. WHO (1982), Sommer A., *Field Guide to the Detection and Control of Xerophthalmia*, Geneva

10.   Diseases of the Uvea

The structure and function of the uvea are described in Chapter 2.

Uveitis

Inflammation is by far the most common disease of the uvea, and this is called 'uveitis'. Uveitis may involve the whole uvea, but is usually confined either to the anterior uvea (the iris and ciliary body) or to the posterior uvea (the choroid). Anterior uveitis is called 'iridocyclitis' (sometimes just 'iritis'), and posterior uveitis is called choroiditis.

Iridocyclitis

Iridocyclitis may be acute or chronic. Acute iridocyclitis is one of the common causes of a painful red eye. The pain may vary from being slight to severe, and there is nearly always some blurring of the vision. Photophobia is also common.

The signs of iridocyclitis are very distinctive. They are best seen with a slit lamp, but some signs can be seen with an ordinary magnifying lens, or even the naked eye.

- The anterior ciliary blood vessels around the margin of the cornea are dilated (*Plate* 13b *and* c).
- The iris constricts and adheres to the anterior capsule of the lens (*Fig.* 10.1) The pupil therefore appears constricted and irregular, even to the naked eye. If the pupil is dilated with mydriatic drops, these adhesions between the iris and the lens may become more noticeable (*Fig.* 10.1, *Plates* 13a *and* 14a).

  After dilating the pupil these adhesions may rupture, leaving deposits of iris pigment stuck to the lens surface (*Plate* 13a *and* f). Even when the inflammation subsides, these adhesions between the iris and the lens persist. They are called 'posterior synechiae'.
- During the acute attack, the anterior chamber contains an inflammatory protein exudate and white blood cells from the iris and ciliary body. With a slit lamp, the protein exudate appears as a 'flare' (*Plate* 13b). The bright beam of a slit lamp will also highlight the white blood cells. In severe inflammation, white cells and fibrin exudate may collect at the bottom of the anterior chamber to form a hypopyon (*Plate* 13c).
- Some of the white blood cells in the anterior chamber form deposits on the back of the cornea. These are called 'keratic precipitates' (*Plates* 13d and 14*a*).

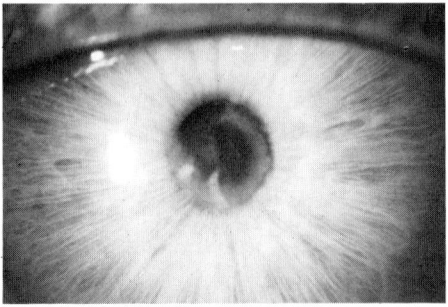

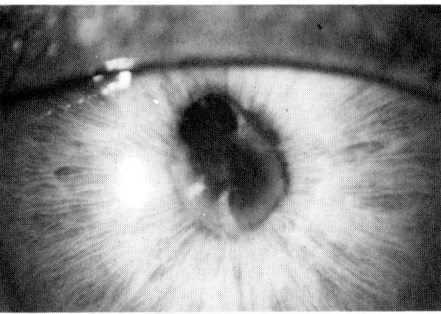

Fig. 10.1 Old iridocyclitis. The pupil is constricted and adherent to the lens. These adhesions become more obvious on attempting to dilate the pupil.

If no slit lamp is available, an ophthalmoscope may help to detect iridocyclitis. It is necessary to use a strongly positive lens in the ophthalmoscope, and to hold it close to the patient's eye. The following signs may then be visible: –
– The shadows of the keratic precipitates may be seen against the red reflex (*Plate* 13e).
– The irregular pupil and pigment deposits from the iris on the lens surface may also be seen (*Plate* 13f).
  An acute attack may occur in one or both eyes, and recurrences are common. This means that there is often a history of previous attacks or evidence of previous inflammation in either eye. After the inflammation subsides, the ciliary vasodilatation and the anterior chamber inflammatory exudate both disappear. The keratic precipitates shrink and become pigmented, and eventually they too usually disappear. However, any adhesions between the pupil margin and the lens or any deposits of iris pigment on the lens surface are both permanent.
  In chronic iridocyclitis the onset of the disease is much more gradual. There is usually little or no pain, and the only significant symptom is blurred vision. The inflammatory changes in the eye are characterized by large, pale keratic precipitates. These are called 'mutton fat' keratic precipitates (*Plate* 14a). There may also be inflammatory granulomatous nodules on, or beneath the surface of the iris.
  Complications of iridocyclitis are frequent, especially if no treatment is given, and may cause permanent blindness.
1. Secondary glaucoma is quite common and may occur in two ways: –

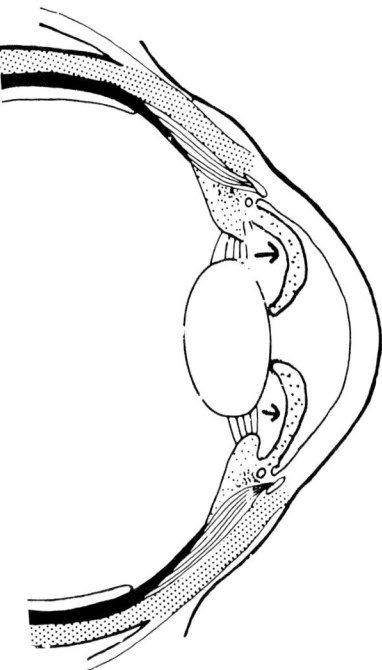

Fig. 10.2 Pupil block glaucoma. The arrows show how the pressure of the aqueous pushes the iris forwards.

- The inflammatory exudate and cells in the anterior chamber may prevent the aqueous fluid from draining out of the eye. The intraocular pressure therefore rises and may damage the optic nerve. As the inflammation subsides, the pressure usually returns to normal, but any damage to the optic nerve and loss of vision is permanent.
- Occasionally, pupil block glaucoma occurs (*Fig.* 10.2). Adhesions between the iris and the lens totally occlude the pupil, and prevent the flow of aqueous fluid through it. Pressure then builds up behind the iris, causing it to bow forwards into the anterior chamber. (This is sometimes called 'iris bombé'.)

Secondary glaucoma is probably the most common cause of permanent visual loss and blindness in patients with iridocyclitis. For this reason, it is important to check carefully the intraocular pressure of any patient with iridocyclitis.

2. Lowering of the intraocular pressure (hypotony) is much less common. It is caused by damage to the ciliary processes which lowers the production of aqueous fluid. Severe hypotony may cause the whole eye to shrink. This is called 'phthisis bulbi'.

3. Cataracts may form, probably because the intraocular inflammation upsets the metabolism of the lens (*Plate* 14b). If the damage is confined to the lens, the cataract should be removed to restore the sight when the inflammation has subsided.

4. Iris atrophy may follow inflammation. The iris becomes thin and depigmented.
5. Band degeneration of the cornea (*see Plate* 10f) is a thin, opaque calcific deposit under the corneal epithelium. It sometimes occurs in chronic iridocyclitis.

Choroiditis

The main symptom of choroiditis is visual loss. This is because any disease of the choroid will always affect the overlying retina. The pattern of visual loss depends on which part of the choroid is affected.
– Choroiditis at or near the macula will cause loss of visual acuity.
– Choroiditis near the optic disc will usually damage the optic nerve fibres, and cause considerable visual loss.
– Choroiditis in the periphery of the choroid may cause very little visual loss in itself. However, inflammatory cells and debris are usually released into the vitreous, and this may cause some blurring of vision.
   Choroiditis is not usually very painful, but a severe attack often causes some discomfort behind the eye.
   It is necessary to dilate the pupil and use an ophthalmoscope to detect the signs of choroiditis. (Debris and cells in the vitreous may blur the fundus details.)
– Areas where the choroid is inflamed become swollen, and there is oedema of the overlying retina (*Plate* 14c).
– After the inflammation has subsided, a characteristic localized scar remains, showing areas both of pigment atrophy and pigment hypertrophy (*Plate* 14d *and* c).
   As the disease resolves, the vision usually improves. However, there will always be a permanent defect in the vision corresponding to the area of the choroidal scar.

Causes of uveitis

There are many possible causes of uveitis. However, in many patients no specific cause can be detected, even after thorough investigations. When laboratory services are not available, it is difficult to find a specific cause in most cases. The known causes of uveitis can be divided into two general groups: infective and non-infective causes.

Infective causes

Many types of organism can infect the uvea.
– Leprosy is an important cause of both acute and chronic iridocyclitis (*see* Chapter 16).
– Tuberculosis is not a common cause of uveitis, but it is much more likely to occur in poor communities. Patients with acute miliary tuberculosis often have small choroidal tubercules, which are visible on fundus examination (*Plate* 14f). These tubercules may be very important in confirming the diagnosis.

Chronic tuberculosis may involve any part of the uvea, and usually presents as a mass with an inflammatory reaction around it. There are 'mutton fat' keratic precipitates in the anterior chamber, and vitreous opacities in the posterior chamber. If the disease is not treated, it may eventually spread to involve the whole eye.

– Syphilis may produce various inflammatory changes in the uvea.

There may be a generalized or localized iridocyclitis or choroiditis. The scars of previous attacks may be visible as iris or choroidal atrophy (*Plate* 14d). Rarely, a localized inflammatory mass called a gumma may be present in the uvea.

(The incidence of leprosy, tuberculosis and syphilis in the community varies greatly from area to area, so the possibility of uveitis from any of these causes will also vary. All three are chronic and progressive diseases which affect other parts of the body also. They are also all three treatable. If a patient has uveitis, especially chronic uveitis, it is very important to take a careful history, and give a general examination to look for signs of leprosy, tuberculosis or syphilis. A routine chest X-ray will help to detect pulmonary tuberculosis, and a blood serology test will help to detect syphilis.)

– Acute bacterial infections of the uvea are not common. The bacteria usually reach the eye after a penetrating injury, or after an intraocular operation. Very occasionally, in cases of septicaemia, the bacteria may enter from the bloodstream. Unfortunately, bacteria multiply very easily in the aqueous and the vitreous and very soon convert the eye into a bag of pus. Systemic and local antibiotic treatment should be given, but it is nearly always too late to save the eye.

– Toxoplasmosis (*Plate* 14c *and* e) is a common cause of choroiditis. It is caused by a common protozoan parasite, which is present in many people. In most cases, the infection is too mild to produce any specific pathological changes at all. However, it is often more severe in newborn babies, who have become infected across the placenta. The organism infects various tissues including the choroid and the overlying retina around the macula and optic disc. When the inflammation subsides, there are characteristic, well-defined areas of choroidoretinal scarring. Some years later, the disease may become active again, often at the edge of a scar from a previous infection. Some rather complicated serological tests are necessary to confirm the diagnosis.

The causative organism is probably sensitive to the anti-malarial drug, pyrimethamine, sulphonamides and the antibiotic clindamycin. Unfortunately, the recommended dose of pyrimethamine (25 mg twice daily) is very toxic to the bone marrow, and clindamycin is toxic to the bowel. These drugs should only be given in very severe cases where the macular vision is threatened, and when it is possible to observe the patient daily in hospital. Like any other type of inflammatory choroiditis, steroid treatment should also be used.

– Onchocerciasis is the most important parasitic worm to cause uveitis (*see* Chapter 15).

– Toxocara is a parasitic nematode worm which is found in domestic animals such as cats and dogs. It is now known to be a significant cause of uveitis or an inflammatory choroidal mass. Young children swallow the eggs, which may then hatch and enter the bloodstream as larvae. The larvae may then

lodge in the choroid and form an inflammatory mass.
- Numerous other parasitic worms whose larvae travel in the bloodstream may rarely cause an inflammatory mass in the uvea.

Non-infective causes of uveitis

In most cases of uveitis, no infective cause can be found. Recent research has shown that people with certain tissue antigens (called 'human leucocyte antigens', or HLA) have a greatly increased risk of developing uveitis. These antigens are hereditary, and this explains why some types of uveitis are common in some communities and uncommon in others.
- Acute recurrent iridocyclitis occurs in people with the B27 antigen. It is often associated with ankylosing spondylitis of the spinal column.
- Behçet's disease is an acute iritis, often with hypopyon, and mouth and genital ulcers. The disease is also associated with certain HLA antigens, and is found especially in the Eastern Mediterranean.

Two other non-infective causes of uveitis are sarcoidosis and sympathetic ophthalmitis: –
- Sarcoidosis is a generalized disease similar to tuberculosis, but without any evidence of infection by micro-organisms. It causes a chronic granulomatous uveitis in the eye.
- Sympathetic ophthalmitis is a rare condition which may occur weeks or even months after a penetrating injury to one eye. The other eye develops a granulomatous uveitis, probably because the body has a hypersensitivity reaction to its own uveal proteins.

Uveitis often occurs following other eye disorders. (These are described in other sections of the book.) Examples are: –
1. Following a virus infection of the cornea, such as herpes simplex keratitis.
2. Following a leakage of lens proteins out of the lens capsule.
3. Following a long-standing retinal detachment.
4. Following intraocular surgery or trauma to the eye.

The treatment of uveitis

The basic treatment for all types of uveitis is corticosteroids.
- Iridocyclitis can be treated locally. Acute iridocyclitis will need steroid drops every hour until the inflammation begins to subside. Alternatively, a subconjunctival steroid injection may be given. For chronic iridocyclitis, steroid drops or ointment should be given 3 or 4 times a day.
- Choroiditis must be treated systemically. This is because local steroid treatment cannot effectively reach the choroid. The basic maintenance dose of systemic steroids is 20 mg of predisone a day, but higher doses may be necessary for a few days in severe cases. Systemic steroid treatment has many possible side effects, so these patients need careful supervision. It is especially important to use systemic steroids very carefully if there is any underlying infection, such as tuberculosis.

Mydriatics should be given to all cases of iridocyclitis to rest the inflamed iris and ciliary body, and to prevent the iris adhering to the lens. Atropine drops 1% once a day are usually effective.

If secondary glaucoma develops, full doses of acetazolamide should be given orally. In the case of pupil block glaucoma (or iris bombé), mydriatic drops may be able to break the ring of adhesions between the iris and the lens. Otherwise an iridectomy operation is necessary.

Other diseases of the uvea

Tumours

Tumours of the uvea are fairly rare.
— Melanomas are the most common form of tumour, but they are very rare in blacks. They usually arise in the choroid, but occasionally in the iris or ciliary body. A melanoma presents in adults as a single solid dark mass in the eye. If it is a choroidal melanoma, it often causes retinal detachment and sometimes glaucoma. The tumour, especially if it is an anaplastic tumour, may also spread to other parts of the body, usually the liver. In the early stages, it may be possible to treat the tumour with radiation therapy, or to excise small tumours of the iris and ciliary body surgically. Unfortunately, in most cases the only treatment is to enucleate the eye.
— Primary tumours from other parts of the body (e.g. carcinoma of the breast) occasionally spread to the uvea.

Degenerative changes

Degeneration and atrophy of the uvea is common. It may occur after uveitis or glaucoma, or it may be part of the ageing process. There are also various rare primary degenerations of the uvea which are usually hereditary.
— Atrophy of the iris affects both the pigment and the muscle cells. The iris appears depigmented, and the pupil is often dilated, irregular and will not react to light.
— Atrophy of the ciliary body may occur. The aqueous secretion will decrease and the eye becomes soft.
— Atrophy of the choroid is especially common in old people, and usually involves the posterior part of the choroid around the macula. Choroidal atrophy also occurs after choroiditis (*Plate* 14e) and onchocerciasis (*see Plate* 22a *and* b). The exact pattern of the choroidal atrophy will vary, but there are usually two features: —
1. Pigment changes. There is atrophy of the choroidal pigment, but sometimes patches of increased pigmentation. The retinal pigment epithelium may also be affected.
2. Blood vessel changes. The fine choroidal blood vessels (called the 'choriocapillaris') atrophy to show the outline of the larger choroidal blood vessels.

11. Diseases of the Lens

The structure and function of the lens are described in Chapter 2. The lens is a unique structure for many reasons: –
– It is transparent, and has no blood or nerve supply.
– It has a higher protein content than any other body tissue.
– It continues to grow throughout life. New fibres form just beneath the capsule, while the older fibres are compressed towards the centre of the lens. A hard nucleus therefore develops with a slightly softer cortex around it.

Various degenerative and ageing changes occur in the lens, probably because of its unusual structure: –
– The lens becomes harder with age, and so has greater difficulty focusing on near objects. This is called 'presbyopia' (*see* page 50).
– The lens becomes more dense, and this may change its refractive power. If the central nucleus becomes more dense (as in nuclear sclerosis), the power of the lens increases and the eye becomes shortsighted. If the outer cortex becomes more dense, the power of the lens decreases and the eye becomes longsighted.
– The lens becomes larger. It may grow so large that the anterior chamber becomes shallow, and acute glaucoma develops.
– The lens becomes more opaque. This is called 'cataract', and is the most important of these ageing changes.

Cataract

Cataract means that the lens becomes opaque, but in the early stages this does not mean that the eye is blind. In fact, most old people have slight opacities in the lens which cause little or no loss of vision at first. Such cataracts are called 'early' (or 'immature') cataracts. As the opacity progresses, however, the vision becomes increasingly blurred. When eventually the lens becomes totally opaque, the eye does go blind, and this is called a 'mature' cataract.

The progression of lens opacities varies very much. Sometimes a patient develops a mature cataract only a few months after the first signs of opacity in the lens. On the other hand, early opacities may be present in the lens for many years with no obvious progression at all. However, if an opacity has formed, it does not normally disappear spontaneously.

Causes of cataract

– Ageing changes in the lens are by far the most common cause of cataract.
– Congenital cataracts may be present at birth.

- Eye injuries often cause cataracts. A perforating injury which damages or even touches the lens will cause a localized opacity at the point of contact. This may then spread to involve the whole lens. A non-penetrating injury may also produce a cataract after a delay of some months, or even years.
- Diabetes seems to be a predisposing factor. Diabetics develop cataracts more often, and at a younger age than non-diabetics.
- Secondary cataracts may develop after almost any other intraocular disease, especially uveitis.
- Corticosteroid drugs used over a long period of time (either locally or systemically) may also cause cataracts.
- Exposure to certain types of radiation sometimes causes cataracts. For example, people working near furnaces may develop cataracts from infra-red radiation. Patients who have received radiotherapy may develop cataracts from X-rays.
- Hypoparathyroidism, Down's syndrome and myotonic dystrophy are rare diseases which are associated with cataracts.

The incidence of cataract

Cataract is a very common disease in all communities, especially in old people. It is always one of the major causes of blindness, and is by far the most common treatable cause. Cataracts seem to be more common and occur at an earlier age in hot countries. The reason for this is uncertain, but there are two possible explanations: –
- Solar and heat radiation. It seems that desert areas, where the summer temperatures are very high and where there is a lot of sunlight have a higher incidence of cataract than tropical rain forests where the heat and sunlight are less. (The wearing of wide-brimmed hats to shield the sun may possibly reduce the incidence of cataract.)
- Dehydration. It is possible that the severe dehydration which occurs during attacks of fever or gastroenteritis may increase the incidence of cataracts.
  There is no definite evidence of any racial susceptibility to cataract.
  The actual number of people who are blind from cataract will also depend on how effective the medical services are in providing treatment. In most rural areas, the incidence of blindness from cataract is quite high (0.2 – 0.5%) and in some places it can be more than 1% of the whole population.

The symptoms of cataract

The main symptom of a lens opacity is a gradual and progressive loss of visual acuity. Eventually, when the cataract is mature, there is only perception of light. In the early stages, however, there may also be other visual symptoms: –
- Dazzling occurs especially when the opacity is mainly in the centre of the lens. In bright light, the pupil constricts and the vision deteriorates. In dim light, the pupil dilates, light enters the eye around the opaque part of the lens, and the vision improves. Dazzling also occurs because the lens opacities scatter the light which enters the eye.
- Refractive changes have already been described.
- Multiple images (ghosting, or polyopia) are caused by poor refraction by the

lens. The patient therefore sees one or more blurred 'ghost' images along with the true image.
- Rainbow-coloured rings (or haloes) around white lights are caused because the light is split into the colours of the spectrum. (Haloes are also a symptom of corneal oedema.)

The signs of cataract

It is necessary to test the pupil light reflexes, then dilate the pupil to examine the lens. Three different types of illumination can be used, and each will give the normal healthy lens a different appearance. These are illustrated in *Plate* 1.
- With diffuse illumination, the normal lens looks black, just as the window of a house looks black when looking into the house from outside. However, some of the light entering the eye is reflected from the lens, especially from its front surface. These reflections from the normal lens are just visible in diffuse illumination (*see Plate* 1a).
- With focal illumination (e.g. a slit lamp), these reflections from the normal lens are much more obvious (*see Plate* 1b).
- With coaxial illumination, using an ophthalmoscope with a + 10 dioptre lens and held a few inches from the patient's eye, the normal transparent lens cannot be seen. Only a clear red reflex from the fundus is seen, without any shadows or distortion (*see Plate* 1c).

Lens opacities develop in different parts of the lens, and their appearance may vary considerably. They also appear different with different types of illumination. Plate 15a *and* b show 8 different cataractous lenses removed from patients' eyes. In *Plate* 15a, they are illuminated from the front, and in *Plate* 15b from behind. Some are mature cataracts, and some are immature. Note how the appearance varies from lens to lens, and also with different illumination.

Recognizing and correctly assessing a lens opacity is very important and should be fairly easy. However, mistakes are often made if a proper examination is not carried out. The pupil should be dilated, and besides looking at the eye externally, the red reflex with an ophthalmoscope should also be observed.

There are three common sites where lens opacities begin: in the lens cortex, the lens nucleus or just inside the posterior lens capsule. These are shown diagrammatically in *Fig.* 11.1. In the early stages, each of these different types of opacity will have a different appearance. Eventually, the entire lens becomes completely opaque and appears as a white opaque mass.

1. Cortical lens opacities are the most common type of cataract. The opacities develop in the outer (or cortical) layers of the lens, and they appear white against the normally dark pupil. *Plate* 15c – e show an eye with typical early cortical lens opacities. At this stage, the patient could still see fairly well.
- With normal diffuse illumination, the white opaque parts of the cortex are visible (*Plate* 15c).
- With focal illumination, the white opaque parts are more obvious (*Plate* 15d).
- With coaxial illumination from an ophthalmoscope, the red reflex is clearly visible. However, the early lens opacities cause some dark areas in the reflex (*Plate* 15e).

Plate 15f shows a more dense cortical lens opacity seen with diffuse illumination. However, with coaxial illumination (*Plate* 16a) some red reflex is

Common types of lens opacity

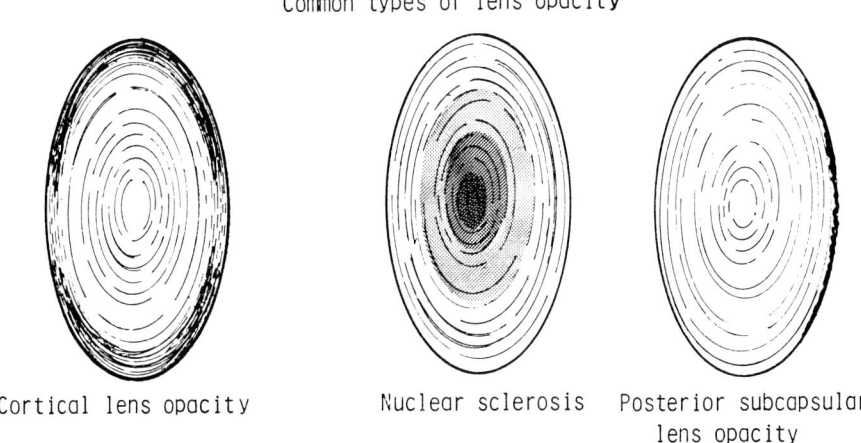

Cortical lens opacity   Nuclear sclerosis   Posterior subcapsular
                                                        lens opacity

Fig. 11.1 A diagram to show the common types of lens opacity.

still present, so the patient still has useful sight. He could see 6/60. Gradually, the lens becomes more opaque. Finally it looks like a solid, white, opaque mass in the pupil (*Plate* 16b). This is the usual appearance of a mature cataract, and the eye is blind at this stage.

2. Nuclear sclerosis means that the nucleus of the lens hardens. At the same time, it becomes darker in colour — first yellow, then brown, and finally black. If the lens cortex has gone white and opaque, these nuclear changes are not visible. Sometimes, however, there are changes in the nucleus, but the cortex remains transparent. *Plate* 16c – e show a lens with early nuclear sclerosis.
  — With diffuse illumination, the dark pupil has a slight yellow appearance (*Plate* 16c).
  — With focal illumination (e.g. a slit lamp), this yellow discoloration of the lens nucleus shows up much more clearly (*Plate* 16d).
  — With coaxial illumination from an ophthalmoscope, the red reflex shows only a slight haze. This means that the cataract is not yet causing too much loss of vision (*Plate* 16e).

Just occasionally, nuclear sclerosis progresses so that the whole lens goes black and opaque (*Plate* 16f). These 'black' cataracts are rather unusual, and are often not diagnosed because of course the pupil also appears black in a normal eye. However, with coaxial illumination, no red reflex is visible.

3. Posterior subcapsular lens opacities are less common. A thin, opaque layer develops just inside the posterior capsule of the lens. Because this opacity is so far back in the lens, it is difficult to see with normal illumination. With the coaxial illumination of an ophthalmoscope, however, the opacity stands out as a grey shadow against the red reflex.

There are other patterns of lens opacity, especially in congenital cataracts, but these are unusual.

Retinal and optic nerve diseases may also be present in the eye as well as cataract. It may be difficult to assess how much of the patient's visual loss is from cataract, and how much from other eye diseases. The following tests may be helpful: –

– Visual acuity. Generally speaking, if any red reflex at all is visible, the patient's vision should be 'counting fingers' or better. Therefore if some red reflex is visible, and the patient's vision is worse than counting fingers, some other eye disease is probably also present.
– The pupil light reflex. A brisk pupil light reflex is a good indication of a healthy retina and optic nerve. However it may be difficult to observe the pupil constriction if there are adhesions between the iris and the lens (posterior synechiae).
– The projection of light. Even a mature cataract will allow some light to reach the retina. The patient should therefore be able to detect the direction the light is coming from. Poor projection of light indicates a retinal or optic nerve disorder.

Complications of cataract

Further degenerative changes may occur in the cataractous lens which can cause other complications in the eye.

1. Sometimes the fibres of the suspensory ligament degenerate, so that a cataractous lens subluxates or dislocates (*see below*).
2. Occasionally, the death and degeneration of lens cells causes the lens cortex to liquefy. The degenerate fluid proteins in the lens capsule absorb even more fluid by osmosis and make the lens swell. This is called a 'hypermature' (or 'intumescent') cataract. Sometimes the solid brown nucleus can be seen inside the milky-white fluid cortex (*Plate* 17a).

– A lens which is swollen in this way becomes larger, and makes the anterior chamber of the eye more shallow. This may provoke angle closure glaucoma.
– Sometimes the fluid lens protein leaks out through the capsule into the anterior chamber. This causes inflammation in the eye and acute uveitis. It is called 'phakolytic uveitis'. The aqueous fluid appears milky because of the leaking lens protein. The treatment is to remove the lens as soon as possible, and to give local steroids. If not treated all the fluid lens proteins are either absorbed or leak out through the lens capsule. All that remains is a small, solid brown nucleus inside a shrivelled capsule. However, by this time, uveitis or glaucoma have usually caused extensive damage to the eye.

Congenital cataract

Congenital cataract is not common, but it is still the most important congenital disorder of the eye. In many cases, it is not possible to discover a specific cause. However, the following are known to cause congenital cataract: –

– Infections of the fetus, especially German measles early in the pregnancy. (German measles may also cause chorioretinitis, deafness and heart defects.)
– Anoxia or trauma to the fetus at birth.
– Congenital cataract is sometimes a genetic disorder, and it may be associated with rare metabolic diseases.

   In severe cases, a congenital cataract may involve the whole lens, producing a dense white opacity. In milder cases, only a certain layer of lens fibres may go opaque. This is called a 'lamellar' cataract. Sometimes the opacity may be confined to the anterior or posterior pole of the lens. These incomplete congenital lens opacities often remain static throughout life.

- If the child has mature congenital cataracts in both eyes, it is best to give surgical treatment as soon as possible.
- If the opacity is incomplete and some red reflex is visible, any treatment should be delayed until the child is old enough to have the vision tested. Mydriatic drops or an optical iridectomy may improve the vision of children with lens opacities localized to the centre of the lens.
- If the cataract is in one eye only, there will nearly always be amblyopia in that eye (*see* page 201). Therefore surgical treatment will not usually improve the vision significantly.

The treatment of cataract

Numerous drops are available which claim either to stop or reverse the formation of cataract, but there is no evidence that any of them work. There is, however some unconfirmed evidence that taking very small doses of aspirin regularly may slow down the progress of cataract.

In the early stages of cataract, it is sometimes possible to improve the vision significantly either with spectacles or by dilating the pupil. However, the basic treatment for cataract is surgical removal of the lens. Modern cataract surgery is a safe and straightforward operation with very few complications.

Many people believe that a cataract should be mature (or 'ripe') before it is removed, but this is not always true. In fact, the correct time for cataract removal is when the loss of vision has become a significant handicap to the patient. Obviously, people have different visual requirements. A middle-aged professional man is likely to need cataract removal at an earlier stage than an old and illiterate villager.

The lens of the eye is a strong convex lens. After a cataract extraction, therefore, the vision is very blurred (less than 6/60) because the eye is out of focus. There are three types of lens which can restore the focus of the lens to normal: —

- A pair of spectacles with a strong convex lens of about + 10 dioptres will give very good visual acuity. Unfortunately, there is some distortion of objects and difficulty in judging distances which some patients find very confusing at first. Another difficulty is that a strong spectacle lens magnifies so that everything appears one-third larger than normal. This does not matter if the patient has had a cataract removed from both eyes. However, if one eye is normal and one eye has had a cataract removed, the images from both eyes will be different sizes. Such a patient will not be able to get binocular vision with a pair of spectacles.
- A contact lens which rests on the cornea causes very little magnification or distortion. It therefore restores the vision to normal. It also means that the patient can have binocular vision if one eye has had a cataract removed, and the other eye is normal. Unfortunately, contact lenses are expensive, and require expert fitting. Many patients, especially if they are old, have difficulty wearing them. Contact lenses cannot therefore be recommended as a general treatment.

– An artificial plastic lens can be implanted in the eye. This too causes no
  magnification or distortion, and so allows binocular vision. However, lens
  implants are very expensive and need a very high level of surgical skill and
  postoperative care. Therefore lens implants also cannot be recommended as a
  general treatment.

Because it is so difficult to restore binocular vision, some people do not
recommend removing a cataract from one eye if the other eye is normal.
However, there is always the risk that a cataract may become hypermature and
permanently damage the eye. This means that it is usually worth while removing a
mature cataract from one eye, when the other eye is normal.

Cataract extraction is the most common of all eye operations, and the general
principles of intraocular surgery are explained in Chapter 4 (*see* pages 44-47).
There are two different ways of removing the lens, intracapsular and
extracapsular extraction (*Fig.* 11.2.) In both cases, it is usual to enter the eye
through an incision at the limbus of just less than 180°, often under the

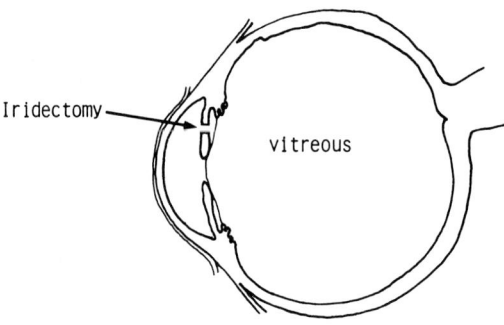

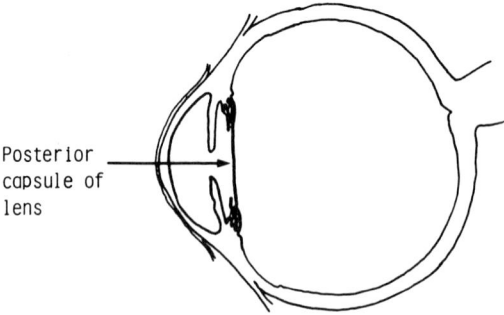

Fig. 11.2 A diagram of the eye after intracapsular and extracapsular cataract extraction.

protection of a flap of conjunctiva. It is then necessary to excise a small segment of the iris, remove the lens, and close the wound with interrupted or continuous sutures.

- In an intracapsular extraction, the entire lens is removed. A small pair of forceps may be used to grasp the capsule of the lens, or else a cryoprobe will adhere to the lens by forming a solid iceball. One common complication of an intracapsular extraction is that the capsule may rupture. Another complication is that some of the vitreous jelly may come out through the wound as well as the lens. Intracapsular extractions are usually only done for old patients.

- In an extracapsular extraction, the posterior capsule and suspensory ligament are left intact. The technique is to incise the anterior capsule with a knife or needle, and express the nucleus of the lens from the eye. A two-way irrigating syringe is then used to remove as much as possible of the rest of the lens matter. The main complication of an extracapsular extraction is that the capsule becomes a thick opaque membrane, so that the patient still cannot see clearly. If any cortical lens matter is left in the eye, this will cause postoperative iridocyclitis. Until recently, extracapsular extractions were only done for young patients. However, modern microsurgical techniques have improved the results of extracapsular extraction. Where suitable facilities are available, extracapsular extraction is now becoming more popular for old patients also.

It is usual to apply a mixture of antibiotics, steroids and mydriatics locally to the eye for about 2 − 4 weeks after the operation. By then the wound should have healed and the eye should be quiet. The complications which may follow any intraocular operation are mentioned in Chapter 4 (page 46). Two complications which occur after about 1% − 5% of cataract operations are retinal detachment and cystoid macular oedema. They may occur some months after the operation.

- Retinal detachment is more likely to occur if there has been any loss of the vitreous at the time of the operation, or if the patient is myopic. Extracapsular extraction reduces the risk of retinal detachment.

- Cystoid macular oedema causes oedema and cystic changes in the macula, so that the patient complains of a loss of visual acuity. The causes of cystoid macular oedema are not clear, and there is no specific treatment. However, it is probable that extracapsular extraction reduces the risk.

An eye which has had the lens removed is called an 'aphakic' eye (*Plate* 17b). It has the following features: −

- The aphakic eye is normally very long sighted, and needs a spectacle lens of about 10 dioptres for normal distance vision.
- The anterior chamber is very deep.
- The pupil appears very black because there is no lens to reflect any of the incident light. (After extracapsular extraction some lens remnants may be seen.)
- The iris often wobbles when the eye moves because there is no lens to support it. This is called 'iridodonesis'.
- The iridectomy, which is the piece of iris removed by the surgeon, is usually visible. Sometimes this involves the complete iris sphincter, so the pupil is U-shaped and not round.

Couching of cataracts

Couching has been the traditional treatment of cataract for thousands of years, and was the only method until the arrival of modern cataract surgery. The coucher inserts a needle or thorn into the eye either at the limbus, or a few millimetres behind it. This ruptures the suspensory ligament and pushes the lens back down into the vitreous. Couching probably originated in India and is still quite common in some isolated rural areas of North and Central Africa and Asia where there are no medical services. Most couchers are uneducated, and travel from village to village, performing a few operations and then moving on.

An eye often looks fairly normal after a couching operation. However, a closer examination will reveal the entry point of the needle (*Plate* 17c). It will also show that the lens, or fragments of the lens, are lying in the lower vitreous (*Plate* 17d). For the first few days after a couching operation, the patient may see quite well. Unfortunately, complications often develop. The most common of these are: –
– Intraocular infection (because many couchers do not sterilize their instruments).
– Uveitis (from rupture of the lens and release of lens matter into the eye).
– Secondary glaucoma.

The results of couching obviously vary according to the skill of the coucher. At best, however, couching will only satisfactorily restore the vision of about one half of the patients, and even these require spectacles.

Other diseases of the lens

The only other important disorder of the lens is caused by rupture of the suspensory ligament. If the rupture is partial, it is called 'subluxation'. If it is total, it is called 'dislocation'.
– Subluxation means that only some of the fibres rupture, so that the lens only shifts slightly from the central axis of the eye. However, the eye becomes astigmatic and myopic, and this is the main symptom of subluxation. It can be quite difficult to detect subluxation, but if the pupil is dilated, it is possible to see the edge of the eccentric lens (*Plate* 17e).
– Dislocation means that all the fibres rupture. The lens nearly always sinks to the lower part of the vitreous where it can be seen with an ophthalmoscope. The cause may be an injury to the eye, or it may be a congenital weakness of the suspensory ligament. Hypermature cataracts also increase the risk of dislocation. An eye with a dislocated lens appears just like an aphakic eye, and needs a strong convex lens to restore the vision.

12. Diseases of the Retina

The structure and function of the retina are described in Chapter 2.

The retina has a very active metabolism. The retinal blood vessels themselves only supply the inner layers with oxygen. The outer layers of the retina obtain their oxygen by diffusion from the blood vessels of the choroid. This means that diseases of the choroid will also affect the retina.

The retina is in fact a part of the central nervous system, and it therefore reacts to injury and disease very like the central nervous system.

- There are no pain fibres, and so the only symptom of retinal disease is visual loss.
- The nerve cells themselves cannot regenerate. (Only the supportive glial cells can.) Any visual loss from retinal cell death is therefore permanent. However, there seems to be a certain amount of reserve function. If only small areas of the retina are damaged or destroyed, there may be no apparent loss of vision.

Retinal diseases are quite common, and a healthy retina is obviously essential for good vision. However, the retina is protected from the environment, and is less susceptible to tropical diseases than many other parts of the eye. Also, many retinal diseases are either unpreventable or untreatable. Therefore, diseases of the retina are not a major concern for most tropical areas.

There are three main groups of retinal disease: –
- Vascular retinopathies (from diseases of the blood or blood vessels).
- Retinal and chorioretinal degenerations.
- Retinal detachments.

Vascular retinopathies

The retina, like the rest of the nervous system, has a high oxygen requirement. Any shortage of oxygen (anoxia) from diseases of the blood vessels will therefore damage the retina. The retinal capillaries are similar to the capillaries of the brain, and are less permeable than in the rest of the body. If protein exudate leaks through diseased capillary walls, it can very easily damage the retina. This is why diseases of the blood and circulation frequently cause complications in the retina. One of the best ways to examine the blood vessels and the circulation is to look into the eye with a direct ophthalmoscope. This gives an image of the retina and its blood vessels about 15 times larger than its actual size.

Like all blood vessel disorders, vascular retinopathies mainly occur in old people. They are also often associated with obesity, and are therefore less common in poor rural communities.

On examining the fundus, the retinal blood vessels will appear abnormal and there may also be haemorrhages and exudates in the retina itself. Most of these changes occur around the optic disc and macula. Some ophthalmoscopes have a green filter in them. This is very useful because it makes the retinal blood vessels much more obvious.

The most common retinopathies are: –
– Hypertensive retinopathy
– Retinal vessel occlusions
– Diabetic retinopathy
– Sickle-cell retinopathy

If possible, the blood pressure should be measured and the urine tested for albumin and sugar. These are two simple screening tests for hypertension and diabetes.

Hypertensive retinopathy

In mild hypertension, the abnormalities are only in the retinal vessels themselves. The walls of the arteries thicken. This causes them to reflect more light from their surfaces, and is called 'silver' or 'copper' wiring. However, the column of blood in the arteries may appear more narrow. The thickened arterial walls also cause kinking and nipping of the thin-walled veins at places where the arteries and veins cross (*Plate* 18e).

More severe hypertension causes damage to the retinal cells, and leakage of protein from the blood vessels (*Plate* 18a). Some or all of the following changes may be seen: –
– Soft (or 'cottonwool') exudates are white patches, usually near the optic disc. These consist of dead or damaged nerve fibres, which are caused in turn by damage to the small arterioles supplying the nerve fibre layer. After a few weeks, soft exudates gradually disappear.
– Hard exudates are denser yellow masses which are often found around the macula. They consist of lipid material which is formed from the products of dying cells and exudates from the blood vessels. This lipid material is contained in the macrophages where it may remain for many months, or even years.
– Flame-shaped haemorrhages may occur, especially from the capillaries and small arterioles in the nerve fibre layer. Occasionally, a haemorrhage spreads into the vitreous body.

In severe hypertension, there is also swelling around the margin of the optic disc. This is called 'papilloedema' (*Plate* 18a).

Hypertension often causes obvious changes in the appearance of the retina, but surprisingly little loss of vision. However, some of the complications of hypertension, especially retinal vessel occlusions, will cause severe visual loss.

Retinal vessel occlusions

Retinal vessel occlusions occur in either the arteries or the veins. A central occlusion involves the whole artery or vein, while a branch occlusion involves only a branch vessel. Sometimes the occlusion is partial, so that there is only partial obstruction of the blood flow.

– Retinal artery occlusions occur mainly in old people with hypertension or atherosclerosis (*Plate* 18b *and* 18c). The most common cause is an atheromatous plaque at the origin of the internal carotid artery. This causes small emboli to pass up and impact in the retinal vessels. Most retinal artery occlusions cause a sudden and severe loss of vision. If it is a central occlusion, there will be total loss of vision. If it is a branch occlusion, only a segment of the vision will be lost. The visual loss is usually permanent, but occasionally an embolus may break up and pass on, so that the loss of vision is only temporary.

A retinal artery occlusion causes the vessels to become thin — sometimes so thin that they cannot be seen through the ophthalmoscope. The part of the retina which the arteries supply becomes white and oedematous. Later, hard white exudates appear in the retina, and the affected vessels appear as thin fibrotic white streaks.

– Retinal vein occlusions (*Plate* 18d) are also associated with hypertension and atherosclerosis. Occasionally, however, they occur in otherwise healthy young people. Very rarely, an increase in the blood viscosity causes a retinal vein occlusion. The symptoms of a retinal vein occlusion are usually less severe than an artery occlusion. The visual loss is more gradual, and is not complete. There may also be some gradual, partial recovery of vision later. The retinal veins become dilated, often with extensive haemorrhages and exudates.

Thrombotic glaucoma is a serious complication which may occur after a central vein occlusion. Shortage of oxygen in the retina somehow stimulates the growth of new blood vessels on the surface of the iris and in the angle of the anterior chamber. This causes a severe type of glaucoma and eventually a painful blind eye.

Diabetic retinopathy (*Plate* 18e *and* 18f)

Abnormal changes in the retina are a common feature of diabetes. It may be many years before these changes eventually appear. On the other hand, people who become diabetic in old age may develop abnormal retinal changes very early in the course of the disease. It is therefore advisable to examine the retina of anyone with diabetes every year.

Diabetes first affects the retinal capillaries. The capillaries may become closed off leading to areas of retinal anoxia. Sometimes the capillary wall may give way to form dilatations known as 'microaneurysms', and these may bleed. The microaneurysms themselves are usually too small to be visible. However, the haemorrhages from them which occur in the deeper layers of the stroma are small and round. They are sometimes called 'dot and blot' haemorrhages. Hard exudates also develop because of lipid degeneration in the anoxic retina. The appearance of these haemorrhages and exudates scattered over the posterior part of the fundus is called 'background diabetic retinopathy', (*Plate* 18e). In itself, background diabetic retinopathy does not usually produce much visual loss. However, there are three common complications which may cause serious visual damage: –

– In diabetic maculopathy, the haemorrhages and exudates occur at the macula, and so cause a loss of visual acuity.
– In proliferative retinopathy (*Plate* 18f), new blood vessels grow (or

proliferate) on the surface of the retina. They are found particularly growing from the optic disc and also along the branches of the retinal vessels. They are narrow and not very easy to see in the early stages. They can be seen much more easily with a green filter in the ophthalmoscope. These new blood vessels probably develop and grow in response to retinal anoxia, caused by the capillaries closing off. Unfortunately, fibrous tissue and glial tissue are also formed along with the blood vessels. Later, when the fibrous tissue contracts, it causes the retina to detach. Eventually, proliferative retinopathy progresses to irreversible blindness.
- Diabetic vitreous haemorrhages are caused when the new retinal vessels formed in proliferative retinopathy bleed into the vitreous. These new vessels are fragile, and easily bleed. They often cause recurrent and increasingly severe vitreous haemorrhages. Diabetic vitreous haemorrhages often progress to irreversible blindness.

Sickle-cell retinopathy

Sickle-cell disease is a disorder of the haemoglobin which causes the red blood cells to become sickle-shaped. The disease is hereditary, and is found in blacks.

Normal haemoglobin is called haemoglobin A. A child whose parents are both haemoglobin A will therefore be genetically AA. Sickle haemoglobin is called 'haemoglobin S', and a child whose parents are both haemoglobin S will be genetically SS. If only one parent has sickle haemoglobin, the child will be genetically AS. This is called the 'carrier state'.

Patients with sickle-cell disease are genetically SS, and all their haemoglobin is abnormal. If the oxygen concentration is low, the red blood cells become sickle shaped. Sickle cells are easily destroyed, causing anaemia. They also cannot flow properly through small blood vessels, causing anoxia and infarction in the tissues. Many children with sickle-cell disease die young. Those that survive often have widespread defects in the body.

Patients who are carriers have no symptoms at all, but may pass on the disease. It seems that the carrier state (AS) gives some resistance to malaria. This would explain why sickle-cell disease has persisted to such an extent in the community.

Two other genetic disorders of the haemoglobin are sometimes found together with sickle haemoglobin: –
- Haemoglobin C is a much milder abnormality than haemoglobin S, and is also found in blacks. Patients whose haemoglobin is half S and half C (genetically SC) are especially prone to eye complications.
- Thalassaemia is another hereditary disorder of the haemoglobin. It occurs mainly in people from the Mediterranean, North Africa and East Asia. Patients who are carriers of both sickle-cell disease and thalassaemia also have quite a high incidence of eye complications.

The most important eye changes in sickle-cell disease occur in the peripheral retina. To detect the changes it is therefore necessary to dilate the pupil. Small peripheral retinal arterioles may become blocked. This causes anoxia of the retina, which in turn stimulates the growth of new blood vessels. These vessels often grow into the vitreous body in the shape of a 'sea-fan' (*Plate* 19a). There may also be patches of increased pigmentation in the peripheral retina. Because all these changes occur in the periphery, which has no visual function, there are

no specific symptoms. Certain complications may, however, cause some loss of vision: –
- The new vessels may bleed, causing a vitreous haemorrhage.
- The new vessels may stimulate the formation of fibrous and glial tissue. When fibrous tissue contracts, it causes the retina to detach.
- Occasionally, a choroidal or posterior ciliary vessel may become occluded. This will produce an area of choroidoretinal ischaemia and later atrophy, which will in turn produce a visual field defect.

Surprisingly, the incidence of retinopathy is highest in people who are genetically SC, less common in people who are S thalassaemia, and least common in SS patients. The reason for this may be that SS patients have the worst general symptoms, and are the most anaemic. Anaemia lowers the blood viscosity, and so prevents vascular occlusions in the retina. Sickle-cell retinopathy is sometimes seen in quite young children, but may regress spontaneously.

A blood test called 'haemoglobin electrophoresis' will confirm the diagnosis of sickle-cell disease, and identify the carriers.

Other vascular retinopathies

Other blood diseases, such as anaemia, leukaemia or collagen diseases may cause retinal haemorrhages and exudates. The best way to test for these disorders is a full blood count and a blood sedimentation rate.

Abnormalities of the retinal blood vessels cause several other rare retinopathies. These may cause localized exudates in the retina, or haemorrhages into the retina or vitreous.

The treatment of vascular retinopathies

General treatment is usually necessary for hypertension, diabetes, sickle-cell disease, anaemia etc.

Unfortunately, there is no really effective local treatment for vascular retinopathies. The only exception to this is diabetic retinopathy, particularly proliferative diabetic retinopathy. However, the treatment involves a technique called 'photocoagulation' using an argon laser or a xenon arc light. The instruments are extremely expensive, and need expert maintenance. The aim of the treatment is to destroy the anoxic peripheral retina, which has very little visual function. This prevents the growth of new blood vessels which causes the blinding complications of proliferative diabetic retinopathy.

Photocoagulation or cryotherapy may also help to destroy the peripheral new vessels in sickle-cell disease.

Surgical treatment can occasionally be effective for a retinal artery occlusion, but only within the first few hours. By suddenly lowering the intraocular pressure, the retinal arteries will dilate. The embolus may then break up and pass on through the circulation. The technique is as follows: –
- Apply local anaesthetic drops.
- Insert a sharp knife or hypodermic needle into the anterior chamber angle, and allow some aqueous fluid to drain out.
- Withdraw the needle, and massage the eyeball.

Retinal degenerations

Retinal degenerations originate either in the retina itself or in the choroid. There are two main groups of choroidoretinal degenerations: genetic disorders and senile degenerations.

Genetic disorders

Many genetic disorders cause choroidoretinal degenerations, and the symptoms usually appear in childhood. The incidence of these genetic disorders varies in different parts of the world, but is likely to be higher in very isolated or inbred communities. The two most common disorders are retinitis pigmentosa and albinism.
- Retinitis pigmentosa particularly affects the peripheral retina. This causes a progressive constriction of the visual field, and difficulty in seeing at night. It may eventually progress to total blindness. Usually there are patches of increased pigmentation along the course of the small peripheral retinal arterioles, as well as narrowing of the retinal arteries and optic atrophy (*Plate* 19b).
- Albinism is a failure to produce the melanin pigment. It usually occurs in the skin, but often in the choroid. Both the skin and the fundus therefore look pale. The visual acuity is diminished because there is poor macular fixation, and there is often nystagmus.

Senile degenerations

Senile degenerations are common in old people, and nearly always occur near the macula. There is a very gradual loss of central vision, while the peripheral vision remains normal. The changes are nearly always bilateral, but are often more advanced in one eye that the other. The usual pattern is for the fine capillary network in the choroid (the choriocapillaris) to degenerate and atrophy. The retina is then affected secondarily. The appearance of the fundus varies, but usually shows pigment degeneration and atrophy both of the retina and the choroid around the macula (*Plate* 19c).

One particular type of degeneration, called 'disciform macular degeneration', may present rather differently with a fairly sudden loss, or distortion of central vision. This is probably due to a defect in the membrane between the retina and the choroid (Bruch's membrane) and in the pigment epithelium. A fibrovascular mass therefore grows between the retina and the choroid, and so destroys the function of the retina.

Onchocerciasis

In certain areas, onchocerciasis is an important cause of choroidoretinal degeneration (see Chapter 15).

There is no effective treatment for any of these degenerative conditions.

Retinal detachments

The normal retina lies in close contact with the underlying pigment epithelium. However, the two layers are not joined together. When a retinal detachment occurs, the retina separates from the pigment epithelium, and protein-rich fluid fills the space in between.

Retinal detachments are not a very common cause of blindness. However, it is one major retinal disease which can be treated and early surgery usually restores the sight. Unfortunately, if surgical treatment is delayed, secondary changes will occur which make the retinal detachment untreatable. Therefore, it is important to be able to recognize a retinal detachment in the early stages.

Why does the retina become detached? There are two predisposing factors, retinal holes and vitreous degeneration. Both these conditions are quite common, but they both have a significant risk of progressing to a retinal detachment.

− Holes or tears in the retina nearly always occur in the thin, peripheral retina, at or beyond the equator of the eye. There must be a hole or a tear for the retina to detach. However, not all retinal holes or tears progress to a detachment. They are much more likely to progress to a detachment if there is also degeneration of the vitreous jelly.

− Vitreous degeneration occurs quite commonly. The vitreous jelly is loosely attached to the retina. If it is firm and healthy, it supports the retina. If fluid degeneration occurs in the vitreous, its fibrils will contract, so that this support is lost. Any vitreous fibrils which remain attached to parts of the peripheral retina will therefore pull on the retina as the vitreous contracts. There is then a risk both that the retina will tear and that it will be pulled away from the pigment epithelium and so become detached (*Fig.* 12.1).

Retinal holes and vitreous degenerations may occur in otherwise normal eyes. However, they occur particularly in three conditions.

1. Myopia stretches the peripheral retina, and makes it more likely to develop holes. Vitreous degenerative changes are also more common in myopic patients.

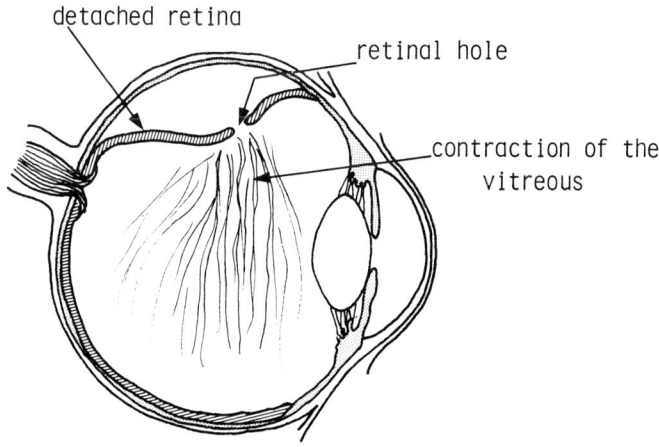

Diagram to show a retinal detachment

Fig. 12.1 Diagram to show a retinal detachment.

2. Cataract extraction deprives the vitreous of the anterior support of the lens. The vitreous may also adhere to the incision. This forward movement of vitreous may pull on the peripheral retina.

3. Blunt injuries to the eye may cause retinal tears or disturbances in the vitreous.

Therefore, myopia, cataract extractions and blunt injuries all predispose to retinal detachments.

Retinal detachments progress at very different rates. The retina may begin to detach almost immediately after a tear. Sometimes, however, a hole or tear may be present for months or even years without progressing to a detachment. Similarly, a detachment may spread to involve the whole retina within a few hours, or remain localized to part of the retina only. There it may spread slowly, or not at all. Retinal holes or detachments usually progress much more quickly in the upper than the lower part of the retina.

When the retina first becomes detached, it is quite mobile and can be re-attached. However, after some weeks, fibroblasts grow over the surface of the retina. These probably come from the pigment epithelium, and pass through the retinal hole. They form a membrane on the surface of the retina, so that it is no longer mobile and cannot be re-attached. In a longstanding detachment, secondary uveitis and a secondary cataract may also develop. It is not clear how this happens.

The symptoms and signs of retinal holes and detachments

'Floaters' and flashing lights are symptoms of vitreous degeneration and retinal holes. A visual field defect and loss of vision is the symptom of a retinal detachment.

— 'Floaters' are black specks seen in front of the eye which move with eye movements, but with a characteristic delay from inertia. They are caused by opacities in the vitreous jelly which cast a shadow on the retina. These 'floaters' are especially noticeable in bright light when the pupil is constricted. They are a common symptom and are often found in otherwise healthy eyes. However, they are particularly common when fluid degeneration of the vitreous has occurred. Therefore it is necessary to dilate the pupil and carefully check the peripheral retina for holes or tears when 'floaters' are first seen.

— Flashing lights are often symptoms of migraine or anxiety. However, they may be caused by spontaneous electrical discharges in the retina. These occur if the peripheral retina tears or the vitreous fibrils are pulling on it. They appear to the patient as a flashing light in the periphery of the visual field.

— A visual field defect is the basic symptom of a retinal detachment. When the retina detaches, it cannot function properly. A retinal detachment starts in the periphery, and so the visual loss starts in the periphery of the visual field. As the detachment spreads, the visual loss spreads centrally like a curtain coming across the vision. The visual field loss relates to the part of the retina which is detached. This means that an upper half retinal detachment will cause a lower half loss of the visual field. If the detachment spreads to the macula, there will immediately be a loss of the visual acuity.

Just occasionally, the retina may tear across a small retinal blood vessel. This will cause a haemorrhage into the vitreous.

Retinal holes and vitreous degenerative changes can be very difficult to detect, even with a dilated pupil. The changes of a retinal detachment are more obvious, and are especially well seen using an indirect rather than a direct ophthalmoscope. Look for the following characteristic features (*Plate* 19d): –

– The retina is displaced forwards. It will therefore be necessary to use positive lenses with a direct ophthalmoscope to bring it into focus.
– The surface of the retina is irregular and wavy. The retinal vessels also appear darker than normal.
– The background pattern of the choroidal vessels and pigment is no longer clearly visible.

It is also important to examine the other eye very carefully. Retinal degenerations and holes are often bilateral, and so prophylactic treatment may be necessary. This is especially important if the first eye has gone blind from a retinal detachment.

The treatment of retinal holes and detachments

Retinal holes or tears (where the retina has not yet detached) should be sealed by producing a localized inflammatory reaction around the hole. This makes the retina adhere firmly to the pigment epithelium and the choroid, and prevents any subsequent detachment. The technique is either to photocoagulate the retina, or to freeze the surface of the sclera with a cryoprobe.

– Retinal detachments can only be treated if preretinal fibrosis has not yet occurred. The same principle of sealing off the retinal hole applies. It is therefore necessary to bring the retina around the hole to rest against the pigment epithelium and the choroid. This means indenting the overlying sclera so that the choroid is pushed up against the retina (*Fig.* 12.2). It is possible to make this indentation by suturing some silicone rubber, sponge or fascia lata to the surface of the sclera over the area of the retinal hole. Another method is to place a tight elastic silicone band or strip of fascia right round the equator of the eye. This will indent the entire peripheral choroid

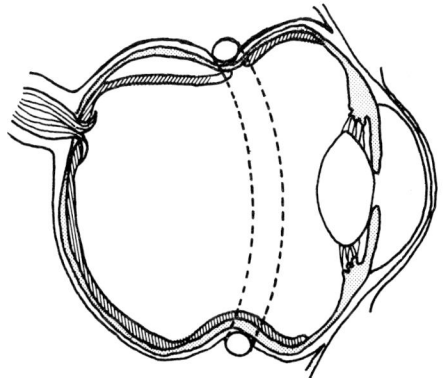

Surgical treatment of a retinal detachment. The retinal hole is sealed off by indenting the outside of the eye. (In this diagram an elastic silicone band is placed around the equator of the eye).

Fig. 12.2 Diagram to show the surgical treatment of a retinal detachment.

and seal it to the equator. Draining the subretinal fluid between the retina and the pigment epithelium may also help the retina and the choroid come together.

Other diseases of the retina

Retinoblastoma

Retinoblastoma is a rare but very malignant tumour of the retina which occurs in infants and young children. The tumour grows between the retina and the choroid and also into the vitreous, forming a white mass in the posterior part of the eye. It may then burst throught the sclera or cornea to form a progressively enlarging fungating mass in the orbit. Alternatively, it may spread down the optic nerve into the brain. It may even spread to the lymph nodes, bones and liver. In the advanced stages of the disease, the diagnosis is usually obvious. However, a tumour which is still confined to the eye is much more difficult to diagnose.

The first indication of a retinoblastoma may be that the eye develops a squint because the child cannot see out of it. The white mass gives off a white reflection in certain lights, which looks rather like a cat's eye. This white mass can be seen behind the pupil with an ophthalmoscope (*Plate* 19e). Unfortunately, it looks similar to various other conditions which occur in infants. The most common of these is congenital cataract. The others are all rare: –
– A parasitic granuloma, especially from toxocara, a nematode worm.
– Tuberculosis, or some other cause of exudative uveitis.
– Retrolental fibroplasia, which is usually caused by giving premature babies too much oxygen.
– Persistent primary vitreous, a congenital disorder.
   The treatment of a retinoblastoma depends upon how far it has progressed.
– If the tumour is still confined to the eye, it will be necessary to enucleate the eye immediately. This usually stops the tumour spreading beyond the eye.
– If the tumour has spread to the orbit, exenteration of the entire orbit may sometimes save the patient's life.
   There is always a high risk that there may be early tumour masses in the other eye. It is therefore necessary to give a general anaesthetic, and examine the entire retina of the other eye. Very early tumours in the second eye can sometimes be treated with radiotherapy and this may save the eye.

Chloroquine retinopathy (*Plate* 19f)

In general, systemic drugs do not harm the retina. However, excessive doses of chloroquine and its derivatives can damage the macula. Chloroquine is a very effective drug against malaria, but must be taken under medical supervision. People who take it excessively (usually for many years) often suffer a loss of visual acuity.

At first, the only changes in the eye are an irregular pigmentation around the macula, and a fine deposit in the cornea. Both these early changes are very slight and are only visible with a slit lamp, but the loss of visual acuity is often quite severe. If the patient is not specifically asked about his consumption of chloroquine, the correct diagnosis may not be made, and the vision will continue to deteriorate. Unfortunately, the visual damage is usually permanent. Eventually, further pigmentary changes around the macula produce the appearance of a target (or 'bulls's eye').

Diseases of the vitreous body

Fortunately, there are very few diseases of the vitreous body.

- Degenerative changes associated with retinal detachments have already been mentioned.
- Vitreous haemorrhages come from the retinal blood vessels. They are most common in diabetes, but may also occur with other vascular retinopathies, after injuries to the eye and sometimes after retinal tears. If the haemorrhage is small, the blood in the vitreous can be seen in front of the retina with an ophthalmoscope. If the haemorrhage is large, the red reflex is completely obscured. Small haemorrhages usually clear gradually. However, a massive haemorrhage may become organized into a pigmented membrane in the vitreous, and may never completely clear.
- Bacteria entering the vitreous during an operation or after an eye injury are extremely dangerous. They multiply rapidly in the vitreous, and the result is usually a disastrous endophthalmitis.

It is now possible to operate in the vitreous cavity, but the equipment is very delicate and expensive.

13. Diseases of the Optic Nerve and Visual Pathways

The optic nerve and visual pathways connect the eye to the brain (*see* page 12 *and Fig*. 2.4). Diseases of the visual pathways can be divided into three groups: –
– Diseases of the optic nerve — common
– Diseases of the optic chiasm — uncommon
– Diseases behind the optic chiasm — uncommon

Diseases of the optic nerve

The optic nerve is susceptible to many kinds of damage, and so diseases of the optic nerve are very common. The damage may be in one or both eyes. However, any optic nerve disease will always cause some loss of vision and some loss of the pupil light reflex.

There are a number of different clinical terms used to describe optic nerve damage. There is often some confusion about these terms: –
– Optic neuropathy is the general term for any damage to the optic nerve.
– Optic neuritis is the general term for any inflammation of the optic nerve. It usually causes considerable visual loss, and also loss of the pupil light reflex. Unfortunately, the optic nerve cannot regenerate, and so optic neuritis nearly always causes some permanent visual loss. However, the vision sometimes improves as the inflammation subsides, because some of the nerve fibres may escape serious damage.

There are two forms of optic neuritis: papillitis and retrobulbar neuritis.
1. 'Papillitis' is the term for optic neuritis in the anterior part of the nerve inside the eye, including the optic disc. It gets its name from the papilla, another word for the optic disc. A fundus examination shows slight oedema of the optic disc, and blurring of its margins (*see Plate* 22c).
2. 'Retrobulbar neuritis' is the term for optic neuritis in the posterior part of the nerve behind the eye. The fundus therefore appears completely normal. Often, the patient complains of a slight pain behind the eye especially when he looks up. The reason for this is as follows. The extraocular muscles take their origin from a fibrous ring at the apex of the orbit. The dural sheath around the optic nerve is attached to this fibrous ring, and especially to the superior rectus muscle.

There is a common saying about optic neuritis: 'The patient sees nothing (at all), and the doctor sees nothing (abnormal).' In papillitis, there is only slight blurring of the optic disc, and in retrobulbar neuritis, the fundus looks normal.

- Papilloedema is oedema of the optic disc (*see Plates* 18a *and* 20a), and it is usually bilateral. At first, the optic disc is swollen with oedema fluid, but there is little or no loss of vision. Eventually, however, the optic nerve degenerates and the vision starts to fail. In long-standing cases, small dilated blood vessels are present on the surface of the disc. The two most common causes of papilloedema are a rise in intracranial pressure or severe hypertension. If papilloedema is diagnosed, it is essential to discover the cause and give treatment as soon as possible.

   Papilloedema is often confused with papillitis. However, in papilloedema there is obvious swelling of the optic disc, but little change in vision. In papillitis, the opposite occurs: the changes in the optic disc are slight, but there is considerable loss of vision. Papilloedema is usually bilateral, while papillitis is usually unilateral.

- Optic atrophy means that a significant number of fibres in the optic nerve have degenerated (*Plate* 20b). This may occur gradually and spontaneously, or after an attack of optic neuritis. There is always some loss of vision, and the pupil light reflex is either diminished or absent. The exact pattern of this visual loss depends upon the cause of the atrophy, and upon which fibres have degenerated in the optic nerve. In mild cases, there may only be a loss of brightness or colour discrimination. However, a careful visual field test will reveal small defects, usually between the blind spot and the centre of fixation. In severe cases, there may be total blindness in one or both eyes.

   The exact appearance of the optic disc will vary according to the cause of the optic atrophy. In the first few weeks after any optic nerve damage, the disc appears normal. After that, the disc appears pale and white because the optic nerve fibres and the small blood vessels nourishing them both atrophy. Often this is the only abnormality that can be seen, and it is sometimes called 'primary optic atrophy' (*Plate* 20b).

   If the optic atrophy follows papillitis or papilloedema, the disc is pale but there is also fibrous tissue or pigmentation around the disc (*see Plate* 22d).

   Sometimes optic atrophy follows massive destruction of retinal ganglion cells, such as in a retinal artery occlusion or retinitis pigmentosa. In this case, the retinal changes can be seen as well as the pale optic disc.

   In optic atrophy following glaucoma, the disc is cupped as well as pale (*see Plate* 20c).

   The optic nerve cannot regenerate, and so visual loss from any form of optic atrophy is permanent.

Causes of optic neuritis and optic atrophy

There are many causes of optic neuritis and optic atrophy (*see Table* 13.1). However, because they all produce very much the same clinical picture, it is often difficult to find a specific cause.

   Some causes of optic neuritis and optic atrophy are especially important in hot countries: –

1. Malnutrition is more likely to damage the optic nerve than any other part of the nervous system. However, malnutrition alone is not a common cause of optic

Table 13.1 — The most common causes of optic neuritis and optic atrophy

Malnutrition	Vitamin B complex deficiency
Toxins	Pipe tobacco Cassava Methyl alcohol
Drugs	Ethambutol Quinine Arsenicals
Infections	Measles Typhoid Meningitis Syphilis Onchocerciasis
Vascular diseases	Ischaemic optic atrophy Cranial arteritis Diabetes Hypertension
Tumours	Orbital tumours Optic nerve gliomas and meningiomas Chiasmal tumours
Head injuries	
Multiple sclerosis	

atrophy. Poor and malnourished people more frequently suffer from optic atrophy, but this is probably because they are more susceptible to optic nerve damage from toxins, infections and other causes. In other words, malnutrition is probably more important as a predisposing factor than a specific cause.

  — Vitamin B complex deficiency was probably the specific cause of optic atrophy among chronically malnourished prisoners of war. The disease was only found in camps where the diet was deficient in vitamin B, and it could be prevented by including yeast extract or other sources of vitamin B in the diet. In normal civilian life, however, vitamin B deficiency alone is not a common cause of optic atrophy. Like malnutrition in general, it is probably more important as a predisposing factor.

2. Toxins can also damage the optic nerve, especially if the patient is also malnourished. The three best documented examples are pipe tobacco, cassava and methyl alcohol.

  — Pipe tobacco contains cyanide, which the body is normally able to detoxify. However, people who are excessive pipe smokers may not be able to detoxify all this cyanide. There is then a risk that the cyanide will destroy any vitamin B_{12} in the bloodstream, and cause vitamin B_{12} deficiency. The patient may complain of poor vision. An eye examination will show a loss of visual acuity, and a central or paracentral visual field defect with early optic atrophy. This condition is called 'tobacco amblyopia', and it is sometimes associated with excessive alcohol consumption.

- Cassava is a cheap staple food in many tropical countries. Because it contains high levels of cyanide, it is necessary to prepare it very carefully so that it is safe to eat. Poor people, who are generally malnourished, and who may often eat badly prepared cassava, sometimes suffer from cassava tropical neuropathy. This condition causes damage to the long tracts in the spinal cord, which makes walking difficult. There is also visual loss from optic atrophy. Sometimes, the visual field defects are in the periphery rather than the centre of the vision.

- Methyl alcohol is sometimes present in home-brewed or illegal alcohol, and can cause blindness. If the patient comes for immediate treatment, it is possible to neutralize methyl alcohol with ethyl alcohol. However, during digestion, methyl alcohol is metabolized into formaldehyde or formic acid. It is probably these metabolic products which cause serious damage to the optic nerve and the ganglion cells of the retina. At first, the patient is prostrate with headache, nausea and delirium. When he recovers, he is either blind or has a severe visual defect.

3. Many drugs can be toxic to the optic nerve. The most important of these are: –
- Ethambutol, which is used against tuberculosis.
- Quinine, which is used to treat malaria, and sometimes to produce an abortion.
- Arsenical drugs, which were once used against trypanosomiasis.

4. Infections can damage the optic nerve, especially in a debilitated or malnourished patient. This may be an acute, generalized infection such as measles or typhoid. All forms of meningitis can damage the optic nerve. Two important chronic infections are syphilis and onchocerciasis.
- Syphilis can damage the eyes in many ways, producing corneal scarring, iritis, chorioretinitis and ocular muscle palsies. However, the most serious and common complication of syphilis in the eye is probably optic neuritis and optic atrophy. This may occur in congenital, secondary, and all forms of tertiary syphilis, especially in tabes dorsalis.
- Onchocerciasis often causes optic atrophy (*see* Chapter 15, page 178).

5. Vascular diseases can also damage the optic nerve.
- Ischaemic optic neuropathy is a condition which is usually found in old people with atherosclerosis. The blood vessels of the optic nerve become occluded, producing optic neuritis and optic atrophy. This causes either sudden or gradual loss of vision. It often produces sector defects in the visual field similar to those of glaucoma. However, the intraocular pressure is normal.
- Cranial arteritis (or giant cell arteritis) is an inflammatory disease of the arterial walls. It is most common in old people, and causes sudden visual loss. It usually involves other cranial arteries too, especially the superficial temporal artery, which therefore feels firm and tender. Cranial arteritis also causes both the blood sedimentation rate and the serum viscosity to rise.
- Diabetic vascular changes can also damage the optic nerve.

6. Tumours, or other space-occupying lesions of the orbit or cranium may press on the optic nerve and damage it. The rise in intracranial pressure will also cause

severe papilloedema. Eventually this will lead to optic atrophy.

7. Head injuries, especially a blunt injury on the temple, occasionally rupture the small blood vessels in the optic foramen. This may cause optic nerve damage.

8. Multiple sclerosis involves the optic nerve more than any other part of the central nervous system. It is an important cause of optic neuritis and optic atrophy all over the world. However, it is more common in temperate than in hot climates. In multiple sclerosis, the nerve fibres lose their myelin sheath. This causes a fairly sudden loss of function, usually followed by gradual partial recovery. At first, there is an attack of acute optic neuritis with severe loss of vision. Over the next few weeks, the vision partially recovers. Further episodes may occur weeks, months or even years later. With each attack, the residual disability increases.

Optic atrophy also occurs after other eye diseases, such as glaucoma, retinitis pigmentosa and retinal vascular occlusions.

Diagnosis

It is often difficult or even impossible to find a specific cause for many cases of optic atrophy. However, it may help to ask about the patient's diet, habits, general health and any drugs he may be taking. A neurological history and examination may also be advisable. Two tests are useful if there is still no explanation. These are the serological test for syphilis and the 'skin snip' test, in areas where onchocerciasis is endemic.

Treatment

Most optic nerve damage is irreversible, and so there is very little treatment for patients with long-standing optic atrophy. However, in less advanced cases, where the cause is known, it may be possible to stop the progress of the disease.

- If there is evidence of malnutrition, it is necessary to give nutritional advice. It may also help to give vitamin B supplements, such as yeast or multivite tablets.
- If cyanide poisoning is suspected (as in tobacco amblyopia or cassava neuropathy), inject large doses of hydroxocobalamin (Neo-Cytamen). This contains vitamin B_{12}. However, it is uncertain how useful this treatment is.
- In optic neuritis, when active inflammatory changes are present in the nerve, systemic steroids may help the inflammation to subside, and may restore some vision. Unfortunately, steroid treatment does not help many cases. If there is no improvement after a few weeks, do not continue the treatment.
- If cranial arteritis is the cause of optic nerve damage, systemic steroid treatment is essential. Such patients must continue on steroid treatment until the symptoms of the disease disappear, and the blood sedimentation rate returns to normal.

Diseases of the optic chiasm

The optic chiasm is much less susceptible to disease than the optic nerve, and so diseases which are localized to the optic chiasm are quite rare. The nasal fibres from each retina which relate to the temporal part of the visual field cross over in the chiasm. A characteristic sign of damage at the chiasm is therefore temporal visual field defects in both eyes. Often, the pattern of visual loss is more complex than this.

Most diseases of the chiasm are space-occupying lesions, such as pituitary tumours, suprasellar cysts, meningiomas or arterial aneurysms. Skull X-rays and more sophisticated neuroradiological tests usually help the diagnosis. Many of these lesions can be treated surgically by a neurosurgeon.

Diseases behind the optic chiasm

Behind the optic chiasm are the remaining visual pathways — the optic tracts, the lateral geniculate body, the optic radiations and the occipital cortex. These visual pathways are also less susceptible to disease than the optic nerve. Diseases behind the optic chiasm are therefore quite rare.

Any disorder of the visual pathways behind the chiasm will affect exactly the same part of the visual field in each eye. This is called a 'homonymous defect'. Disorders of the left side of the brain produce defects in the right visual field of each eye, and vice versa. The most common defect is when one complete half of the visual field is lost in each eye. This is called a 'homonymous hemianopia'. Sometimes, however, only a quadrant or a small sector of the visual field is lost. The 'edge' of these visual field defects is always well-defined and distinct, rather than gradual.

Damage to the visual pathways behind the chiasm is usually the result of a cerebrovascular accident or stroke. Occasionally, however, the cause is a space-occupying lesion in the cerebral cortex. If the damage is in the occipital cortex, the patient is sometimes unaware of any visual loss. This is called 'cortical blindness'. Complete cortical blindness may occur in young children after an attack of encephalitis. Occasionally, it also occurs in old people with bilateral ischaemic changes in the occipital cortex.

14.   Glaucoma

Chapter 2 (page 11) explains how the aqueous fluid circulates and maintains the pressure in the eye. Glaucoma is a pathological rise in the intraocular pressure, which damages various structures in the eye, especially the optic nerve.

There are two main types of glaucoma: open angle glaucoma and angle closure glaucoma.

Open angle glaucoma (Chronic simple glaucoma)

In open angle glaucoma, the aqueous fluid is produced and circulates normally. However, for reasons which are not clear, the aqueous cannot drain through the trabecular meshwork properly. There is therefore a very gradual rise in the intraocular pressure.

About 1% of the world's population suffer from open angle glaucoma. The incidence rises with age, so that it is uncommon under the age of 30, but quite common over the age of 60. The disease often runs in families. Relatives of a patient with open angle glaucoma are therefore more likely to develop the disease than other people. Open angle glaucoma is more severe in blacks, and also develops at a younger age.

The normal intraocular pressure is 10 – 20 mmHg There are slight variations during the day, and a large fluid intake causes the intraocular pressure to rise. However, a pressure of 20 – 30 mmHg increasingly indicates that glaucoma is likely, and above 30 mmHg is definitely abnormal.

The signs and symptoms of glaucoma

The rise in intraocular pressure does not cause any pain or any inflammation in the eye. The first and most important structure to be affected is the optic nerve where it enters the eye. Here the optic nerve is supplied by small choroidal blood vessels which are damaged by the rise in intraocular pressure. This causes gradual and progressive atrophy of the optic nerve head which can be seen with an ophthalmoscope. The optic disc looks pale and has a hollowed out or cupped appearance called 'glaucomatous optic atrophy' (*Figs*. 14.1 and *Plate* 20c-e). In severe cases, the blood vessels disappear at the edge of the optic disc, and reappear out of focus at the bottom of the disc (*Plate* 20c).

The only important symptom is a very gradual loss of vision from the optic nerve atrophy. This visual loss progresses slowly in a characteristic pattern. Arcuate-shaped defects in the visual field (called 'scotomas') spread out from the

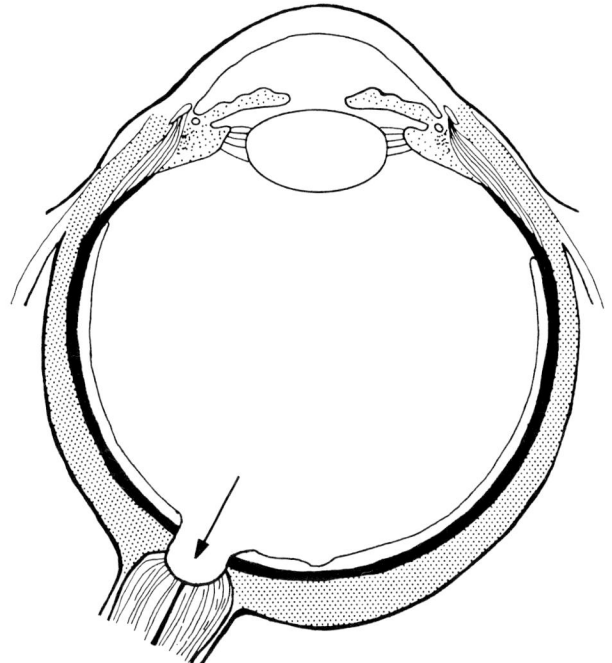

Fig. 14.1 A diagram to show the shape of a cupped optic disc (Compare with *Fig.* 2.1).

blind spot. These scotomas gradually enlarge until the only vision left is in the macular area, and the extreme temporal periphery (*Fig.* 14.2 *and* 3.1d). Eventually even this vision is lost. However, it is usually several years from the first signs of visual loss to the development of blindness.

Open angle glaucoma may be very far advanced by the time it is first diagnosed, and not just because the patient has delayed seeking medical advice. The truth is that in the early stages of the disease, the patient is often unaware of anything wrong with his sight. The visual field defects are not noticed by the patient for three reasons: –

– They are in the periphery of the field of vision.
– Like the normal 'blind spot', the patient is often not conscious of them.
– They progress very gradually.

There is also no pain or inflammation.

Advanced glaucoma causes more extensive damage to the eye. The sphincter muscle of the iris atrophies, so that the pupil becomes dilated and non-reactive. Glaucoma comes from the Greek word for dark blue, possibly because the early Greek scientists thought that the inside of the eye looked dark blue through the dilated pupil. If the pressure in the eye is very high, the corneal endothelial cells may be unable to keep the cornea dehydrated. The cornea will then look hazy from oedema (*Plate* 20f). At this advanced stage, there may be slight discomfort in the eye.

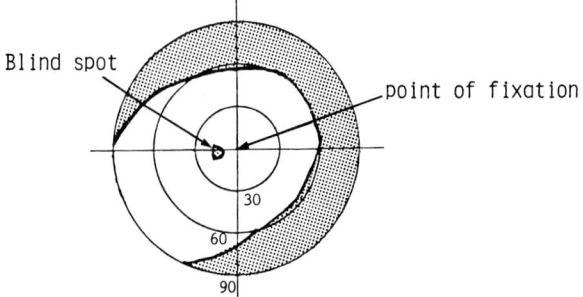

The normal visual field

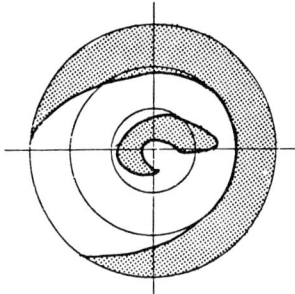

Typical visual field defect in early glaucoma

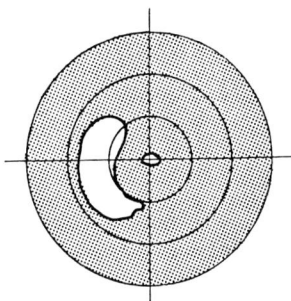

Typical visual field defect in advanced glaucoma

Fig. 14.2 Visual field changes in glaucoma.

The diagnosis of open angle glaucoma

Glaucoma is a progressive disease, and any visual loss is permanent. Early diagnosis and early treatment are therefore essential to prevent permanent blindness.

There are three basic changes in open angle glaucoma.
− a rise in the intraocular pressure,
− atrophy and cupping of the optic nerve head,

- loss of vision from visual field defects.

Each of these changes can be easily detected in advanced cases when the patient is blind or almost blind. They are very hard to detect in early glaucoma.

- The intraocular pressure can only be measured accurately with the right equipment. A slight rise in pressure (from 20 – 30 mmHg) may damage the optic nerve in some patients but not in others. For both these reasons, it is difficult to diagnose early glaucoma from the intraocular pressure alone.
- Advanced glaucomatous atrophy is obvious (*Plate* 20c), but the early changes are not obvious (*Plate* 20d). As the glaucoma advances, the optic disc becomes more and more cupped and pale. The problem is that the appearance of the normal disc varies from person to person. In many normal patients a small part of the optic disc is pale and cupped on the temporal side. This is called 'physiological cupping' (*Plate* 20e). If less than half of the total disc diameter is pale and cupped, the disc is usually normal. However, if more than half of the disc is pale and cupped, or if the cups in both eyes are different sizes, early glaucoma is very likely.
- Visual field defects need careful examination with special apparatus to detect them in the early stages. They also need an alert and co-operative patient.

Glaucoma is a slowly progressive disease. If you are not sure whether the patient has early changes of glaucoma, you should examine him again 6 months or a year later.

Occasionally, the optic disc and the visual field show definite changes of glaucoma, but the intraocular pressure is normal. This is a condition called 'low tension glaucoma'. Some disorder of the circulation (e.g. arteriosclerosis or anaemia) has caused ischaemic atrophy to the optic disc, even though the intraocular pressure is normal.

The treatment of open angle glaucoma

The aim of treatment is to reduce the intraocular pressure to normal levels, and so prevent further damage to the optic nerve. There is no purpose in treating eyes which are already blind. It wastes the patient's time and money and only raises false hopes.

Open angle glaucoma is nearly always a bilateral disease, but one eye is often more damaged than the other. One eye may be blind, while the other still has some useful vision. Generally speaking, it is worth treating 'counting fingers' vision looking straight ahead. If the vision is worse than this, treatment is not worth while.

It is possible to lower the intraocular pressure either medically or surgically.

MEDICAL TREATMENT.

Chapter 3 describes the drugs used in medical treatment. The usual plan of treatment is to start with: –

either pilocarpine drops, 2% – 4%   4 times a day,
  or adrenaline drops, 1%   2 times a day,
  or timolol drops,   0.25% – 0.5% 2 times a day.

If the control of pressure is adequate after a month, the treatment should continue the same. If there are side effects, it will be necessary to use a different drop. If the pressure control is still inadequate, a combination of these drops can be used. Acetazolamide tablets can also be given but they have several long term complications.

Medical treatment for open angle glaucoma should continue for the rest of the patient's life. There should also be regular supervision to make sure that the intraocular pressure is under control, and that there has been no further loss of vision. It is therefore necessary to examine the visual field, the optic disc and the intraocular pressure every 6 months at least.

Unfortunately, there are many reasons why long term medical treatment is often impossible: –
– First, patients cannot always afford treatment for the rest of their life.
– Second, the patient may not be able to use the drops properly, or apply them regularly.
– Third, it may be impossible to check the patient's progress with regular follow-up visits.
– Fourth, the necessary drugs may not be available.

Ideally, one should only recommend surgery to patients who have not responded well enough to medical treatment. In practice however, for any of the above reasons, surgery is often preferable.

SURGICAL TREATMENT.

1. Drainage operations. In most glaucoma operations, a small fragment of corneoscleral trabecular tissue is excised in order to improve the flow of aqueous fluid out of the eye. The aqueous fluid can then pass straight into the subconjunctival space, where it is slowly absorbed (*Plate* 21a *and Fig.* 14.3). Traditional operations use a knife, a trephine blade or a cautery to excise a full thickness segment of limbal sclera. However, a recent modification of this technique, called a 'trabeculectomy', excises only the deeper layer of the corneoscleral trabecular meshwork. The remaining flap of superficial sclera acts as a slight barrier to the flow of aqueous fluid from the eye. There is therefore less danger that the aqueous fluid will drain away too quickly and cause postoperative complications.

After any glaucoma operation, the eye may be soft for a few days, but usually the pressure stabilizes at a normal level. As the aqueous fluid leaves the eye, it forms a small bleb under the conjunctiva at the operation site. The aqueous fluid is eventually absorbed by the subconjunctival veins or lymphatics, or passes slowly through the conjunctiva into the tears.

Complications of drainage operations There are the usual short term complications of any intraocular surgery (*see* page 46). There are also four important long term complications which may occur after glaucoma drainage operations: –
i. Sometimes fibrosis and scarring block the aqueous drainage pathway during the first few months after surgery. The glaucoma then recurs. Blacks are more likely to form scar tissue, and so are probably more susceptible. Local steroid treatment for some weeks after the operation may help to prevent this fibrosis and scarring.

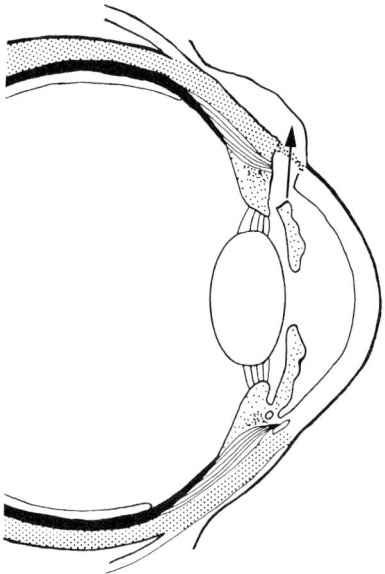

Fig. 14.3 A diagram to show the passage of aqueous fluid after a glaucoma drainage operation.

ii. Bacteria can enter the eye from the conjunctival sac through the drainage pathway, and cause endophthalmitis. This is a rare but very serious complication.

iii. Glaucoma surgery increases the incidence of cataract formation, possibly because of damage to the lens at the operation.

iv. The pressure in the eye may become too low.

2. Other surgical procedures. It is possible to lower the production of aqueous fluid by the ciliary processes, rather than improve the drainage. The usual technique is to apply either diathermy or cryotherapy superficially to the sclera overlying the ciliary body. Unfortunately the results are not very reliable. Recent research has shown that argon laser treatment can lower the intraocular pressure.

Ideally, one should follow up all patients who have had a glaucoma operation for the rest of their lives. However, this is just as difficult as following up patients on medical treatment. Fortunately, a glaucoma drainage operation which functions successfully after the first few months, nearly always continues to function successfully for the rest of the patient's life. The overall success rate for glaucoma surgery is about 80%.

Angle closure glaucoma

Angle closure glaucoma usually comes on suddenly with severe symptoms. Therefore it is very different from open angle glaucoma. The mechanism is that the iris bows forward so that the iris root touches the back of the cornea (*Fig.* 14.4). This closes the angle of the anterior chamber and prevents the aqueous reaching the trabecular meshwork. Therefore the intraocular pressure rises. As the pressure rises the iris root gets pushed forward even more, and closes the

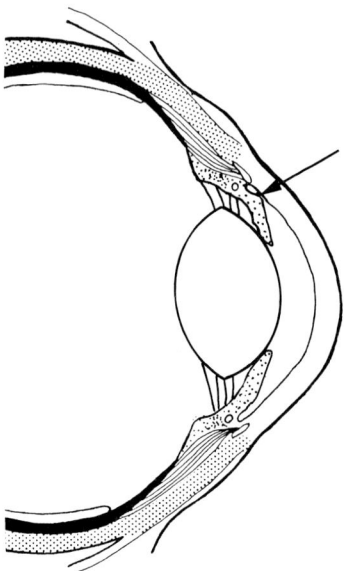

Fig. 14.4 A diagram of an eye with a shallow anterior chamber angle. The arrow shows where the iris root has come forward to touch the back of the cornea.

anterior chamber angle completely.

Angle closure glaucoma only occurs if there is a shallow anterior chamber. This means that the root of the iris lies very close to the back of the cornea. The depth of the anterior chamber varies from person to person. It may become more shallow in older people because the lens continues to grow throughout life. Therefore angle closure glaucoma only occurs in middle or old age. Rarely a cataractous lens may become very swollen and precipitate angle closure glaucoma (*see* page 138).

The other factor which sometimes starts the attack of angle closure glaucoma is a slight dilatation of the pupil. This causes the iris root to bunch up and close off the angle. Different stimuli make the pupil dilate.
– seeing in the dark,
– excitement,
– mydriatic drops,
– medicines with an atropine-like action (some antidepressants and gastrointestinal sedatives).

However, the patient must have a shallow anterior chamber.

Angle closure glaucoma is slightly more common in women than in men. It is, however, rare among blacks, probably because the heavily pigmented iris is more rigid and will not easily dilate or bow forwards.

The signs and symptoms of angle closure glaucoma

In a typical case, there is sudden loss of vision and an acute, severe pain in the eye. There may also be nausea and vomiting. The acute attack usually occurs in one eye only. However, the other eye will also have a shallow anterior chamber, and so will always be at risk of developing the disease later.

Examination of an eye with acute angle closure glaucoma shows these features (*Plate* 21b): –
– The ciliary blood vessels are dilated.
– The cornea is hazy from oedema.
– The anterior chamber is shallow.
– The pupil is semi-dilated, non-reactive, and often slightly irregular.
– The intraocular pressure is very high, and so the eye feels stony hard and acutely tender.
– There is usually severe loss of vision. This is partly from the corneal haze, but mainly from the acute rise in intraocular pressure, which causes ischaemia to the optic nerve.

With immediate treatment, there is a chance of partial or complete recovery of sight. Without treatment, ischaemia rapidly progresses to permanent optic nerve damage and permanent blindness (especially in old people). Eventually the pain and inflammation subside, leaving the features of absolute glaucoma — a hard eye with a dilated pupil, atrophy of the iris and total atrophy of the optic nerve.

Occasionally, the attack of glaucoma aborts spontaneously, and the angle reopens again before the damage has become permanent. In these cases a segment of the iris has usually atrophied, and so distorts the pupil. There may also be partial optic disc atrophy.

Angle closure glaucoma does not always present so acutely, and there may be minor attacks with spontaneous recovery. Typically, the patient feels some ocular discomfort, and has blurred vision with rainbow coloured rings (or haloes) around lights. These haloes are from corneal oedema. Small drops of fluid in the cornea split white light into its spectral colours, so that a rainbow halo is seen.

Just occasionally, angle closure glaucoma presents chronically with a very gradual rise in intraocular pressure and no symptoms at all. There is a very gradual visual field loss similar to open angle glaucoma. The only difference is that the anterior chamber angle is closed rather than open. It is possible to see the anterior chamber angle with a slit lamp and a special mirrored contact lens called a gonioscope.

The treatment of angle closure glaucoma

The aim of treatment in acute glaucoma is to lower the intraocular pressure as quickly as possible by medical means. It is then necessary to perform an iridectomy operation to prevent the periphery of the iris blocking the angle of the anterior chamber. There is a high risk that the other eye may develop acute glaucoma later. For this reason, the operation should always be on *both* eyes.

The diseased eye should receive pilocarpine drops 2% – 4%. The drops should be given intensively: 1 drop every 5 minutes for an hour, then every hour for 12 hours. The other eye should receive pilocarpine drops 4 times a day. Pilocarpine constricts the pupil and makes the iris taut. The iris pulls away from the back of the cornea, and opens up the angle of the anterior chamber.

A dose of 250 mg acetazolamide (Diamox) 4 times a day will lower the production of aqueous fluid. The first dose can be given by injection. In very severe cases, osmotic diuretics may help to lower the intraocular pressure (*see*

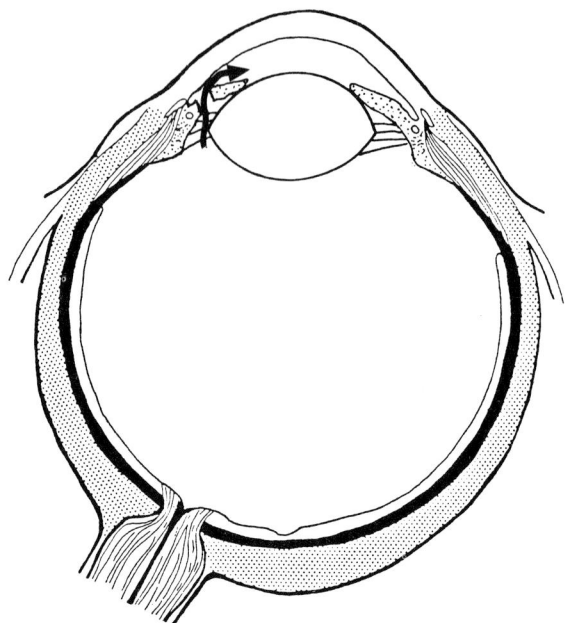

Fig. 14.5 A diagram to show the flow of aqueous fluid after an iridectomy operation.

page 42).

As soon as the intraocular pressure has returned to normal, and the ocular inflammation has subsided, an iridectomy should be performed on both eyes.

An iridectomy is a fairly simple operation. A segment of peripheral iris is excised through a small limbal incision. The aqueous fluid can then flow freely from either side of the iris. The operation thus prevents the iris from bowing forward and closing the angle (*Fig.* 14.5). After a successful iridectomy, there is no risk that acute angle closure glaucoma will develop.

Just occasionally, severe attacks cause the iris root to adhere permanently to the back of the cornea. Much of the angle is permanently blocked, and there is a persistent rise in the intraocular pressure. The treatment for this is the same as for open angle glaucoma.

If a patient with acute glaucoma has a swollen, hypermature cataract, it is best to remove the cataract.

Secondary glaucoma

Sometimes complications of other eye diseases cause a rise in the intraocular pressure. This is called secondary glaucoma.

Secondary glaucoma following iridocyclitis is quite common (*see* Chapter 10).
Thrombotic glaucoma is a complication of certain vascular disorders of the retina, especially after a retinal vein thrombosis or in diabetic retinopathy.

In both these conditions new blood vessels grow on the retina. For some reason, this stimulates new blood vessels to grow on the surface of the iris also.

This is called 'rubeosis of the iris'. The new blood vessels also obstruct the drainage of the aqueous, and produce a very severe type of glaucoma. Most of these eyes are blind, and the aim of treatment is only to relieve pain. Local corticosteroid drops may do this but an injection of 1 ml· of alcohol into the retrobulbar space is often a cheaper and more permanent method of pain relief in a blind eye (*see* page 44).

Malignant glaucoma is a rare complication of any intraocular surgery. The aqueous fluid does not pass into the anterior chamber, but collects either behind the vitreous body or behind the iris and lens. The iris is pushed forward against the back of the cornea and so blocks the aqueous drainage pathway. Urgent and rather complex surgery is necessary, as well as mydriatic drops.

Steroid induced glaucoma occurs in certain individuals as a complication of local steroid treatment. The pressure returns to normal when the treatment stops.

Congenital glaucoma

Congenital glaucoma is a rare condition, in which the angle of the anterior chamber does not develop normally in the embryo. A mesodermal membrane covers the trabecular meshwork, and so the intraocular pressure rises excessively. The fetal and neonatal eye is less rigid than an adult eye, and it stretches in response to the pressure. The eye, and especially the diameter of the cornea, increase in size. This condition is called 'buphthalmos', which means ox-eye (*Fig.* 14.6). As the cornea stretches, it causes splits in the Descemet's membrane. These splits produce faint white lines on the cornea. The cornea is also hazy or oedematous, and the corneal oedema causes photophobia. The characteristic

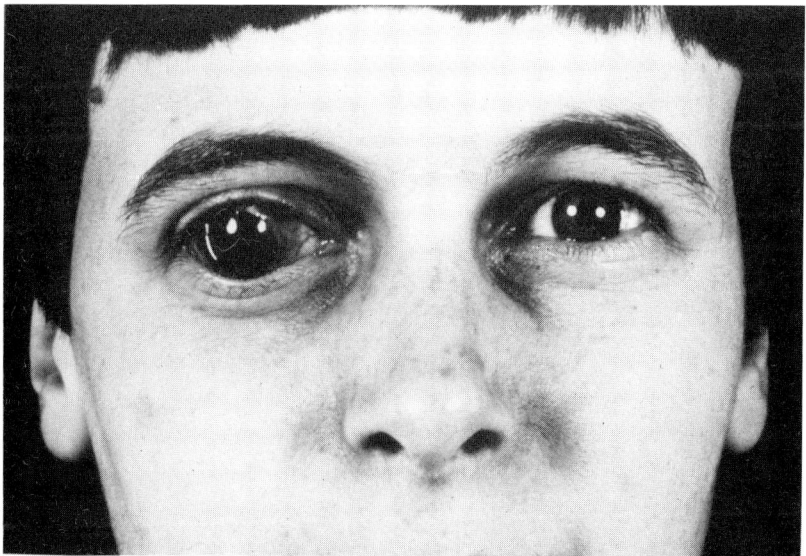

Fig. 14.6 Congenital glaucoma in the right eye.

presenting symptoms of congenital glaucoma are in fact photophobia and the large eye.

Congenital glaucoma is usually bilateral, but one eye is often more diseased than the other. It is important to examine an infant very closely under general anaesthetic, and to check the intraocular pressure before diagnosing congenital glaucoma. It is usual to give pilocarpine drops and acetazolamide to lower the intraocular pressure before surgery. The treatment is then to incise the mesodermal membrane in the angle of the anterior chamber. This technique is called 'goniotomy'.

The prevention of blindness from glaucoma

Glaucoma, and especially open angle glaucoma, is an important cause of blindness all over the world, especially in old people and blacks. Early detection is the only way to prevent blindness from open angle glaucoma. In this way, patients can receive treatment before they have become almost blind. However, even in areas with good ophthalmic services, patients sometimes go blind from glaucoma. Planning an early detection scheme for glaucoma in an area with too few doctors is therefore a serious challenge, and must involve non-specialists.

Sometimes patients do not seek early treatment because they mistake glaucoma for cataract. (It is not usual to treat cataracts surgically until the vision is considerably reduced.) Old patients with glaucoma often wait until they are almost blind before they come for treatment.

The best way to screen for glaucoma is to examine the optic disc with an ophthalmoscope, and to measure the intraocular pressure. It is possible to measure the intraocular pressure either with a portable applanation tonometer or a Schiotz tonometer (see Fig. 3.12). Both of these instruments are fairly cheap, and can be used by non-specialists. A screening test for glaucoma should be part of the routine eye test for any patient over forty. Relatives of glaucoma patients and people over sixty are especially at risk.

It is impossible to prevent angle closure attacks, which come on suddenly in otherwise normal eyes. However, it is simple to perform an iridectomy operation. This guarantees complete protection from acute glaucoma to the second eye.

15.   Onchocerciasis and Loaisis

Onchocerciasis is a parasitic disease caused by the filarial worm, *Onchocerca volvulus*. Large numbers of larval microfilaria are found in the skin and eye, and it is these microfilaria which produce the symptoms. *Fig.* 15.1 shows where onchocerciasis is found. The main focus is in the savanna zone of West Africa, spreading across Central Africa and into the Yemen. Onchocerciasis is also a problem in parts of Central America, and may have arrived with the slave trade.

Onchocerciasis is spread by the black biting fly, Simulium damnosum. This fly breeds in fast flowing rivers, and explains why the disease is commonly called 'river blindness'. Local names for onchocerciasis often describe the symptoms. For example, 'craw – craw' in West Africa describes the itching of the skin; 'sowda' (black) in the Yemen describes the increased pigmentation.

About half a million people in the world are blind or partially blind from onchocerciasis, and up to 50 million have some symptoms. Onchocerciasis is a problem mainly in isolated and rural communities in less developed countries. For this reason, attempts to eradicate the disease have made little progress until recently. However, WHO has now organized control and research programmes, and is especially active in the Volta river basin, one of the most heavily infected areas.

The life cycle of Onchocerca volvulus in man and the Simulium fly (*see Fig.* 15.2)

The adult worms are mainly found in the subcutaneous tissues, but they may also occur in deep structures. Several worms usually coil together in a mass surrounded by fibrous tissue, and are called an 'onchocercoma'. The male is about 4 cm long and 0.2 mm in diameter. The female is larger, up to 40 cm long and 0.4 mm in diameter. The worms may live for up to 20 years, and during that time the female produces living larvae (microfilaria) which are 300 μ long and 8 μ wide. These microfilaria can live for up to a year in the human host.

The microfilaria move actively, and spread throughout the skin and into the eye by their own movements. They are often found in the urine and sputum of infected patients, and almost certainly spread into the bloodstream and lymphatics also. If the microfilaria remain in the human host, they die without further development. They must pass through the insect vector to complete their life cycle.

The insect vector is a biting black fly of the genus Simulium which is commonly called the 'buffalo gnat'. Different species can carry the disease, but the most important species is Simulium damnosum. The fly lays its eggs in well-oxygenated

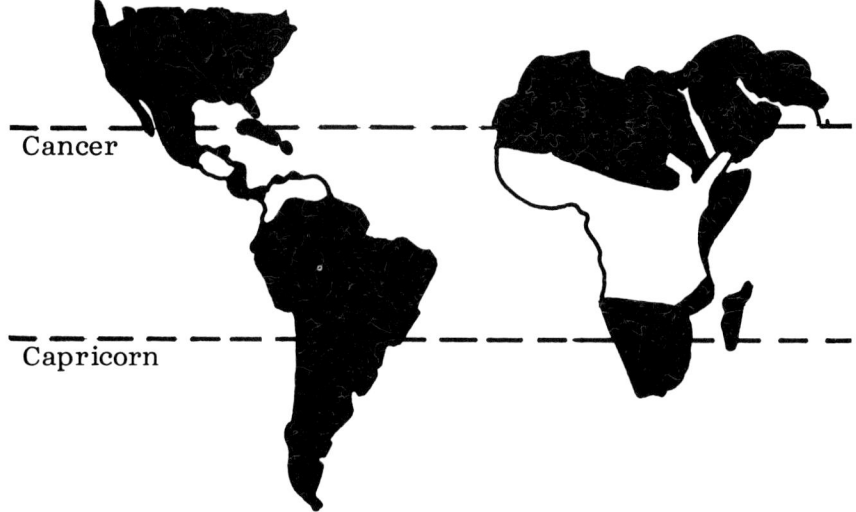

Fig. 15.1 Areas of the world where onchocerciasis is found (shown in white).

water, such as fast flowing rivers and streams. Here larvae hatch and eventually develop into adult flies.

Female flies feed on human blood. They feed during the day, and they cut the skin open in a messy way which explains the description 'open-cast mining'. If the fly feeds on blood from an infected person, it may also ingest some microfilaria. These microfilaria can escape digestion by migrating to the thoracic muscle of the fly. Over a period of about a week, the microfilaria undergo further development, and migrate from the thoracic muscle to the haemocele in the head of the fly. They are now infective microfilaria, and are ready to enter another human host when the Simulium fly bites again.

It is not at all clear how the infective microfilaria develop into adult worms in the human host. Somehow the worms congregate, the female is fertilised and starts to produce microfilaria. People who live or work in areas where the black biting fly and the disease are found are at risk of contracting onchocerciasis. The risk increases with the number of infected flies in the area.

Clinical signs and symptoms

The symptoms of onchocerciasis are caused much more by the microscopic larval microfilaria than by the adult worms. These microfilaria may be found all over the body. However, they are concentrated in the skin and the eye, and it is here that they cause the most damage. People who are heavily infected can often tolerate the living microfilaria surprisingly well. It seems to be the dead microfilaria which cause inflammation and the characteristic symptoms.

It is usual to consider onchocerciasis a disease of the eye and skin. However, heavily infected people have lower than average body weight, and there is often some regional lymphadenopathy.

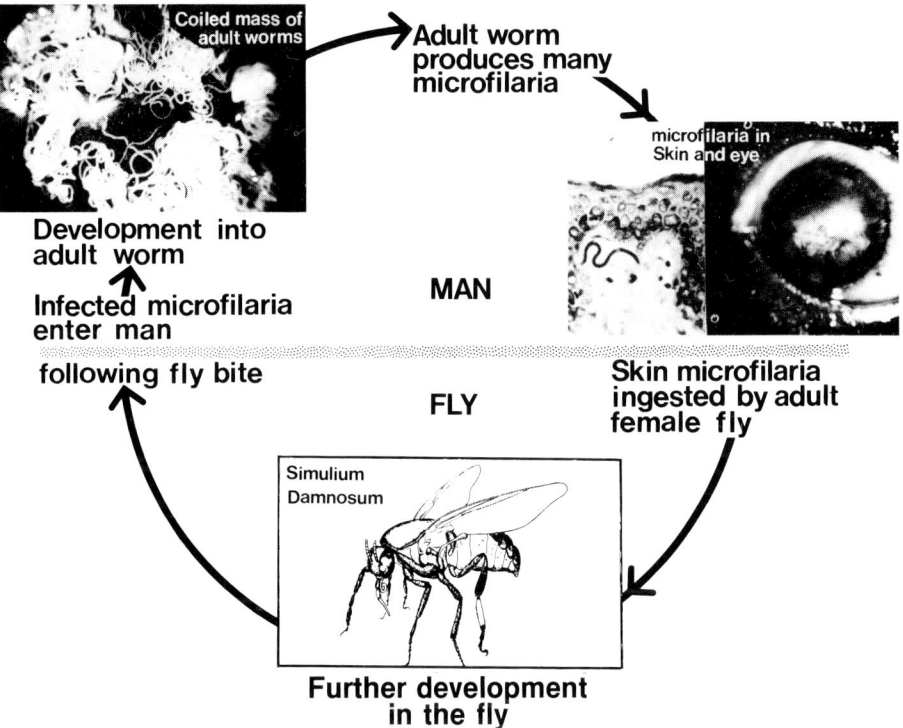

Fig. 15.2 The life cycle of Onchocerca volvulus.

Skin changes

1. Onchocercomata are collections of adult worms, coiled together and surrounded by fibrous tissue (*Figs.* 15.2 *and* 15.3). These onchocercomata are firm, well-defined, subcutaneous nodules. They vary from 0.5 to 10 cm in diameter, are painless and rarely produce any other symptoms. An average adult in a highly infected area might have about ten of these nodules. In Africa, the nodules are usually around the pelvis and on the body, and only occasionally on the limbs, head and neck. In Central America, however, about half of the nodules are on the head and neck. It is not yet known what percentage of the total adult worm load is in these nodules, and what percentage lies free in the subcutaneous tissues or in deeper structures, where they cannot be palpated. Adult worms may also occur in other sites such as the brain, and this would explain the association of onchocerciasis with epilepsy.

2. Dermatitis usually causes itching, which can vary from being mild to very severe and persistent. A number of skin changes may occur: –
   i. A papular rash is especially associated with itching, and the skin may show scratch marks (*Fig.* 15.4). Dead microfilaria in the dermis produce an inflammatory reaction, which then causes a papular rash.

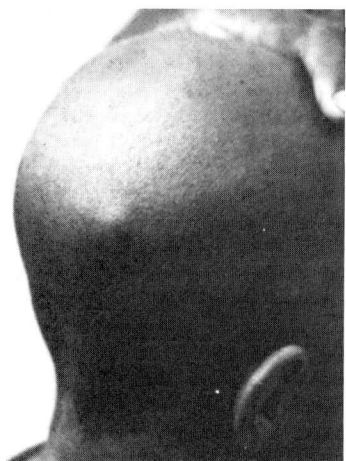

Fig. 15.3
Onchocercal nodule on the head.

 ii. Patchy depigmentation (or 'leopard skin') usually presents on the shin, but it may present anywhere on the legs or the genitalia (*See Fig.* 15.5). This patchy depigmentation is not diagnostic of the disease, but is very common in patients with long-standing onchocerciasis.

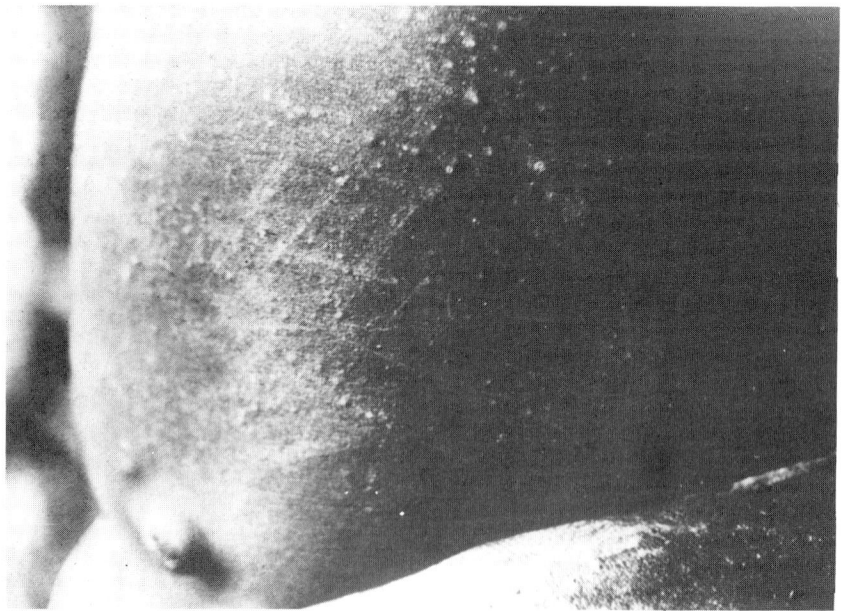

Fig. 15.4 A papular rash, and scratch marks.

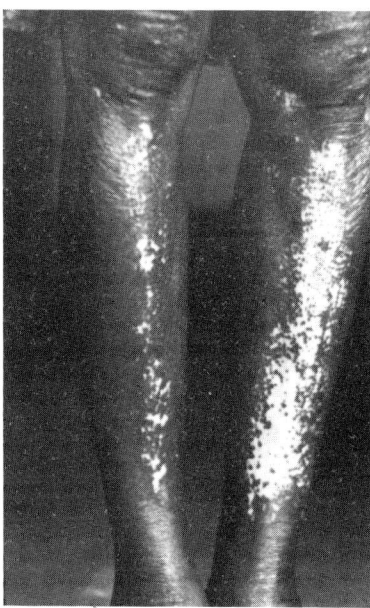

Fig. 15.5 Patchy depigmentation of the shin.

   iii. Atrophy and scaling of the skin (or 'lizard skin') is especially common on
      the buttocks and thighs. Sometimes the whole skin changes, and gives the
      appearance of early ageing (*Fig.* 15.6).
   iv. Lymphoedema makes the skin thick and oedematous, so it looks like the
      skin of an orange. There may be greater tissue oedema especially in the
      groin. This is called 'hanging groin', and is associated with chronic
      inflammation of the inguinal nodes.

Eye changes

The microfilaria are found in nearly every part of the eye, but it is not certain how
exactly they enter. One route is likely to be from the skin and conjunctiva into the
cornea. It is also probable that they enter from the periocular tissues, along the
ciliary vessels and nerves. Another possibility is that the microfilaria enter the eye
in the bloodstream or the cerebrospinal fluid along the optic nerve sheath.

There is a great difference between the presence of living microfilaria, and the
inflammatory reaction which they apparently produce when they die. It is quite
common to see an eye which contains many microfilaria, but which shows very
little evidence of inflammation. The pathological changes develop slowly. Even in
an area which is heavily infested with Onchocerca volvulus, it usually takes many
years of exposure to cause serious visual loss.

Most of the early changes in the anterior chamber need a slit lamp to see them
properly, but the advanced changes are visible to the naked eye. An
ophthalmoscope will show the changes in the fundus.

The clinical signs in the different parts of the eye are as follows: –

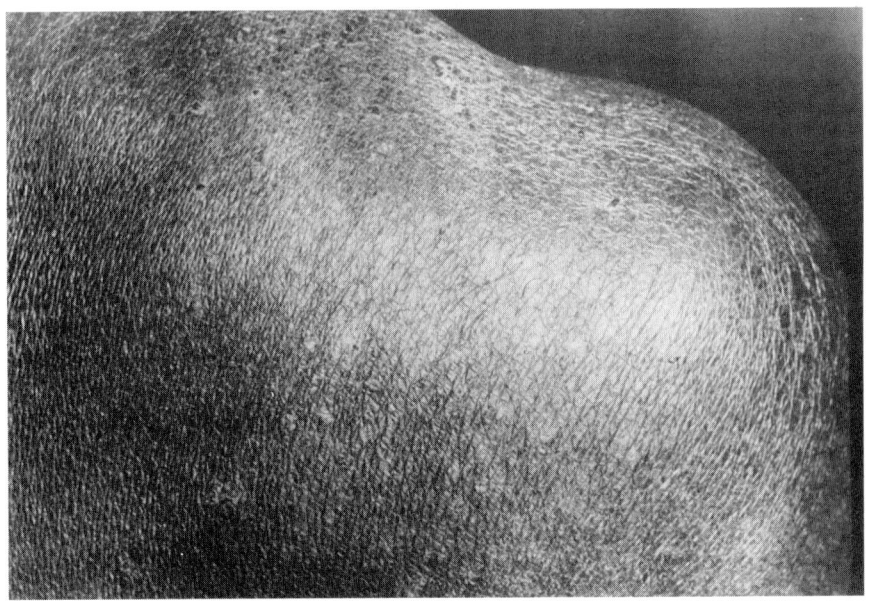

Fig. 15.6 'Lizard skin' atrophy of the back.

— The cornea may contain large numbers of living microfilaria. They are usually
   only visible with a slit lamp at high magnification and with retro-illumination.
   Dead microfilaria are slightly more obvious than living ones. Moreover, soon
   after death an inflammatory reaction around the larva produces a small, faint
   punctate opacity in the stroma of the cornea. This opacity is up to 0.5 mm in
   diameter, and usually requires a slit lamp to see it. However, with good
   illumination, it is just occasionally visible using a hand lens, or even the naked
   eye. These are called 'snowflake', 'fluffy' or 'cracked-ice' opacities after their
   appearance (*Plate* 21c), and will apparently disappear without scarring.

   Patients who have been exposed to heavy infestation of microfilaria for a
   long time develop a pattern of corneal scarring called 'sclerosing keratitis'.
   This scarring is mainly peripheral, and is clearly visible to the naked eye,
   especially in the interpalpebral fissure and the lower cornea. Sometimes the
   scarring spreads to the centre and may eventually cover the whole cornea.
   There is often irregular pigmentation associated with the scarring (*Plate* 21d
   and e. *Fig.* 15.2 also shows advanced sclerosing keratitis). It may also be
   possible to see calcification and other secondary changes. It is uncertain
   whether the changes of sclerosing keratitis are due to the death of individual
   microfilaria, or are a reaction to the large numbers of living microfilaria.

   Patients with sclerosing keratitis usually have a very strongly positive skin
   snip (*see below*), but in old patients the microfilaria may have died.

   Sclerosing keratitis may be confused with other corneal diseases (*see*
   Chapter 20, page 229).

   If the whole cornea is scarred, the inner eye is also likely to be damaged.

Corneal grafting cannot help such an eye.
- The anterior chamber often contains living microfilaria, which move vigorously. These microfilaria may adhere either to the endothelium of the cornea, or occasionally to the lens. They may also be visible in the anterior vitreous body behind the lens. It is sometimes possible to increase the number of microfilaria in the anterior chamber by asking the patient to bend his head down between his knees for one minute.

  It really needs a slit lamp to see these microfilaria. However they can sometimes just be seen with an ophthalmoscope if a slit lamp is not available. Hold the ophthalmoscope very close to the patient's eye using a + 25 or + 30 dioptre lens in order to focus on the anterior chamber. If the pupil is dilated, and there are no significant opacities in the cornea or lens, the clear red fundus reflex will appear in the pupil. The microfilaria may be just visible as moving shadows against this red background.
- The lens very rarely contains microfilaria. Even when microfilaria are present, they are probably not responsible for any lens changes or for the formation of a cataract.
- The iris and ciliary body are often inflamed in heavily infected patients. There is nothing specific about this inflammation, but it is usually chronic and non-granulomatous. The usual features of onchocercal iridocyclitis are: –
  - fine pigmented deposits on the back of the cornea, or the front of the lens. (These deposits can usually only be seen with a slit lamp.)
  - atrophy of the iris,
  - irregularity of the pupil, which may be visible to the naked eye (*Plate* 21d).
- Glaucoma is not a common complication, but it may cause blindness. It can develop as a complication of the iridocyclitis, because anterior and posterior synechiae block the pathway for aqueous circulation. Eventually, aqueous production may fall, causing low intraocular pressure (ocular hypotony).

  Glaucoma sometimes occurs in young patients with fairly quiet eyes, but large numbers of microfilaria in the aqueous fluid. These microfilaria probably cause inflammatory changes in the trabecular meshwork which block the aqueous flow. There is no proof of this yet.
- Fundus changes such as choroido-retinal degeneration and optic atrophy are common, and may cause serious visual loss. Both changes appear to be mainly inflammatory reactions to the microfilaria. It is not certain how the microfilaria enter the posterior part of the eye. However, it seems likely that they move from the orbit to the choroid along the scleral canals for the ciliary vessels. Certainly it is at these sites that the choroido-retinal changes usually first appear. Fundus changes are usually bilateral, but not always symmetrical.
- Choroido-retinal atrophy usually starts as a mottling of the retinal pigment epithelium (*Plate* 21f). This mottling may then progress to atrophy of the pigment epithelium, and atrophy of the choroidal capillaries (*Plate* 22a). Increased pigmentation, sub-retinal fibrosis and sheathing of the retinal vessels may also be visible (*Plate* 22b). Typically, the changes first develop lateral to the macula, then spread around, but not usually over, the macula itself. Finally, however, these changes cover the entire posterior retina.

  Onchocercal chorioretinal atrophy may appear similar to senile or degenerative changes in the retina, such as senile macular degeneration (*See*

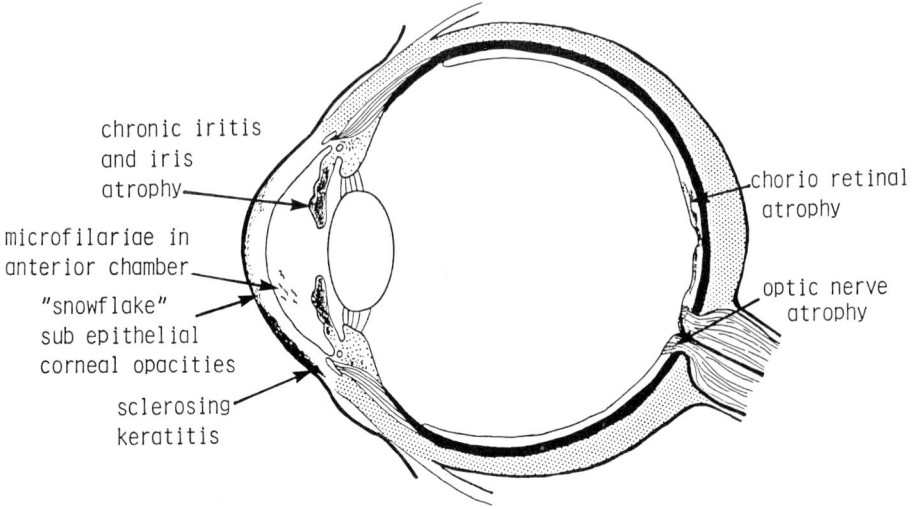

chronic iritis
and iris
atrophy

microfilariae in
anterior chamber

"snowflake"
sub epithelial
corneal opacities

sclerosing
keratitis

chorio retinal
atrophy

optic nerve
atrophy

Fig. 15.7 A summary of the effects of onchocerciasis on the eye.

Plate 19c). Other types of choroiditis produce more localized, well-defined lesions (*See Plate* 14e).
– Optic atrophy. Occasionally there may be active inflammation of the optic nerve called optic neuritis. The inflammation causes swelling and oedema of the optic disc (*Plate* 22c). However, it is more common to see the changes of optic atrophy. The optic disc is pale, indicating atrophy of the optic nerve, and there is also evidence of previous inflammation such as: –
    – gliosis of the disc,
    – sheathing of the retinal vessels,
    – pigmentation around the disc (*Plate* 22b *and* d).
    In a few cases, the optic atrophy may just be secondary to the choroido-retinal degeneration. It is also possible for previous glaucoma (*see above*) to produce secondary optic atrophy. Primary optic atrophy with no signs of any previous inflammation is not usually onchocercal.
– Visual loss (*Fig.* 15.7) may result from pathological changes either in the anterior or the posterior segment of the eye, and often there are changes in both. The changes in the anterior segment of the eye are sclerosing keratitis, and iridocyclitis and its complications. The changes in the posterior part of the eye are choroido-retinal and optic atrophy. These two types of changes are about equally important in causing visual loss.
    In the fundus, choroido-retinal atrophy is usually more obvious than optic atrophy, but optic atrophy is probably a more important cause of visual loss. This visual loss can follow any pattern. Most commonly, however, the optic nerve fibres which go to the peripheral retina are damaged, and cause constriction of the visual fields ('tunnel vision') and night blindness. If there is only choroido-retinal atrophy, and the optic nerve is healthy, the macula and the peripheral retina may be undamaged, and some useful vision may remain.
    Any kind of visual loss from onchocerciasis is nearly always irreversible.

Diagnosis

In advanced cases, the characteristic changes in the eye and skin are enough to make a clinical diagnosis. However, it is often necessary to demonstrate the microfilaria or the adult worms in less advanced cases. It is especially important in younger patients, who may be quite severely infested without any obvious clinical changes.

There are a number of different methods of demonstrating the microfilaria. Some of these methods can also indicate how severe the infection is. This is very important both for the treatment and the prognosis.

A slit lamp can be used to see the microfilaria in the eye. It is easier to see living microfilaria moving in the anterior chamber, or dead microfilaria in the cornea.

A 'skin snip' examination is the best laboratory test for onchocerciasis (*Fig.* 15.8). In this test, a small piece of skin is suspended in water or saline. After a few minutes, the microfilaria emerge, and it is possible to see them moving actively under the low power of a microscope.

It is only necessary to excise a small piece of skin (1 mg). However, the sample should include the outer part of the dermal papillae, where the microfilaria are most concentrated. There should therefore be faint blood staining of the wound after a few seconds. If possible, take samples from more than one site. A skin snip from just outside the lateral canthus will give the best indication how many microfilaria are in the eye. Another recommended site is the iliac crest. In Africa, this is the area with the highest concentration of microfilaria. Raise the skin with

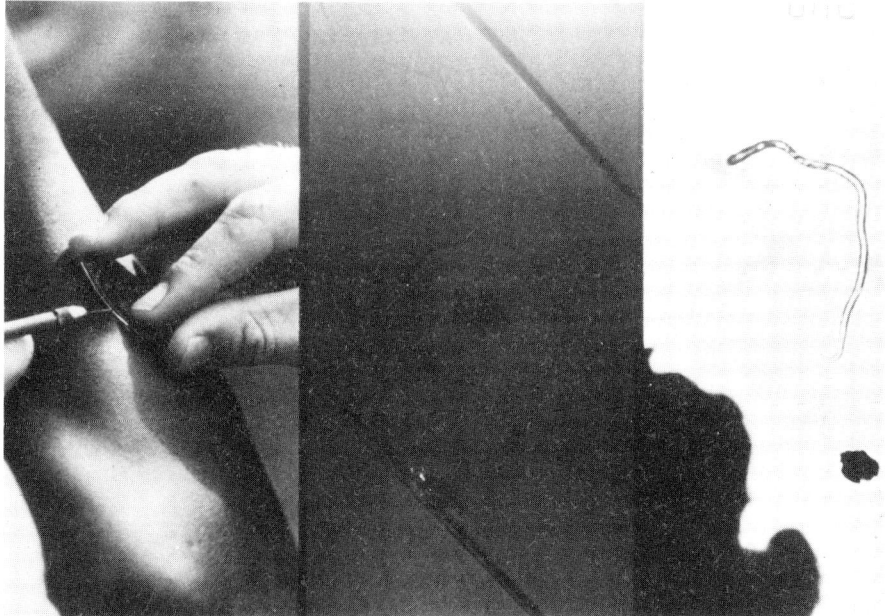

Fig. 15.8 A skin snip: –
a. Taking the skin with a needle and razor blade
b. Mounting the skin on a microscope slide
c. A microfilaria emerging from the skin under the microscope

the point of a needle, and cut a tiny fragment with a blade, fine scissors, or with a corneoscleral punch. Leave the fragment on a slide in a drop of normal saline. If no microfilaria have emerged after a few minutes, tease the skin sample and re-examine it after half an hour. It is possible to adapt this method and use it for counting the numbers of microfilaria.

Unfortunately, other microfilaria may be present in the skin, especially Dipetalonema streptocerca. These other filarial worms do not seem to produce any specific pathological changes in the body. To identify the microfilaria, it may be necessary to stain them and examine them under the high power of a microscope.

The Mazotti test assesses the concentration of microfilaria by the patient's reaction to the drug diethylcarbamazine (DEC). A dose of 50 mg kills the microfilaria and produces a reaction in the patient. Patients with slight infections have mild reactions. However, as the number of microfilaria increase, so the reaction becomes more severe. Within an hour after taking the drug, a patient with many microfilaria will begin to react strongly. At first there is itching, which may progress to erythema, and often progresses to skin oedema and a papular eruption. In severe reactions, there is fever, malaise, headache, joint pains and lymphadenopathy. The reaction subsides after $1-2$ days. It is not certain whether the microfilaria become antigenic and so stimulate an inflammatory response, or whether their increased movement causes the reaction.

The Mazotti test is both specific and sensitive, and is useful in cases where the diagnosis is not clear. There is usually no such uncertainty in heavily infected patients, however, and the test should not be necessary. If it is performed for any reason, a smaller dose is recommended to lessen the reaction.

It is sometimes possible to demonstrate microfilaria in the urine by giving a small dose (25 mg) of DEC.

Histological examination of tissue from a skin nodule will detect adult worms.

Epidemiology

According to numerous surveys, very nearly 100% of the population in hyperendemic areas suffer from onchocerciasis which they acquire at an early age. Significant visual loss from the disease is rare below the age of 15, but the incidence rises gradually with age. Moreover, males are more likely to develop visual loss than females.

The usual definition of blindness is visual acuity worse than counting fingers at 3 metres. By that definition, in a typically hyperendemic area, 5% of the whole community will be blind, and 30% of males over 40. This very high incidence of blindness is in fact found in particular areas of the savanna zone of West Africa. However, blindness rates vary very much from community to community. In the forest zone of West Africa, the black biting fly is just as common, and the incidence of onchocerciasis about the same as in the savanna zone. However, the blindness rate is usually much lower (1.5%) and often not much more than in non-onchocercal areas. Similarly, in America, the incidence of blindness from onchocerciasis is higher in Guatemala than in Venezuela. Even between neighbouring villages, both the infection and blindness rates are often very different.

It is not always clear why the incidence and severity of the disease should vary so much in different communities. However, many different factors are important in the life cycle of the parasite. Obviously, even a slight alteration to one of these factors can change the local pattern of the disease. For example, neighbouring villages may have different infection rates because one village is nearer to a breeding site for the fly. Then again, clothing, especially thick clothing, is likely to give some protection.

Onchocerciasis is spread by different species of Simulium, and some of these are more efficient vectors than others. In Guatemala, the main vector is Simulium ochraceum. This species prefers to bite man rather than animals, and prefers the upper parts of the body. In Venezuela, however, the fly Simulium metallicum bites man and animals but prefers the lower parts of the body. In some parts of Africa, the vector is Simulium naevei, a species which is easier to eradicate than Simulium damnosum.

There is also evidence that there are different strains of onchocerca, and that some of them are more virulent than others. This may explain why the disease is more severe in the savanna areas of Africa. The climate too may be an important factor. Certainly in the savanna, the cornea is more exposed to sunlight, dust and drying, and sclerosing keratitis is more severe. Males possibly have a higher incidence of blindness because they are more likely to work outside in the fields. However, this is not true in all communities, and it may be that men have a specific susceptibility to onchocerciasis. Racial and nutritional differences between communities may also be important factors, but there is no direct evidence for this.

Immunology

The immunological responses of the body to the parasite are not fully understood. It seems likely that there is a reaction to the adult worms, because they are usually surrounded by inflammatory and fibrous tissue. However, the microfilaria have a protective mechanism against the host antibodies and do not seem to provoke an inflammatory reaction until they die. DEC does not apparently kill microfilaria *in vitro*. Presumably it kills them in the body by interfering in some way with the protective mechanism. Even a small dose of DEC seems to be enough to make the microfilaria antigenic, and this in turn stimulates the rapid and severe reaction in the body.

The immunological reaction of the body to the infective microfilaria transmitted from the fly is even less clear. It is not certain how many of these infective microfilaria survive the body defences to develop into adult worms.

It is possible that microfilaria in pregnant women may invade the fetus across the placenta. This would change the immunological reaction to later infection by the parasite.

Treatment

Blindness is by far the most important feature of onchocerciasis. Most of the pathological changes in the eye are irreversible, and so the basic aim of treatment is to stop the disease and prevent any further loss of sight. To stop the disease, it is necessary to kill as many of the adult worms and microfilaria as possible.

The traditional treatment for onchocerciasis is a course of DEC and suramin.

DEC kills the microfilaria, but not the adult worms. Suramin kills the adult worms and some of the microfilaria. Unfortunately, drug treatment has many serious problems.

DEC is in itself a relatively non-toxic drug. It seems to kill the microfilaria by interfering with their protective mechanism against the host antibodies. Without this protection the microfilaria die, and it is the dying microfilaria which stimulate the reaction in the body. The usual course of treatment starts with a daily dose of 50 mg The dose gradually increases during the first week to at least 250 mg twice daily, and then continues for about two more weeks. Heavily infected patients usually suffer severe side effects after taking DEC. For this reason, these people should also receive systemic steroid therapy to suppress the worst of the side effects. If possible, start giving a daily dose of 20 mg of prednisone the day before the DEC is given, and continue for a week. Antihistamines may also be helpful. However, even with all these precautions, there is always a risk that the sudden death of many microfilaria may precipitate further damage to the eye.

DEC may clear the body of microfilaria, but there is no real benefit if the adult worms continue to produce microfilaria. To be really effective, it is also necessary to kill the adult worms. Intravenous injections of 1 gm of suramin, given weekly for four weeks will kill most adult worms and microfilaria. However, suramin is a very toxic drug. It can produce nausea, circulatory collapse, renal damage and even death. For this reason, it should only be given after a previous course of DEC has effectively cleared the body of microfilaria, and after all reactions have subsided. It should not be given to debilitated patients, and the following precautions are also advisable: –
– Give a small test dose first.
– Give all the injections very slowly.
– Check the urine for albumin.

Fig. 15.9 summarises the drug treatment for onchocerciasis.

According to all the available evidence, a course of DEC and suramin succeeds

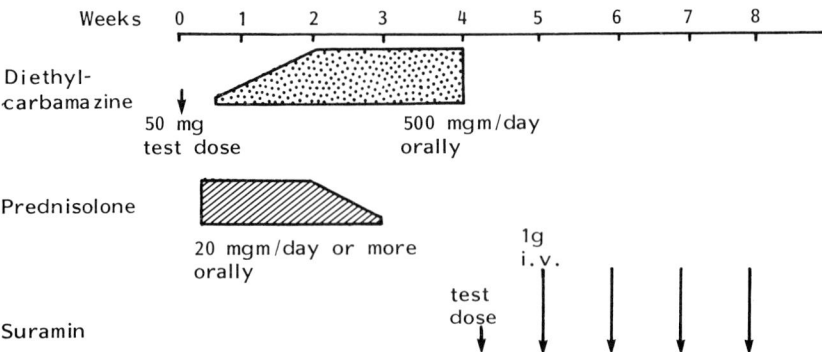

Fig. 15.9 The drug treatment of onchocerciasis.

fairly well either in stopping, or at least slowing down the progress of visual damage. This is true even for patients who live in areas where there is a risk of re-infection. However, the treatment is long, uncomfortable and dangerous, and so is not suitable for everyone with onchocerciasis. It is unsuitable for patients who are already blind, and for patients who are only lightly infected and are unlikely to develop eye complications. The group most suitable for treatment are patients who are heavily infected, but who have no significant eye damage. It is often difficult to decide whether or not to treat patients who are heavily infected and already have some eye damage. Without treatment, eye damage in these patients is most likely to deteriorate. With treatment, the sudden death of many microfilaria in already damaged tissues is most likely to cause complications.

There is an urgent need for new and more effective drugs to treat onchocerciasis. At present, several new drugs for onchocerciasis are being tested. The most promising are ivermectin and flubendazole. They appear to have some action in stopping the adult worms producing microfilaria. Therefore their action lasts longer than DEC, and there are less side effects from the sudden death of many microfilaria. Ivermectin is given orally, and flubendazole by intramuscular injection.

In certain areas, it is the practice to excise onchocercal nodules. This is called 'nodulectomy'. Nodulectomy is probably worth while in areas where most of the onchocercomata are on the head and neck. Otherwise it is probably not beneficial.

Patients who have onchocerciasis and glaucoma are especially difficult to treat. There is a high risk that the death of the microfilaria may make the glaucoma worse. It is best to give local steroid treatment to the eye. If the glaucoma does not respond, it may then be advisable to perform glaucoma surgery. Only then can medical treatment begin.

Onchocerciasis control programmes

Blindness from onchocerciasis is only a problem in certain, fairly limited areas of the world. However, the personal suffering which it causes is enormous, and so there is an urgent need for programmes to control the disease. Because the drug treatment for onchocerciasis is so unsatisfactory, there is little chance of eradicating the parasite in the human host. Most control programmes therefore try to control the insect vector.

At the moment, a lot of effort and money is going into a programme of Simulium fly control in the Volta River basin. The Simulium fly breeds in fast flowing rivers, and the fly larvae feed on particles in the water. By spraying the breeding sites of the fly with insecticide in particle form, it should be possible to eradicate the new generation of flies, and so interrupt the life cycle of Onchocerca volvulus. Unfortunately, the Simulium fly can travel distances of up to 50 miles. This means that any programme must cover a large area to be effective. Another problem is that the adult worms can live for up to 20 years. The programme must therefore continue for a long time before no active carriers of the disease remain.

An alternative scheme is still in the experimental stage. In this scheme, long-term doses of DEC are used to control the number of microfilaria in the body. There is less damage to the tissues, and the disease is more difficult to transmit. DEC may also kill the infective microfilaria. DEC eye drops are also being tested.

One challenge in onchocerciasis control is to find the appropriate technology. Perhaps the greatest challenge, however, is to find suitable skilled workers who are prepared to devote their skills and energy to these unfortunate parts of the world.

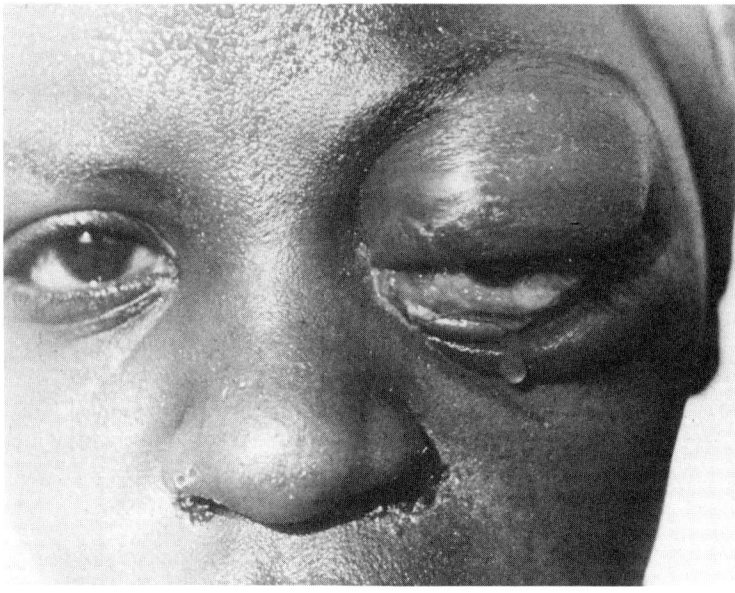

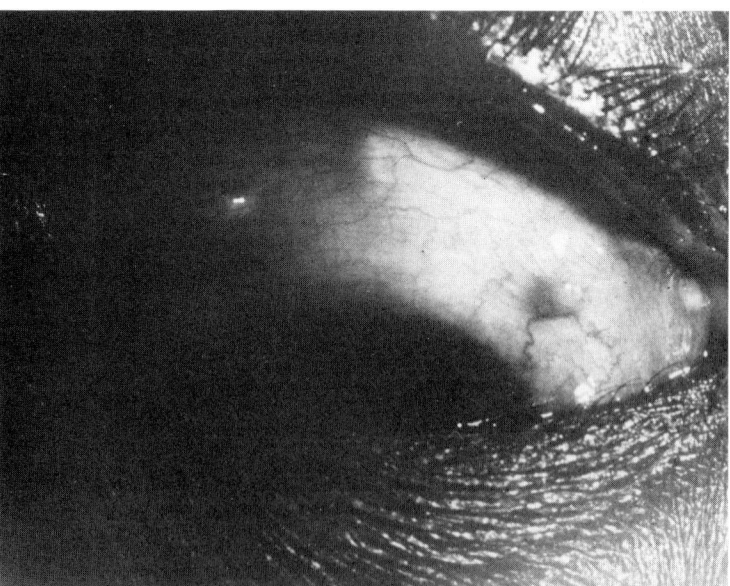

Fig. 15.10 *a*, Calabar swelling. *b*, After a few days the swelling subsided, and the fragments of a dead worm were visible under the conjunctiva.

Loaisis

Loaisis is only found in the equatorial rain forests of Central and West Africa, and it is caused by the filarial worm, Loa loa. It is the only other filarial infection with specific complications in the region of the eye.

The life cycles of Loa loa and Onchocerca volvulus are in many ways similar. A biting fly of the genus Chrysops ingests microfilaria when it bites, and transmits them when it bites another person. The microfilaria develop into adult worms, which move around fairly freely in the connective and subcutaneous tissues. Unlike onchocerciasis, however, it is the adult worms which cause the symptoms, and not the microfilaria.

The Loa loa worms often appear under the conjunctiva (*Plate* 22e). They can move quite vigorously, and may even cause severe pain, irritation or itching. Sometimes the body reacts to the worms with an acute attack of localized inflammatory oedema, called 'Calabar swelling'. A common site for Calabar swelling is the orbit and eyelids, and usually means that the worm is dying. The characteristic feature is a sudden and severe episode of oedema (*Fig.* 15.10), but the patients feel well in themselves. After a few days, the oedema subsides, and the tissues return to normal. Calabar swelling looks alarming, but it does not seem to damage the vision or leave any permanent scarring.

The diagnosis of loaisis is usually obvious from the history and the physical evidence. Blood samples may show variable numbers of microfilaria, and the eosinophil count usually increases, especially during an attack of oedema.

The treatment for loaisis is oral DEC, which kills the microfilaria, and probably the adult worms too. It is wise to start with a small dose and gradually increase to 150 mg 3 times a day for 3 weeks. Sometimes it is possible to catch a worm moving across the conjunctiva. Instill local anaesthetic drops, make a small incision in the conjunctiva and remove the worm with forceps.

For further reading

1. WHO (1974) A. A. Buck, ed. *Onchocerciasis: Symptomology, Pathology and Diagnosis*. Geneva. An overall account of the disease with illustrations.
2. Anderson J. and Fuglsang H., Ocular onchocerciasis. *Tropical Diseases Bulletin* 74 (4): 257 − 272. A review of research and current trends on the disease.

16. Leprosy and the Eye

Leprosy is a chronic infectious disease caused by *Mycobacterium leprae*. The disease was known and feared in ancient times, but the cause remained unknown until in 1873, Hansen, a Norwegian doctor, first demonstrated the bacteria which cause the disease. For this reason, leprosy is sometimes called 'Hansen's disease'.

There are probably at least ten million leprosy patients in the world, mainly in Africa, Asia and South America. The highest incidence is in Central and West Africa, but the disease is also common in East Africa and the Indian sub-continent. Leprosy involves the eyes more frequently than any other systemic disease, and often leads to blindness.

It is still not clear how leprosy is contracted. However, in most cases there is close contact, usually in childhood, with an active 'open' case. These open cases may excrete large numbers of organisms, especially in their nasal discharges. There are a number of possible theories as to how the organisms may enter the body. They may enter directly through the skin. They may be inhaled as droplets in the air. It is just possible that the organisms are carried by mosquitoes or biting flies, but there is no proof of this.

It seems that the organisms can only survive at temperatures below the normal body temperature, and so prefer the surface tissues. After they have entered the body, the organisms multiply and spread in the superficial nerves (especially the Schwann cells), the skin, and superficial organs such as the testis, nose, mouth and eye. In the eye, the organism is only found in the anterior parts — the iris, cornea, sclera and eyelids.

The incubation period before symptoms appear seems to be 2 – 7 years. When symptoms do eventually occur, the clinical appearance varies very much according to the cell mediated immunity (CMI) of the patient towards the organism (*Fig.* 16.1): –

– In patients whose CMI is low, the organisms spread and multiply throughout the tissues. They are engulfed, but not killed by the macrophages. This is the clinical picture of lepromatous leprosy.

– At the other extreme, where the CMI is high, there is a localized inflammatory reaction in the infected tissues, with thickening of the superficial nerves and depigmentation of the skin. A histological examination will reveal very few organisms, or none at all. This is the clinical picture of tuberculoid leprosy. (In people whose resistance is very high, the disease may even heal itself spontaneously without producing any symptoms or signs at all. Many people in endemic areas have probably overcome an infection with leprosy in this way.)

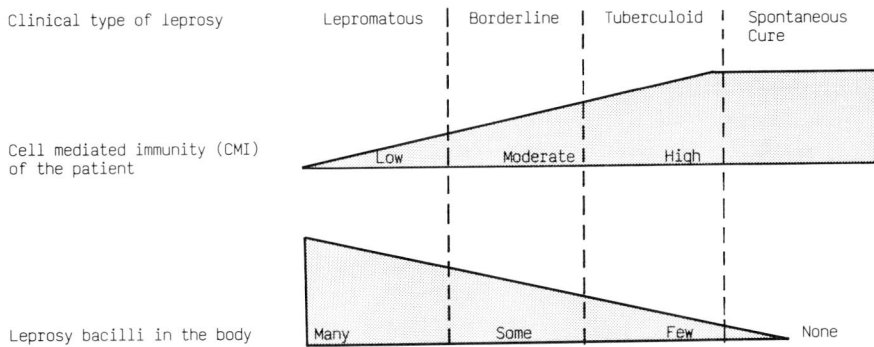

Fig. 16.1 A diagram to show the different types of leprosy and the immune reactions of the patient.

— Most patients are somewhere between these two extremes of tuberculoid and lepromatous leprosy, and may show varying degrees of resistance to the organism. These are called 'borderline cases'. Leprosy specialists divide these borderline cases into several different sub-groups. There is 'borderline lepromatous' leprosy which tends towards the lepromatous end of the spectrum, and 'borderline tuberculoid' which tends towards the tuberculoid end of the spectrum. There is also 'borderline borderline' in the middle.
— One common and important feature of leprosy is called the 'reactional state'. There are several different types, but in all of them the symptoms fairly suddenly become worse. They are usually caused by changes in the CMI, and may occur spontaneously or during treatment. As far as the eye is concerned, the two important changes produced by a 'reactional state' are a facial palsy and acute iritis.

Since the introduction of dapsone (DDS) in 1940, effective chemotherapy has been available for leprosy. The standard dose is 50 – 100 mg per day for several years in tuberculoid cases, and probably for life in lepromatous cases. Dapsone is still the basic drug for treating leprosy, but other newer drugs are often used as well, especially rifampicin, and clofazimine. Clofazimine has slight anti-inflammatory properties also, but unfortunately it causes a reddish discoloration of the skin and conjunctiva. For patients towards the lepromatous end of the spectrum more than one drug should be given to prevent drug resistance.

The basis of modern leprosy control is early diagnosis and treatment. By identifying and treating open active cases in the early stages, there is less danger that leprosy will spread in the community. There is also less danger that the patient will suffer the severe mutilation of long standing leprosy. The most exciting prospect for leprosy control in the future is the development of a vaccine. The organism has recently been grown in the armadillo, and a vaccine produced. Local trials of this vaccine are now being carried out.

Eye changes in leprosy

Leprosy does not always involve the eye, and so not all leprosy patients have ocular leprosy. The lowest reported incidence of ocular leprosy is 6%, while the highest is 90% of all leprosy patients. There are many reasons for this wide variation: –

– Patients who have had leprosy for a long time are more likely to develop complications. The complication rate in chronic patients in a leprosy settlement is therefore much higher than in a group of less advanced cases who are receiving treatment as out-patients. Earlier diagnosis and more effective treatment of leprosy in recent years has lowered the incidence of ocular complications and blindness.
– The clinical pattern of leprosy may differ from area to area.
– Many of the early eye changes are not obvious to the naked eye. Some cases of ocular leprosy can only be diagnosed by a careful examination with a slit lamp.

In areas where leprosy is endemic, it is essential for anyone seeing eye patients to know the eye signs of leprosy. This is because undiagnosed leprosy patients may first present with eye lesions. It is equally essential for anyone seeing leprosy patients to know the eye signs. This is because it is especially important to care for the eyes of known leprosy patients to prevent blindness.

Early diagnosis is essential for leprosy. Unfortunately, the early changes are as difficult to detect in the eye as in the rest of the body. The advanced changes are obvious, but by then the damage is irreversible. (One study in the USA found that patients who first went to the doctor with eye symptoms waited an average of 6 years before leprosy was correctly diagnosed!)

The word 'leprosy' always makes patients feel anxious and afraid, and the course of treatment is long. For both these reasons, in doubtful early cases it may be wise to wait until a second opinion, further investigations or the progress of the disease itself confirms the diagnosis.

There are a number of specific eye changes in leprosy: –

Loss of eyebrows and eyelashes

This is called 'madarosis' and it is one of the most common eye changes in lepromatous leprosy. Madarosis is usually symmetrical and it is more common in the lateral part of the eyebrows (*Fig.* 16.2). Loss of the eyelashes is slightly less frequent (*Plate* 22f).

Skin changes

In lepromatous leprosy, the facial skin may be diffusely thickened and inflamed, or there may be nodules on the skin. These changes are often found on the eyelids or the eyebrows. After treatment, baggy folds of skin may persist on the lids or brows.

Facial nerve palsy (*Figs.* 16.2 – 16.4)

The facial nerve is a motor nerve supplying all the facial muscles and in particular the orbicularis oculi which closes the eyelids. The branches of the facial nerve run fairly superficially under the skin. They are therefore very susceptible to damage, especially in tuberculoid or borderline leprosy. It is common for these, and other superficial nerves, to thicken, and so it is often possible to feel them just under the surface of the skin.

If a facial palsy is unilateral, the whole face is pulled over to the undamaged side, and the defect is usually obvious. However, facial palsy in leprosy is often bilateral and incomplete. This means it only weakens the facial muscles but does not completely paralyse them. Also the face looks symmetrical, and so the clinical changes are much less obvious. The face loses much of its expression and character because of the general weakness of the facial muscles. This is called a 'leprous stare'

The most important defect in a facial palsy is the failure to close the eyelids. This may be obvious in a complete palsy, but in an incomplete palsy, three simple tests will demonstrate the weakness.
- Tell the patient to close the eye gently as in sleep. The eyelids may not come together properly.
- Tell the patient to close the eyes tightly. This will usually reveal any weakness in the orbicularis oculi muscle (*Figs.* 16.2 *and* 16.3).
- In doubtful cases, hold the patient's eyes open, and get him to close his eyes against this resistance.

When a patient with a facial palsy attempts to close his eyes, the eyeball usually turns upwards spontaneously. In this way the cornea is protected under the upper eyelid. This is probably a protective reflex to prevent corneal damage during sleep. It is called 'Bell's phenomenon'.

In a complete facial palsy, the lower eyelid will sag, and may eventually become everted. This is called an ectropion.

Often, the eye waters in facial palsies. The lower eyelid loses its tone and the lower punctum draining the tears does not rest against the eyeball. The pumping action of the orbicularis oculi which helps to drain the tears into the nose is lost. Another reason for a watering eye may be leprosy changes in the nose which obstruct the nasolacrimal duct.

A facial palsy will prevent blinking and this prevents the precorneal tear film from forming. The exposed part of the cornea becomes dry, and is therefore very susceptible to damage. The eye may also be dry because occasionally leprosy involves the lacrimal glands.

The conjunctiva

The conjunctiva may show non-specific conjunctivitis or exposure changes.

The cornea

The cornea may show a variety of changes: –
- Beading and thickening of the corneal nerves is an early and specific sign of leprosy which is only visible with the magnification of a slit lamp.
- Punctate keratitis is a similar localized inflammatory reaction to leprosy bacillae in the superficial layers of the cornea.
- Interstitial keratitis is a more extensive inflammatory reaction to leprosy organisms in the corneal stroma. It may subside to leave a diffuse corneal scar or pannus (*Plate* 22f).
- Secondary corneal ulceration and scarring (*Figs.* 16.2 *and* 16.4).
    This is by far the most important cause of corneal changes in leprosy. It occurs because the protective corneal reflexes are damaged or destroyed

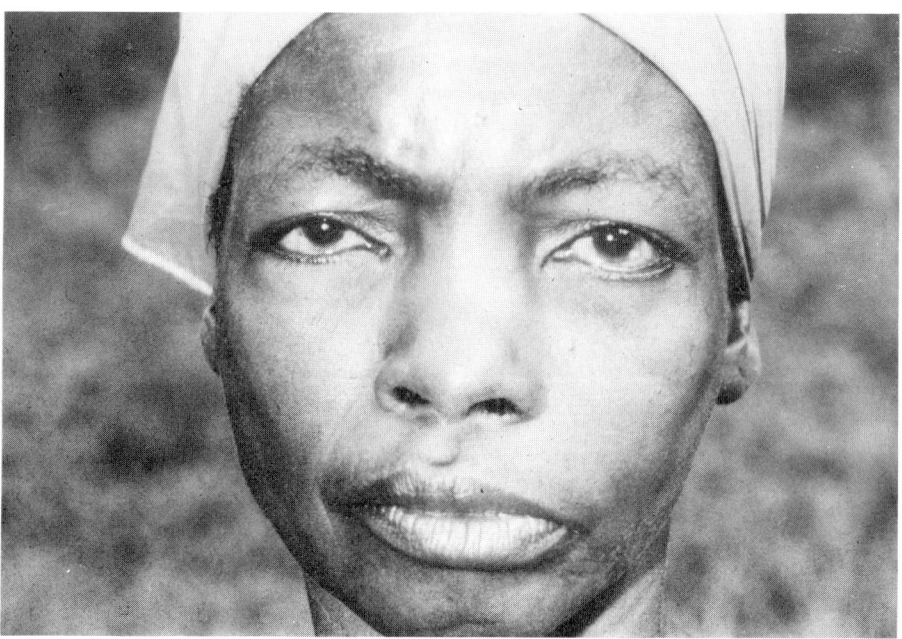

Fig. 16.2 A patient with a partial facial palsy from leprosy. Note that the face appears fairly normal at rest. When the patient attempts to close her eyes the left-sided weakness of the face becomes obvious and the eyelids do not close properly. There is a faint scar at the lower margin of the left cornea. This is from exposure damage.

because leprosy affects the superficial nerves. The fifth cranial nerve (trigeminal nerve) supplies the sensation of the cornea. This is sometimes damaged by leprosy, causing corneal anaesthesia. The loss of corneal sensation destroys the sensory part of the reflex. The facial palsy which prevents blinking and eyelid closure destroys the motor part of the reflex. If there is either corneal anaesthesia or a facial palsy, secondary corneal damage is common. If both are present, then secondary corneal damage is inevitable.

The exposed lower cornea is most at risk. Keratitis and corneal ulceration will progress to corneal scars or total destruction of the eye.

The iris

Iritis is also a common and damaging ocular complication, especially of lepromatous leprosy. The first sign that leprosy bacilli have spread into the iris is usually that the dilator muscle becomes too weak to oppose the action of the sphincter muscle. The pupil therefore becomes progressively more and more constricted (*Plate* 22f). Whitish lepromatous nodules may appear on the iris, which are probably diagnostic of leprosy. They are called 'iris pearls'. There may also be a chronic granulomatous iridocyclitis with 'mutton fat' keratic precipitates on the back of the cornea. All these changes occur slowly and insidiously in a quiet, white eye.

However, acute iritis often develops in lepromatous leprosy as a reaction between systemic antibodies and antigen, which is released when the micro-

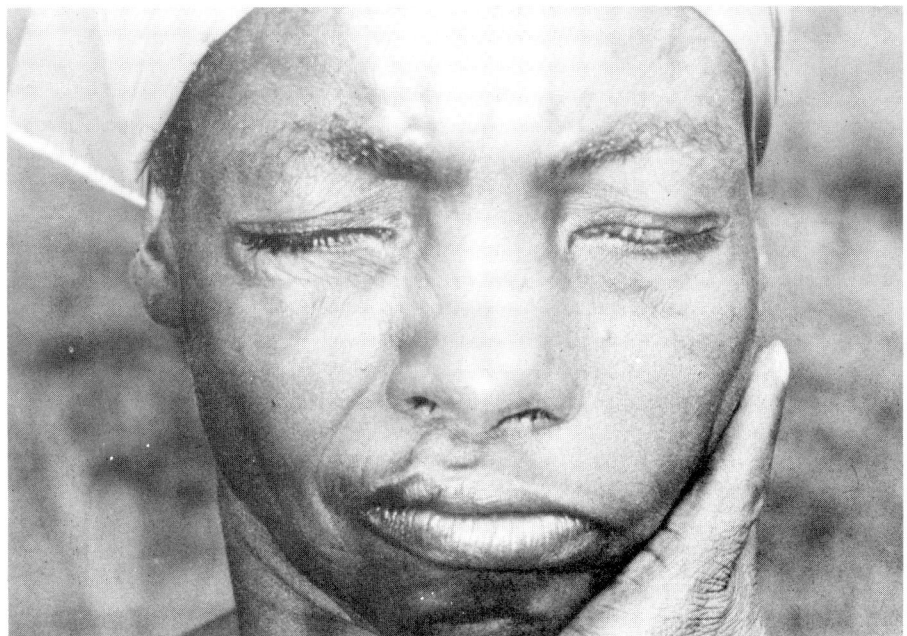

Fig. 16.3 Note the asymmetry of the face when the same patient tries to close her eyes. The left eyelids do not close properly.

organisms break up. This reaction often occurs during treatment, but it may occur in untreated cases. There is an acute iridocyclitis with a red painful eye, ciliary vasodilatation, and protein exudate and inflammatory cells in the anterior chamber. Any of the complications of acute iritis may develop e.g. secondary glaucoma, pupil block and iris bombé, diminished secretions of aqueous fluid, and phthisis bulbi.

Other eye changes

Any part of the anterior segment of the eye may be invaded by the leprosy bacilli, and show inflammatory or degenerative changes. Scleritis and episcleritis are often found (*Plate* 22f). Nodules in the sclera may occur in lepromatous leprosy. Cataract change in the lens is quite common in leprosy patients (*Fig.* 16.4), and is probably a complication of iridocyclitis.

There is unfortunately a high incidence of blindness in long-standing leprosy. Surveys of settlements may show blindness rates of 10% or more. The two most common causes of blindness are iridocyclitis and its complications, and corneal scarring from facial palsy and corneal anaesthesia. An eye which is blind from cataract, but which has no other serious damage, is of course treatable.

The diagnosis of leprosy

The diagnosis of leprosy is basically clinical. However, if the facilities are available to examine skin smears and nasal discharges, they will detect the

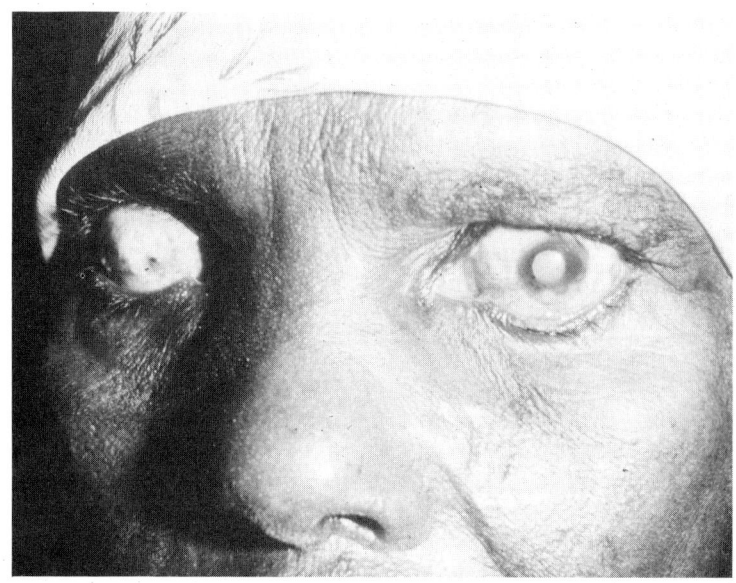

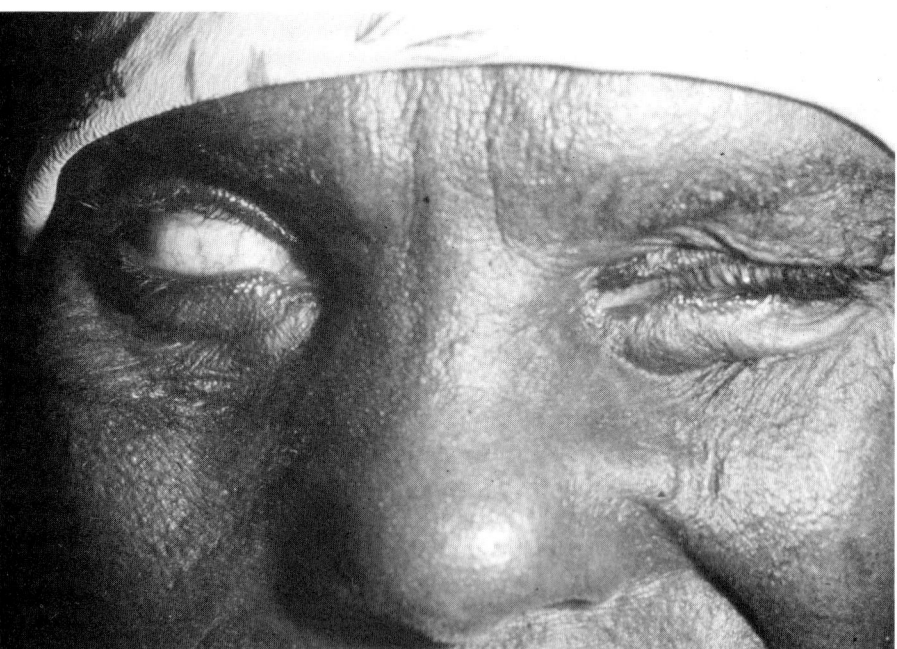

Fig. 16.4 Advanced facial palsy and corneal scarring from leprosy. On attempting to close the eyes, the right eye will not close at all and has a completely opaque cornea. The left eye shows scarring of the lower cornea and there is also a mature cataract.

presence of leprosy bacilli. This is more important in lepromatous cases where large numbers of bacilli are present. It is not usual to find any bacilli in tuberculoid cases, but the thickened paralysed nerves and the skin changes make the clinical diagnosis easier. The lepromin test may also be helpful. This test assesses the cell mediated immunity of the body to antigen from leprosy bacilli.

The treatment of ocular leprosy

To treat ocular leprosy, it is of course necessary to give local treatment to the eye. However, it is also necessary to treat the systemic disease generally. There are specific drugs for leprosy which should be given in the recommended doses. If possible, someone who is experienced in the management of leprosy should supervise the treatment.

Iritis

The chronic low grade iritis in a quiet eye which is found in lepromatous leprosy is very difficult to treat. Steroid drops are probably not advisable because the inflammation is slight and prolonged steroid drops cause so many complications. The long term use of mydriatics (eg atropine 1% daily) to try to keep the pupil dilated is probably beneficial. Acute iritis and its complications need the same basic treatment as any other type of acute iritis, with local corticosteroids and mydriatics (*see* page 132).

Cataracts

Cataracts should be treated by lens extraction. However, there must be some evidence of light projection to make it worth operating. Cataract extraction should only be performed in lepromatous leprosy when all the organisms have been killed by drug treatment. This may take some years, and can be confirmed by a skin smear examination.

Damage to the corneal protective reflex

Damage to the corneal protective reflex (either from a facial palsy or corneal anaesthesia) carries a high risk of corneal ulceration or scarring. It is advisable to examine the eye regularly, and ask the patient to report at the first sign of a red or watering eye. Frequent applications of a water based lubricant eye drop (e.g. methyl cellulose) help to preserve the precorneal tear film. If the eyelids do not close in sleep, either methyl cellulose or antibiotic ointment will help to protect the eye at night. If the cornea has ulcerated, immediate treatment is required with intensive antibiotic drops and ointment. Also the eyelids must be held together in order to protect and cover the cornea. This can be done either with adhesive strapping or else the eyelids can be sutured together until the ulcer heals.

Facial palsy

If the facial palsy has come on recently, it is probably due to inflammatory changes in the facial nerve from a 'reactional state'. It should be treated urgently

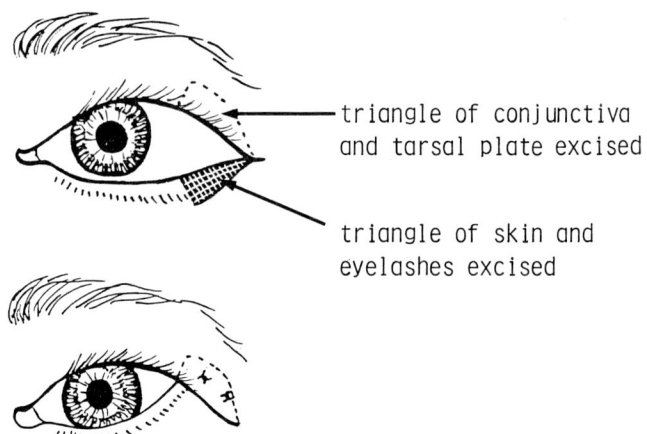

Fig. 16.5 Diagram of a lateral tarsorrhaphy.

with systemic steroids, and will probably recover. (The starting dose is up to 50 mg of prednisolone a day for 2 weeks, and then a maintenance dose of 15 – 20 mg a day for up to 3 months.)

A facial palsy which is permanent and complete must be treated surgically. Even if the palsy is temporary or partial, surgical treatment is often advisable. If corneal anaesthesia is also present, the risk of corneal ulceration increases, and the need for surgical correction of the facial palsy becomes more urgent. Many techniques can be used to correct a facial palsy. Some of these are very sophisticated and are only possible in special centres. However, in nearly all cases a simpler operation called a 'tarsorrhaphy' produces very satisfactory results.

A lateral tarsorrhaphy is the simplest and often the most effective way to correct a facial palsy. The technique is to sew together the lateral margins of the eyelids, and so shorten the interpalpebral fissure (*Fig.* 16.5): –

– Inject local anaesthetic and adrenaline into the eyelids.
– Incise along the margins of the lateral part of both upper and lower eyelids so as to split the eyelids into two parts. The anterior part contains the skin, eyelashes and orbicularis muscle. The posterior part contains the tarsal plate and conjunctiva. It is usual to split about a third of the lid margin. However, it is better to do a large tarsorrhaphy than a small tarsorrhaphy. A large tarsorrhaphy may not look so elegant, but it will adequately protect the cornea. A small tarsorrhaphy may look cosmetically better, but it may not protect the cornea so well.
– Remove a small triangle of the posterior part of the upper lid containing tarsal plate and conjunctiva.
– Remove a small triangle of the anterior part of the lower lid containing skin, eyelashes and orbicularis muscle.
– Overlap and secure these two triangles with mattress sutures so as to narrow and shorten the interpalpebral fissure.
– If the lower lid has stretched and is sagging, it is possible to excise a V-shaped wedge at the same time as the tarsorrhaphy.

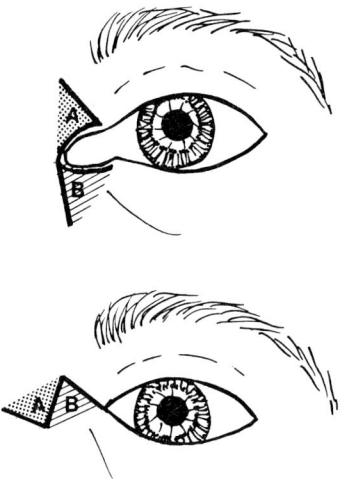

Fig. 16.6 Diagram of a medial tarsorrhaphy.

A medial tarsorrhaphy may also be necessary for severe cases. The basic technique is a modification of the Z-plasty: –
– Dissect two small triangular flaps of skin A and B (*Fig.* 16.6). Take great care not to injure the underlying lacrimal canaliculi.
– Sew together the conjunctival edges of the wound at the inner canthus.
– Suture the two triangular skin flaps as shown. Flap B is rotated up, and flap A is rotated down. This narrows the inner end of the interpalpebral fissure, and tightens the lower lid.

The temporalis muscle and tendon transplant is a more advanced plastic surgical procedure for total facial palsies, but it is only possible in special centres. The technique is to use a segment of the temporalis muscle which has strips of the overlying temporalis fascia attached. If the fascia are threaded in the lid margins and round the medial canthal tendon, they hold the eyelids close together. When the patient shuts his mouth firmly, the temporalis muscle contracts and the eyelids close completely.

Madarosis

Madarosis can be treated by performing an eyebrow graft. A free graft of hair skin is used from the nape of the neck. However, this is a skilled technique which requires considerable experience to perform well.

For further reading

1. Fritschi E. P. (1971) *Reconstructive Surgery in Leprosy*. Bristol, John Wright.
2. Jopling W. H. (1984) *Handbook of Leprosy* (Third edition). London, Heinemann.
3. WHO *Expert Committee on Leprosy*. Technical Report Series 675 (1982), Geneva.

17.   Squint

A squint means that the eyes are looking in different directions, because their visual axes are not parallel. Squints are quite common all over the world, and are usually classified according to the direction in which the eye turns.

Horizontal squints are more common than vertical squints. A convergent squint (sometimes called 'esotropia') means that the eye turns inwards (*Fig.* 17.1), and a divergent squint (sometimes called 'exotropia') means that the eye turns outwards (*Fig.* 17.2).

If there is a vertical squint, one eye will turn upwards, or the other eye will turn downwards (*Fig.* 17.3). The eye that turns upwards is sometimes called 'hypertropic', and the eye that turns downwards 'hypotropic'.

Sometimes one eye is always straight and the other eye always squints. Sometimes the squint may be in either eye, and this is called an alternating squint. Then again, the squint may only appear in certain situations. For example, it may appear for near vision only, for distance vision only, or when the patient looks in a certain direction. Squints may cause double vision, and this is called 'diplopia'.

Squint is a very complex disease, because the control of the eye movements is very complex. Also the assessment and care of squint is a very complex subject. Fortunately, squints are not usually an important cause of blindness, and most of them can be treated by following a few basic rules.

Causes of squint

Normally, a complex set of reflexes, called the 'binocular reflexes' keep the two eyes always pointing in the same direction. These reflexes involve both the sensory and the motor parts of the nervous system: −
- The sensory part of the reflex takes the two images produced by the two eyes and joins them together in the brain. This makes one stereoscopic image, so that everything appears in three dimensions.
- The motor part of the reflex makes sure that the two eyes always move together, so that they are always pointing in the same direction.

The binocular reflexes are much weaker in children, and therefore squints usually start in early childhood. Most squints occur when something goes wrong with these reflexes. Disorders of the vision will affect the sensory part, and disorders of the eye movements will affect the motor part. Refractive errors are also an important cause of squint in children.

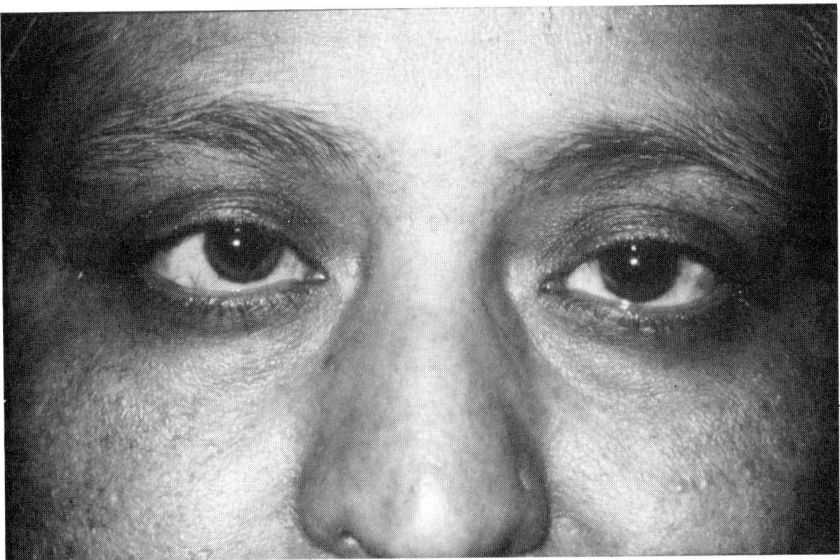

Fig. 17.1 A small right convergent squint. Note how the corneal light reflex from the right eye is not central.

Disorders of the vision

If one eye is diseased, then the image from that eye is blurred. The brain may not be able to join this blurred image with the normal image from the healthy eye. There is no stimulus for the diseased eye to remain pointing in the same direction as the healthy eye, and so the diseased eye develops a squint. Any disease which affects the vision of one eye (e.g. a corneal scar, cataract, a disease of the retina or optic nerve) may cause a squint in that eye.

In early childhood, convergence is very active. This means that a young child with defective vision in one eye usually develops a convergent squint. However, in later life, an eye with defective vision is more likely to develop a divergent squint.

Disorders of the eye movements

Defective eye movements will obviously cause a squint. The defect may be in the extraocular muscles themselves, or in the cranial nerves which supply the muscles: –

– The six extraocular muscles are shown in *Fig.* 2.7. They pass from the wall of the orbit to the sclera of the eyeball. The actions of these muscles are quite

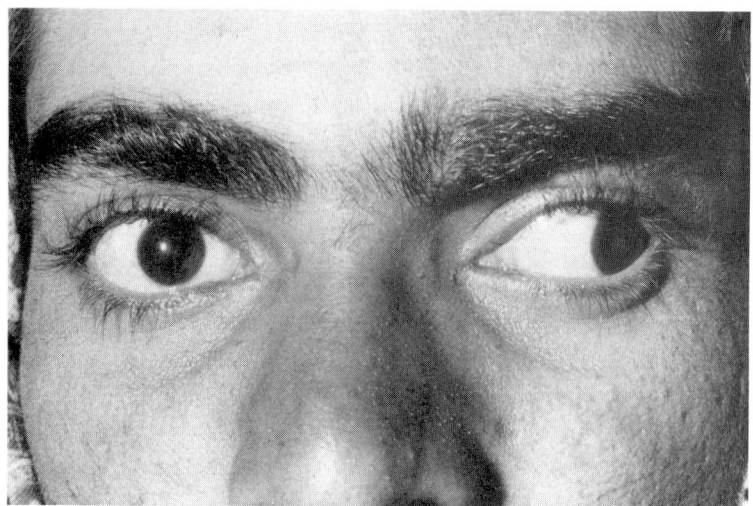

Fig. 17.2 A large left divergent squint. The left eye is so divergent that there is no corneal light reflex visible from the left eye.

complex, but *Fig.* 17.4 shows the main action of each muscle in a simplified way. There are many possible disorders of the extraocular muscles, but the four most common are as follows: –
1. Congenital abnormalities.
2. Fractures of the orbital walls, causing adhesions to the muscles.

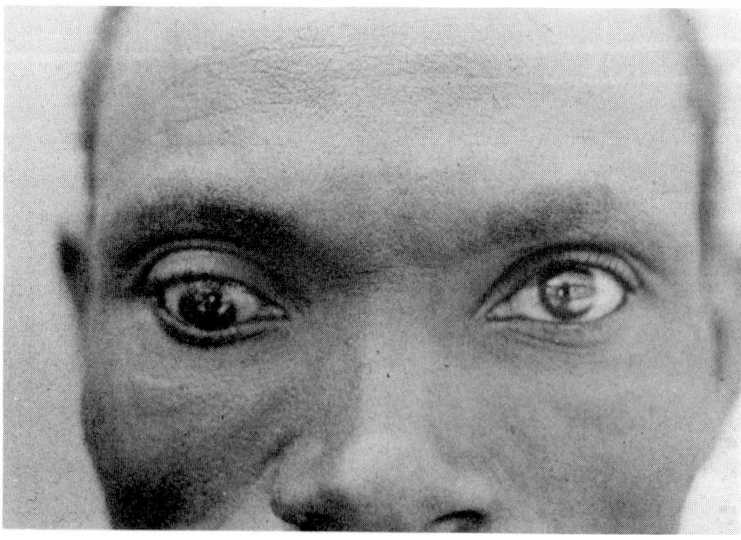

Fig. 17.3 A vertical squint.

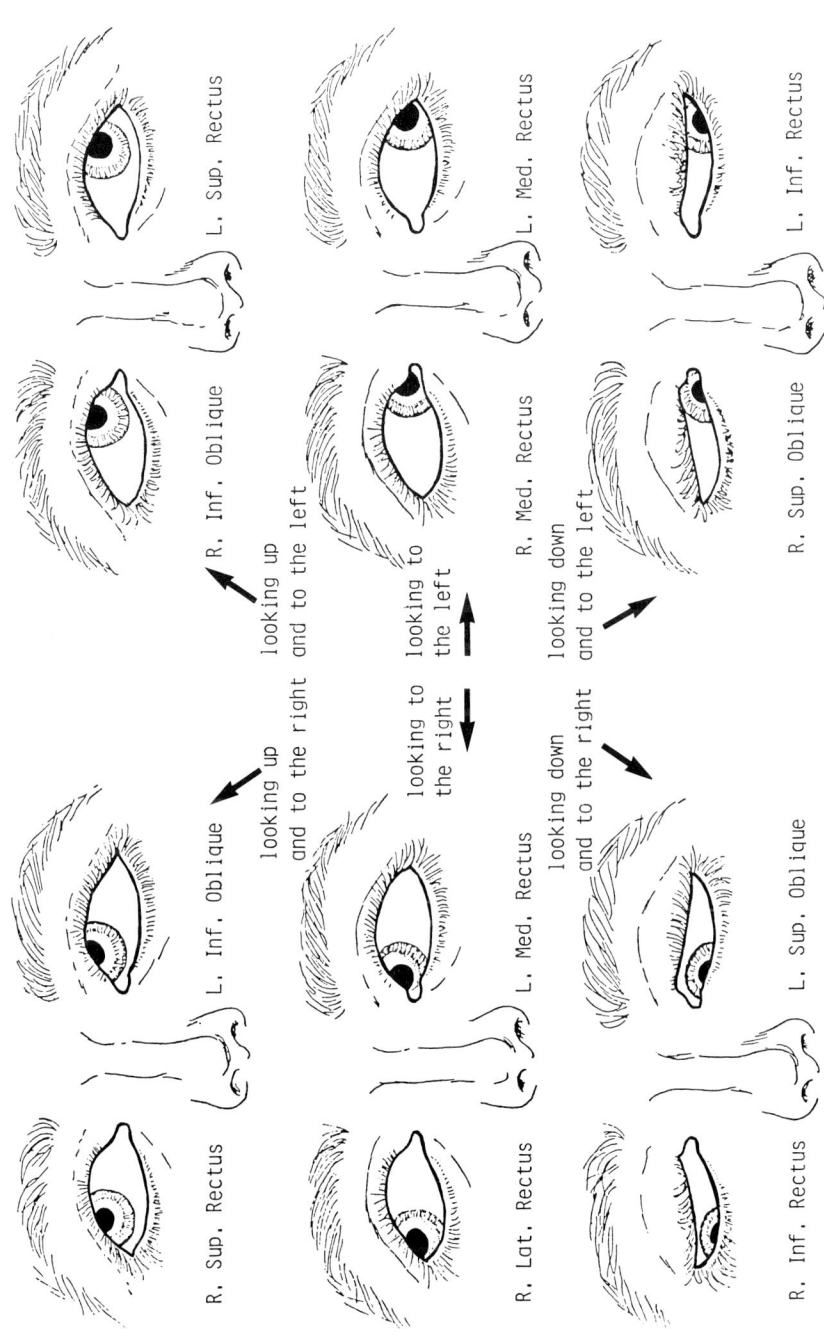

Fig. 17.4 A diagram to show the six directions of gaze and the main action of each extraocular muscle

L. Sup. Rectus

L. Med. Rectus

L. Inf. Rectus

R. Inf. Oblique

R. Med. Rectus

R. Sup. Oblique

looking up and to the left

looking to the left

looking down and to the left

looking up and to the right

looking to the right

looking down and to the right

L. Inf. Oblique

L. Med. Rectus

L. Sup. Oblique

R. Sup. Rectus

R. Lat. Rectus

R. Inf. Rectus

Table 17.1 Squint from cranial nerve palsies affecting the eye muscles

Nerve	Eye muscles affected	Defect in movement	Main symptoms
III Oculomotor	Superior, medial and inferior rectus. Inferior oblique (also supplies levator of upper lid and pupil constriction)	No movement at all except abduction of the eye. Sometimes partial lesion may only involve selected muscles	Ptosis, constant diplopia when eyelid elevated. Dilated pupil. Affected eye diverges
IV Trochlear	Superior oblique	Limitation of downward movement when eye is abducted	Vertical diplopia on looking down especially reading. (If bilateral the two images may be tilted)
VI Abducent	Lateral rectus	Limitation of abduction	Horizontal diplopia when looking to the affected side

3. Dysthyroid eye disease, causing inflammation and fibrosis in the muscles.
4. Generalized muscle disease (e.g. myopathy and myasthenia gravis), which often affects the eye muscles.
- The III, IV and VI cranial nerves supply the extraocular muscles, and so damage to these nerves will also cause a squint. The VI cranial nerve is most likely to be damaged, because it has a long intracranial course and is very thin. The effects and symptoms of the different nerve palsies are shown in Table 17.1.

Cranial nerve palsies are the most important cause of squints which develop in adults, and they may cause squints in children. At first, a squint from a cranial nerve palsy is only in the direction in which the affected muscle acts. The movements in all other directions are normal. This is called a 'paralytic squint'. However, after some months, secondary changes often take place in the innervation and action of the other extraocular muscles, so that the squint occurs in all directions. This is called a 'concomitant squint'.

Cranial nerve palsies can have many causes. The most common are: –
- head injuries
- space-occupying lesions inside the skull
- meningitis
- arteriosclerosis ⎫
- diabetes   ⎬ (these three causes are common in old people)
- hypertension   ⎭

Refractive errors

A refractive error in one eye only will obviously blur the vision in that eye and therefore may cause a squint.

Long sight (hypermetropia) in both eyes is also a common cause of childhood squints. To focus on a near object, the eyes must accomodate and also turn inwards so that they are both looking at the object. These two reflexes, accomodation and convergence, are linked in the brain. A long-sighted child, who must accomodate even to see distant objects clearly, must accomodate even more to focus on near objects. Excessive accomodation produces excessive convergence, and therefore a convergent squint.

Other causes of squint

Squints sometimes develop in children when there is no obvious defect or refractive error in the eye. The squint may come on when the child is tired at the end of the day. Alternatively, the squint may first appear during a generalized illness or emotional upset.

The effects of a squint

The effects of a squint are very different in adults and children.

If the squint starts in adult life, the patient will develop double vision (diplopia) and abnormal head postures: –
- When the squint first begins, the patient sees everything double. This is very confusing, and in order to prevent it, the patient may shut or cover one eye. Double vision may be present only when the patient looks in certain directions, especially with a paralytic squint. The patient then turns his head in order to avoid looking in the direction which produces diplopia. In this way an abnormal head posture develops.

If the squint starts in childhood, the child often develops a 'lazy eye' (amblyopia): –
- When the squint begins in early childhood, the child probably experiences some double vision just like an adult. However, after a short time, the brain somehow ignores the image from one eye, so that the double vision stops. Eventually, the brain somehow permanently ignores this image causing a loss of vision in the squinting eye. This is called 'amblyopia'. Amblyopia does not affect the overall visual field, but only the visual acuity. In severe cases, the visual acuity may fall to only 'counting fingers'.

Amblyopia only develops in infants and young children. Anything which prevents a clear image in one eye may also cause amblyopia. For this reason, the same disorders which cause squint in children also cause amblyopia. Indeed, most children with a squint in one eye develop amblyopia. For example: –
- A cataract in one eye will prevent a clear image in that eye. Even if the defect is corrected in later life, the eye will not see well.
- A refractive error in one eye will blur the vision. Even if the refractive error is corrected at a later age, the visual acuity of that eye may still be poor.

Even prolonged application of an eye pad can cause amblyopia in an infant. This is why the eyes of young children should only be padded when it is absolutely necessary.

Clinical examination and assessment of squints

The corneal light reflex

This is the best and simplest test of squint. The cornea is transparent, but its front surface reflects enough light to act as a convex mirror. If the patient looks at a bright light, such as a torch or an ophthalmoscope, a reflection of that light can be seen from the corneal surface. If the two eyes are straight, then the two corneal light reflexes are central and symmetrical. If one eye squints, then the reflex deviates from the centre of that cornea (*Figs.* 17.1 *and* 17.2).

The cover test

The cover test helps to demonstrate a small or intermittent squint which may not be obvious with the corneal light reflex. The patient must look at a small object. The examiner covers each of the patient's eyes in turn. If there is a squint, the eye which is not covered will move to take up fixation of the object.

Testing the ocular movements

There are six extraocular muscles, and each one produces most of the movement in a particular direction. There are therefore six main directions of gaze (*Fig.* 17.4). If the diplopia or squint only occurs in certain directions of gaze, it is possible to detect a defect in an individual muscle.

Assessing squints in children

It is necessary to examine the eye very carefully for any disease which might explain the squint. Two tests are especially important: –
– The visual acuity should be tested in both eyes to see if there is any eye disease or amblyopia. This requires both skill and patience, especially in young children, but it is very important.
– The refraction of the eyes should also be measured. Cycloplegic drops (atropine or cyclopentolate) will dilate the pupil and paralyse the ciliary muscle which is very active in young children. A retinoscope and a set of trial lenses can now be used to measure the refraction.

Epicanthus

It is important not to mistake epicanthus for a squint. Epicanthus is a prominent fold of skin on the nasal side of the eye (*Fig.* 17.5). It occurs because the ethmoid sinuses develop before the other sinuses, so that many young children have a broad nasal bridge. The fold of skin covers much of the white sclera nasal to the iris. This looks like a convergent squint, especially when the child looks to one side or the other. However, the corneal light reflex and cover tests will both show that this is not a true squint.

The management and treatment of squints

The management and treatment of squints is very different in children and in adults.

Squints in children

It is necessary to correct any refractive errors and amblyopia before straightening the squint surgically.

- Refractive errors should be corrected with spectacles. Young children will usually wear spectacles happily if they see better with them.
- Amblyopia develops because the brain rejects the image from one eye. The aim of treatment is therefore to force the brain to accept that image by patching over the good eye for about two weeks. After successful treatment, a constant squint in one eye will become an alternating squint. There is never amblyopia in alternating squints. Unfortunately, it is not always possible to correct amblyopia in this way: –
    1. Children often resent this treatment because they cannot see well when the good eye is covered.
    2. The treatment is most effective in children under 5. With increasing age, it becomes less effective and is useless in children over 8.
    3. Patching over the good eye does not always work, and is useless if there is any disease in the squinting eye. If there is no improvement after two weeks, it should be stopped.

    It is not possible to test the vision in very young children, and so it is difficult to diagnose amblyopia. However, if a child has a constant squint in one eye and no apparent eye disease, there is probably amblyopia in the squinting eye.
- Surgical treatment can straighten the eye by either weakening, strengthening or re-aligning the extraocular muscles. However, it is not usual for the patient to recover binocular vision. The main reason for surgery is to improve the cosmetic appearance. In some cultures, a squint is a serious defect, while in others it is ignored.

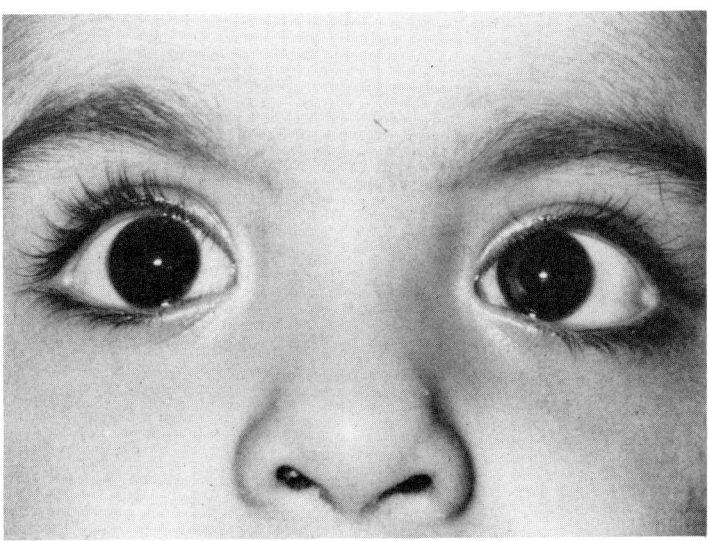

Fig. 17.5 Epicanthus. The child appears to have a left convergent squint, but the corneal light reflexes are central.

Squints in adults

If the squint first started in childhood, cosmetic surgery is the only treatment.

If the squint is recent, look for a cause. There may be a serious neurological or general medical disease.

— Double vision can be temporarily relieved by covering one eye.
— Small squints can be corrected with prism glasses.
— Large squints may need extraocular surgery to re-align the two eyes, and cure the diplopia. However, spontaneous improvement sometimes occurs from the regeneration of damaged nerves. For this reason, it is necessary to wait six months before surgery.

18. Orbital Diseases

Orbital diseases are not very common. However, they are often serious, and may cause blindness or even death. The three main types of orbital disease are: –
– space-occupying lesions in the orbit,
– acute orbital cellulitis,
– dysthyroid eye disease.

Space-occupying lesions in the orbit

Space-occupying lesions in the orbit are perhaps the most difficult of all eye diseases to diagnose and treat. There are many different possible causes, and it is difficult to both choose and perform the correct treatment.

The common presenting feature is forward displacement of the eye. This is called 'proptosis'. It is possible to assess proptosis with an instrument called a 'proptometer' (*Fig.* 18.1). This measures how far forward the cornea is in relation

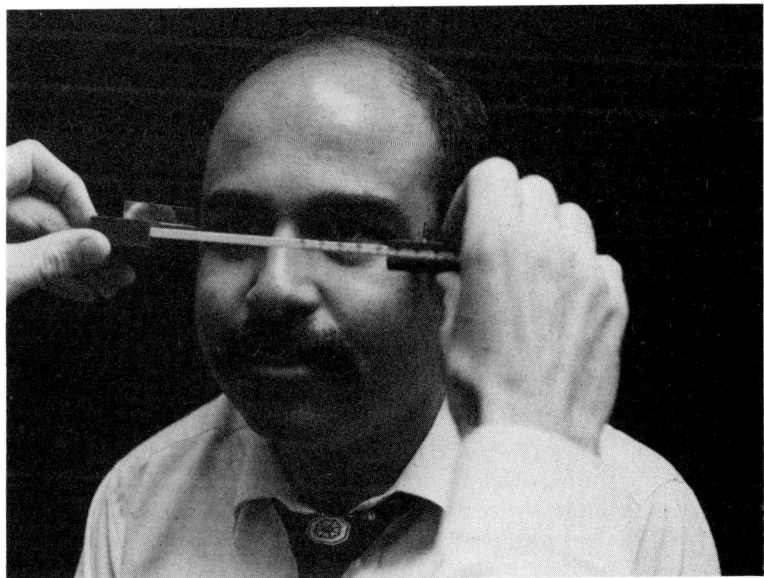

Fig. 18.1 Examining a patient with a proptometer.

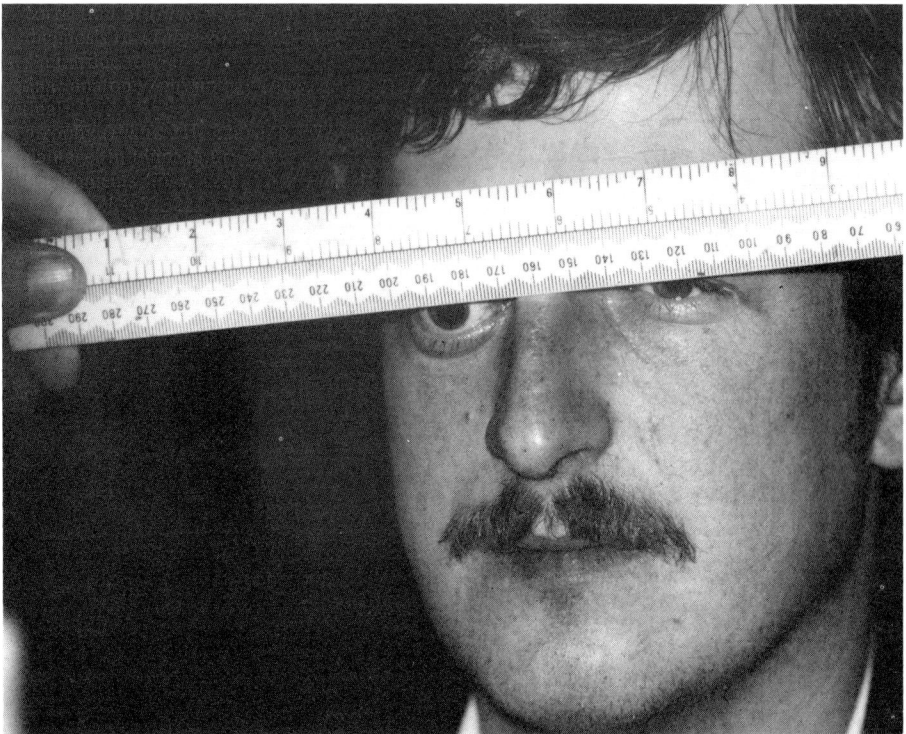

Fig. 18.2 Using a ruler to measure any vertical or horizontal displacement of the eye. This patient had a lacrimal gland tumour causing proptosis and also displacing the right eye downwards and inwards.

to the bony orbital rim. Without a proptometer, the best way to assess proptosis is as follows: –
– Sit the patient down.
– Stand over him, and look down at his forehead from above.
– If one eye is proptosed, it will appear to be displaced forwards in relation to the superior orbital rim.

It is also necessary to check for any vertical or horizontal displacement of the eye. Hold a plastic ruler between the centre of each pupil. If this is not level, it will indicate vertical displacement. Then measure the distance from the bridge of the nose to the centre of each pupil. This will detect any horizontal displacement (*Fig.* 18.2). Lesions inside the extraocular muscle cone usually displace the eye forwards only (*Fig.* 18.3). Lesions outside the muscle cone or in the wall of the orbit usually displace the eye in the opposite direction to the lesion. For example, a lesion of the frontal sinus in the roof of the orbit usually displaces the eye downwards (*Fig.* 18.4).

It is important to check that the optic nerve and extraocular muscles are functioning properly. Severe proptosis from any cause carries the risk of ischaemic pressure changes in the optic nerve and exposure ulceration of the cornea. Both of these conditions can cause permanent damage to the sight (*Fig.* 18.5). It is also necessary to examine the eye carefully for any sign of inflammation, such as dilated conjunctival blood vessels, or conjunctival chemosis.

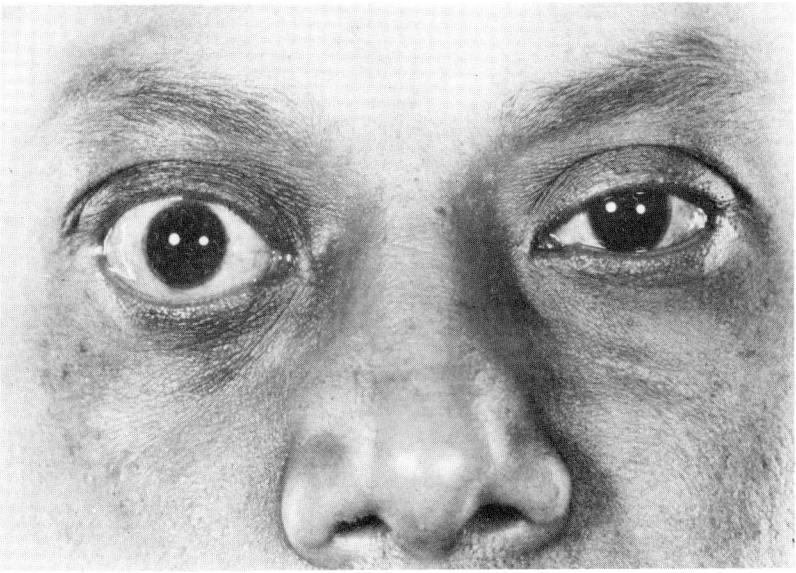

Fig. 18.3 Proptosis of the right eye. This patient had a haemangioma inside the extraocular muscle cone, pushing the eye forwards.

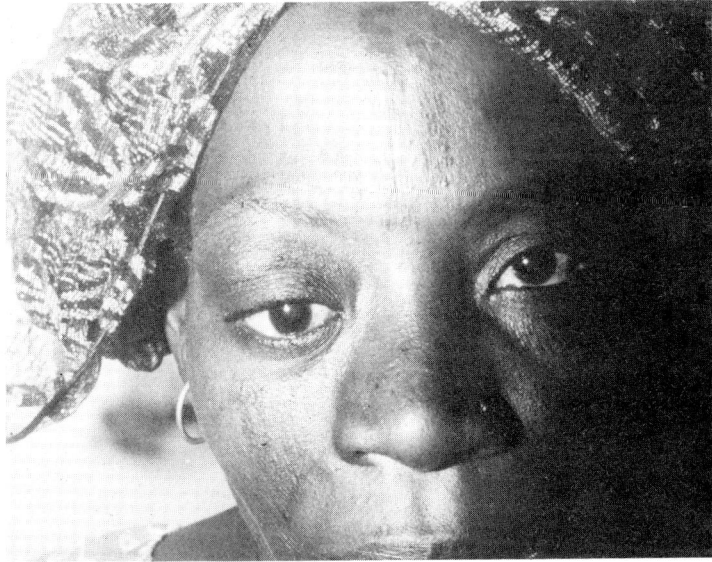

Fig. 18.4 Proptosis of the right eye. This patient had a mucocoele of the frontal sinus, pushing the eye downwards.

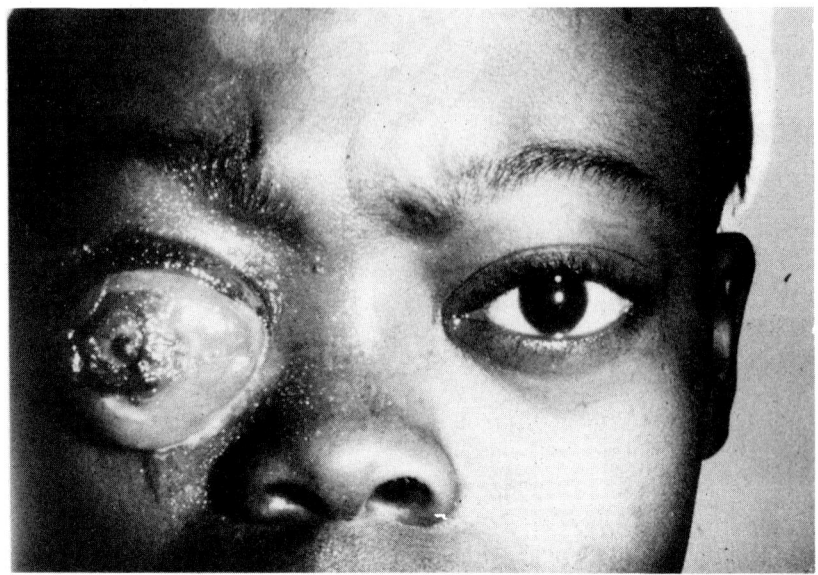

Fig. 18.5 Leukaemic deposits in the orbit in a young boy. The right cornea has ulcerated away completely, and there is chemosis of the conjunctiva.

Orbital lesions are much easier to identify and diagnose using certain X-ray techniques — tomograms, orbital venograms and especially a soft tissue scan. Unfortunately, most of these techniques are only available in specialized medical centres. However, even a plain X-ray can be useful, especially in detecting any underlying nasal sinus disease.

The most important space-occupying orbital lesions are: –
– tumours,
– cysts,
– inflammatory orbital masses.

Tumours

There are many kinds of orbital tumour, both benign and malignant, but none of them are common.

The most frequent benign tumours are haemangiomas, lacrimal gland tumours and neurofibromas. They all present with a very slow and gradual proptosis. Very rarely, abnormal blood vessels may rupture and cause a sudden orbital haemorrhage.

Malignant orbital tumours grow more rapidly. They may infiltrate and destroy the surrounding tissues, or spread to other parts of the body. The most frequent malignant tumours are: –
– A neglected retinoblastoma which has spread outside the eye.
– Lymphoma or leukaemic deposits which may occur in the orbit. Burkitt's lymphoma usually starts around the maxilla in children (*Fig.* 18.6). It is an important cause of orbital tumours in central Africa.

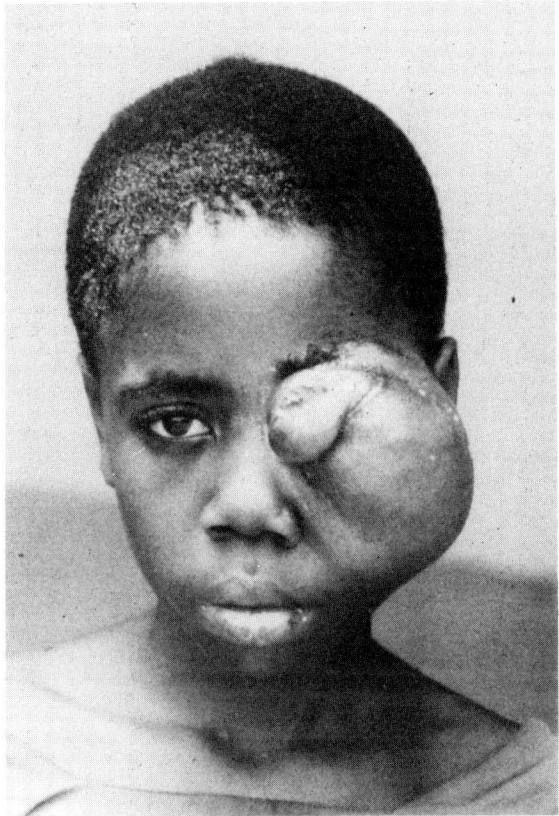

Fig. 18.6 A child with Burkitt's lymphoma. The tumour started in the maxilla, and spread to the orbit.

– A carcinoma of the conjunctiva or lacrimal gland (*Fig.* 18.7).
– A rhabdomyosarcoma arising from the extraocular muscles.
– Malignant tumours of the nasal sinuses which may spread into the orbit.

Cysts

Cysts present clinically in the same way as benign orbital tumours. These may be dermoid or epidermoid cysts, or parasitic cysts such as a hydatid cyst.

Inflammatory orbital masses

Some orbital masses are inflammatory in nature. However, they present clinically just like orbital tumours, and so are often called 'pseudotumours'. In most cases, there is local evidence of inflammation such as pain in the orbit, or oedema of the eyelids or conjunctiva. There may be a specific cause for the inflammation, such as a parasitic worm.

Chronic nasal sinus infections may cause inflammatory masses in the orbit.

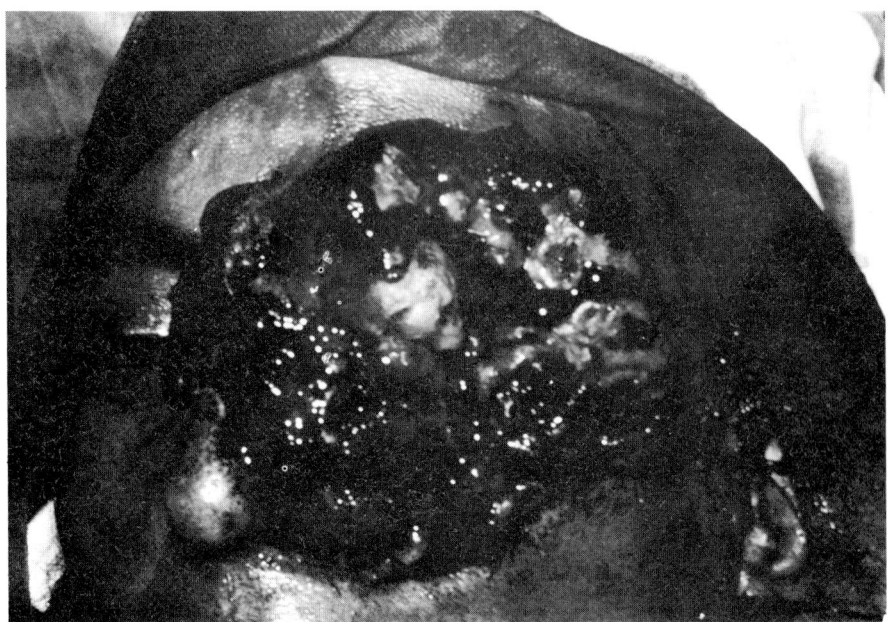

Fig. 18.7 Advanced conjunctival carcinoma. This was successfully removed with an exenteration of the orbit.

The treatment of space-occupying lesions in the orbit

Planning treatment for these lesions is not easy. There are three decisions to be made: –

1. Does the disease originate in the nasal sinuses? If it does, the nasal sinuses should be explored surgically. Sinus infections and mucocoeles need to be drained, and nasal tumours need a biopsy.

2. If the disease originates in the orbit itself, is surgical treatment necessary? Orbital surgery is difficult. Lesions which do not appear either to be growing or harming the eye can often be left untreated.

3. If surgery is necessary, what operation should be performed?

– Benign tumours and cysts should be removed completely. It is possible to enter the orbit by removing the bony lateral wall. The tumour can then be removed without disturbing the eye. However, there is a risk of damaging important orbital structures during the operation.

– Suspected malignant tumours or inflammatory masses need a biopsy. It is usual to enter the orbit through the skin or conjunctiva for this. Further treatment depends on the result of the biopsy.

– Some malignant tumours (e.g. most carcinomas) are best treated by removing the entire orbital contents. This is a mutilating operation called an exenteration, but it may save the patient's life.

– Malignant tumours like lymphoma should be treated with chemotherapy or radiotherapy.

- Inflammatory lesions may need systemic steroids or other specific medical treatment.

Acute orbital cellulitis (*Fig.* 18.8)

Acute orbital cellulitis is nearly always a complication of a nasal sinus infection. The infection spreads through the very thin bone between the nasal sinuses and the orbit. Young children are especially at risk. This is because upper respiratory tract infections are very common in young children, and the walls of the sinuses are less well developed. The common presenting features are: –
- proptosis,
- inflammation and oedema of the eyelids,
- all the systemic signs of an acute infection, e.g. fever, malaise etc.

Sometimes, the infection resolves without treatment, or an abscess forms and discharges itself through the skin at the orbital margin. However, there is a danger that the infection will spread backwards along the orbital veins into the cavernous sinus at the base of the brain. There is then a risk of septicaemia or intracranial infection. Inflammation and oedema in both orbits indicates that the

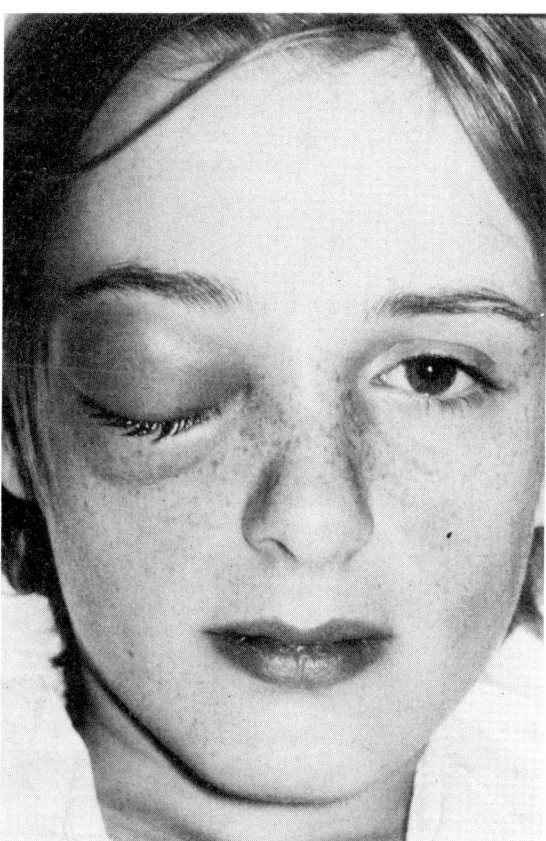

Fig. 18.8 Acute orbital cellulitis. Note the inflammation and oedema of the eyelids.

infection has reached the cavernous sinus. The treatment for orbital cellulitis is systemic antibiotics in large doses.

Orbital cellulitis can also be caused by allergic reactions to parasites in the orbit or eyelids, especially the Loa loa worm (*see Fig.* 15.10 page 184). In parasitic infections, there is also lid oedema and proptosis. However, the patient usually feels well and there is very little localized pain or tenderness. A white cell count will show increased neutrophils in acute orbital cellulitis of bacterial origin, but increased eosinophils in parasitic infections.

Dysthyroid eye disease (*Fig.* 18.9)

Dysthyroid eye disease is associated with primary thyrotoxicosis. An auto-immune inflammatory reaction occurs in the orbit, but it is not known why this happens. The orbital tissues swell, and there is some degree of proptosis. Often, the most severe signs in the orbit are seen in patients with only mild thyrotoxicosis.

Apart from the proptosis, there are two special features of dysthyroid eye disease.
- The eyelids retract so that the palpebral fissure widens and the patient appears to be staring. This is caused by contracture of the sympathetic muscle fibres in the eyelids.
- The eye movements may be restricted, and this produces diplopia. It is caused by inflammation and contracture in the extraocular muscles.

In severe cases, there may be a risk of blindness either from pressure damage to the optic nerve, or from ulcers in the exposed cornea.

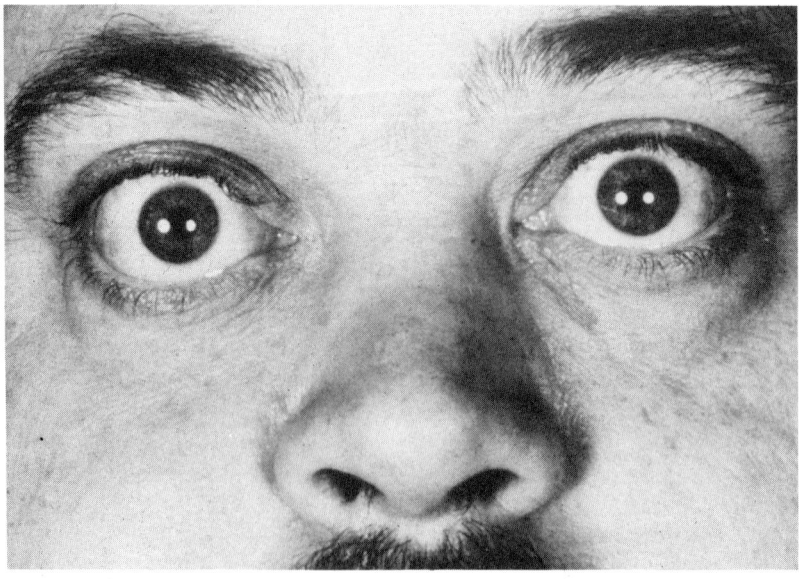

Fig. 18.9 Dysthyroid eye disease. Note the proptosis in both eyes, and the retraction of the eyelids.

Dysthyroid eye disease is usually, but not always bilateral. Eventually, the disease burns itself out, but the patient may be left with serious damage to the eye, or a squint or diplopia.

Treatment

Methyl cellulose drops and antibiotic ointment may prevent any exposure changes in the cornea. The diplopia may require either patching of one eye, prism spectacles or ocular muscle surgery. Appropriate plastic surgery can sometimes improve retraction of the eyelids.

In severe cases, where the sight is threatened, it is necessary to reduce the pressure in the orbit. This may be done surgically by removing the roof of the maxillary antrum. This allows the orbital contents to expand into the empty space of the antrum. Alternatively, a short course of very high doses of systemic steroids (up to 100 mg of prednisolone a day) will shrink the inflamed orbital tissues.

19. Eye Injuries

The eye is an external organ, and so it is easy to injure. For this reason, eye injuries are common amongst people all over the world. All medical workers should be able to treat minor eye injuries, and should know something about serious eye injuries. Serious injuries, however, may require specialist surgical treatment. The eye is so complex, that occasionally a minor injury may have serious complications.

It is helpful to try to answer three questions to assess an eye injury properly: –
- What caused the injury? Most patients will explain what happened. Just occasionally, however, the patient is unaware of any injury, especially if a small, sharp fragment has penetrated the eye at high speed.
- When did the injury occur? In some areas, patients may arrive days, or even weeks after the injury. This further complicates the treatment.
- Which parts of the eye are injured?

There are basically seven common patterns of eye injury: –
- corneal and conjunctival foreign bodies, and corneal abrasions,
- burns,
- non-penetrating, or blunt injuries to the eyeball,
- penetrating injuries to the eye,
- injuries to the eyelids,
- orbital injuries,
- cranial nerve injuries.

Corneal and conjunctival foreign bodies, and corneal abrasions (*Plate* 23a – d *and Fig.* 19.1)

These are the most common eye injuries. They are especially common where there is dust, sand or other particles in the air. Because the cornea is so sensitive, most patients are aware of any foreign body or abrasion.

A corneal foreign body may be on the cornea, or embedded in the cornea. Normally, it is easy to detect, but if it is dark-coloured, it may be more difficult to see against the pupil or a dark iris (*Plate* 23a). Most corneal foreign bodies are very easy to remove. First instill local anaesthetic drops in the eye.
- If the foreign body is on the cornea, gently remove it with the edge of a sterile hypodermic needle.
- If the foreign body is embedded in the cornea, it may be necessary to use the point of a needle to pick it out.
- Very occasionally, the foreign body penetrates deeply into the corneal stroma.

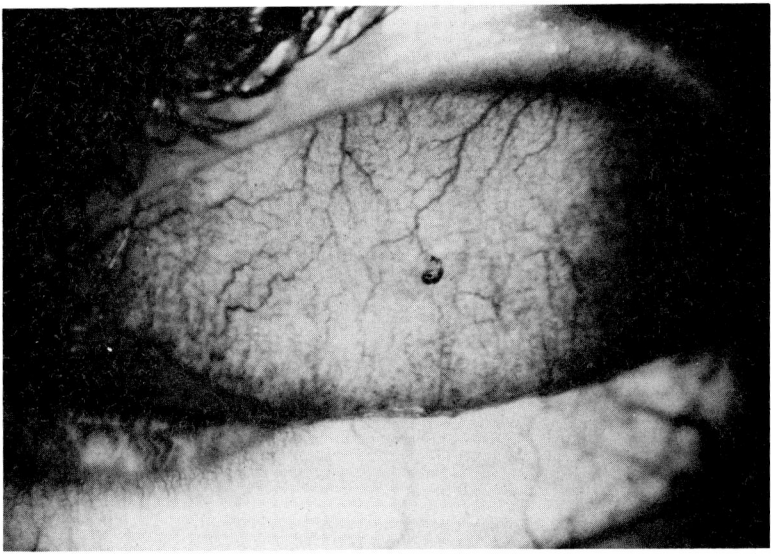

Fig. 19.1 A conjunctival foreign body under the upper eyelid.

It may then require specialist treatment.

− If a fragment of iron is embedded in the cornea, a small superficial rust ring may develop. It may even develop after the fragment has been removed. This rust ring will eventually disappear spontaneously. However, a small dental burr will remove the rust and may help the cornea to heal quicker.

A conjunctival foreign body is usually easy to see. It may however be stuck to the inside of the upper eyelid, where it will scratch the cornea each time the patient blinks. It is always a good idea to check for foreign bodies by everting the upper lid (*Fig.* 19.1). A cottonwool bud can usually be used to wipe off a conjunctival foreign body.

A corneal abrasion occurs when something rubs or scratches the eye, and removes some of the epithelial cells. It is a common injury especially amongst people who work in thick forests, and always produces severe pain and photophobia. There may be some redness in the eye, but otherwise it looks normal to the naked eye. However, fluorescein drops will immediately stain the abraded area of the cornea (*Plate* 23b − d).

The treatment of abrasions and foreign bodies is essentially the same. Instill antibiotic drops or ointment, and pad the eye until the corneal epithelium has regenerated. This usually takes one or two days. In severe cases, mydriatic drops may help to relieve the pain. If there is any risk of injury with vegetable matter, in a hot humid climate, it is wise to apply a fungicide as well, if available (*see* page 99).

Burns

Burns to the eyelids and eyes may be caused by open fires or chemicals. Most fire burns occur in the home, when small children or epileptics fall into the fire.

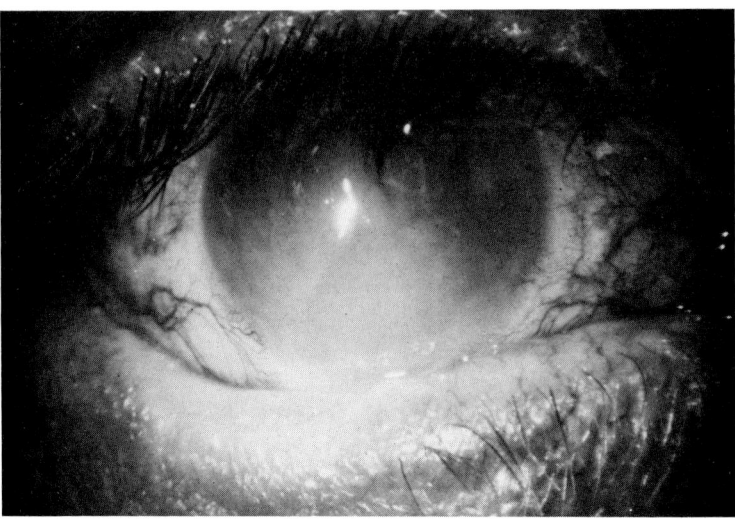

Fig. 19.2 A corneal scar following a lime burn.

Chemical burns are common in industries which use irritant fluids such as acids, alkalis, cement or lime.
– An eyelid burn may require local or systemic antibiotics. It is best not to pad the eye, but to let a firm scab develop. Severe burns will cause secondary skin contractures, and will need skin grafting later (*see Fig.* 5.6, p. 57).
– Any burns to the cornea and conjunctiva, and especially alkali burns, need urgent and careful treatment. It is necessary to irrigate the eye very thoroughly, and then instill antibiotic drops or ointment frequently. Unfortunately, a common complication of any burn to the eye is corneal and conjunctival scarring (*Fig.* 19.2). Local steroids will help to prevent excessive scarring. They can be used as soon as the risk of infection has passed, but the eye will need very close observation.

Non-penetrating, or blunt injuries to the eyeball

Blunt injuries may occur in many different circumstances. However, the force of any blunt injury is great enough to compress the eyeball from front to back, so that it stretches at the equator (*Fig.* 19.3). There is then a risk that this stretching deformity of the eye will tear the delicate intraocular structures. Other complications are the direct result of concussion damage to the cells. In most blunt injuries, there is usually some bruising or haemorrhage of the eyelids, conjunctiva or orbit (*Plate* 23e).
    There are several complications of blunt injuries: –
– Bleeding into the anterior chamber (hyphaema) is the most common complication. Usually the blood comes from small blood vessels which have torn in the root of the iris and ciliary body. At first, the red blood cells diffuse throughout the anterior chamber. Later they sink to the bottom of the anterior chamber, and are eventually absorbed. In a very severe hyphaema,

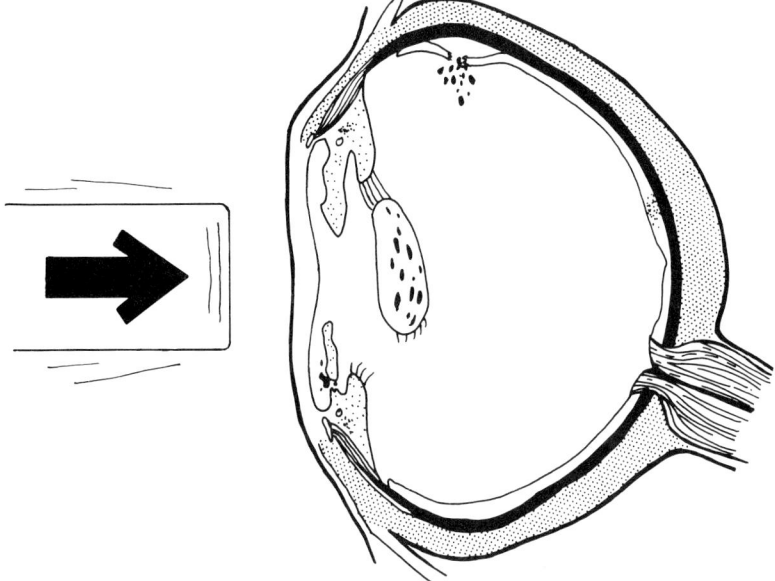

Blunt injury causing sudden stretching and deformity of the eye

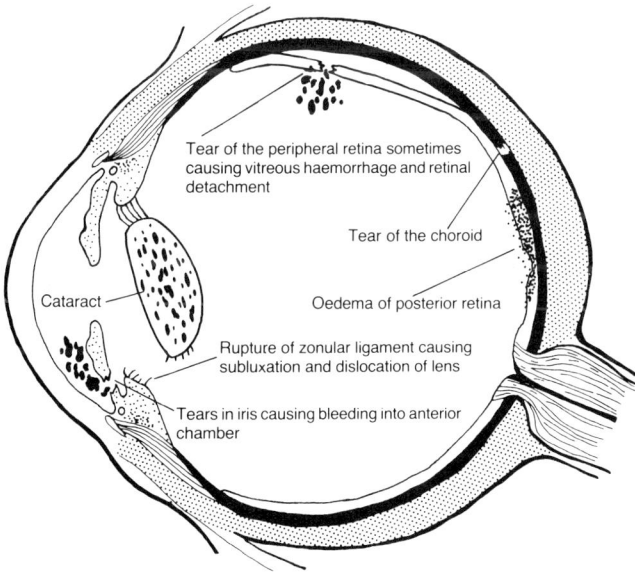

Tear of the peripheral retina sometimes causing vitreous haemorrhage and retinal detachment

Tear of the choroid

Cataract

Oedema of posterior retina

Rupture of zonular ligament causing subluxation and dislocation of lens

Tears in iris causing bleeding into anterior chamber

Results of blunt injury

Fig. 19.3 The complications of a blunt injury to the eye.

the whole of the anterior chamber may be full of blood clot. It will appear as a black opaque mass which obscures the iris and pupil, and is called a 'blackball' hyphaema (*Plate* 23f). Excessive blood may also obstruct the drainage of aqueous fluid, and so cause secondary glaucoma. A blackball hyphaema together with a rise in intraocular pressure is a very bad sign. If red blood cells and their breakdown products enter the cornea and other eye structures, they leave deposits of blood pigment and cause permanent loss of function.

– The suspensory ligament supporting the lens may rupture. Minor tears will partially dislocate the lens, so that it tilts and lies asymmetrically in the eye. Refractive changes will result, especially astigmatism and myopia. Severe tears may dislocate the lens completely, so that it comes to lie in the vitreous body.

– Delayed cataract sometimes follows a blunt injury, and is a result of concussion damage to the lens cells. It may develop months or even years later.

– The retina may tear at its periphery. In itself, a torn retina produces few symptoms, if any, but it may provoke a haemorrhage into the vitreous body, or progress later to a retinal detachment. After any blunt injury, it is necessary to examine the peripheral retina very carefully to make sure that no tears or dialyses are present.

– Retinal oedema may occur as a result of concussion injury to the retina. The retina appears white and shiny, and because it cannot function normally, there is blurring of the vision. Retinal oedema usually recovers fully, but if it is near the macula, there may be some permanent macular damage.

– The choroid may tear, causing a choroidal haemorrhage, which will damage the overlying retina.

– Rupture of the eyeball is very rare. However, if the force of the blunt injury is sufficient, it is usually the sclera which tears, near the equator. In this case, the prognosis for recovery of sight is poor.

The treatment of blunt injuries

Most blunt injuries do not require any special treatment. However, it is probably beneficial for the patient to rest until any hyphaema, vitreous haemorrhage or retinal oedema has subsided. If the eye is very inflamed, mydriatics and local steroids may help to reduce the inflammation.

If there is *both* a blackball hyphaema *and* a rise in intraocular pressure, it will be necessary to: –
– make a limbal incision to open the anterior chamber,
– gently milk or irrigate the semi-solid blood clot out of the anterior chamber of the eye.

Urgent cryotherapy will be necessary to prevent any tears of the peripheral retina from progressing to retinal detachments.

Penetrating injuries to the eye

Any sharp object or fragment which hits the eye can cause a penetrating injury. In urban communities, industrial and road accidents are the most common causes, but in rural communities, thorns or twigs may penetrate the eye. Most penetrating eye injuries are fairly easy to recognize (*Plate* 23f). Occasionally, however, a very small fragment penetrates the eye at great speed. The fragment is

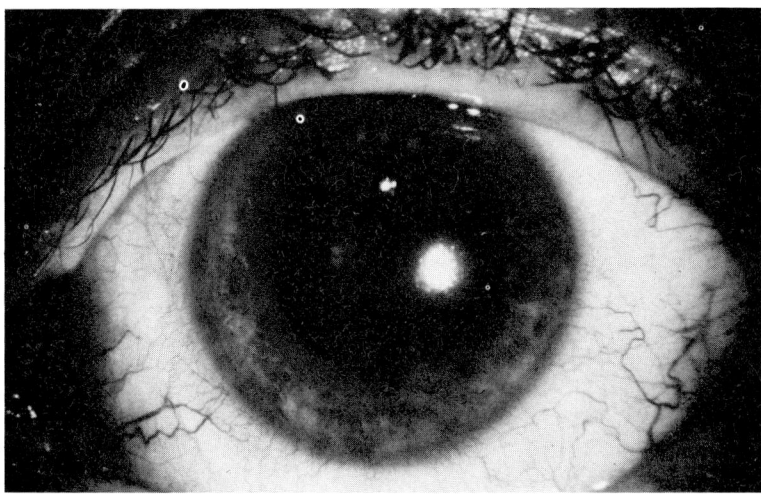

Fig. 19.4 A small penetrating wound in the iris which is very difficult to see.

usually of metal or stone and comes from grinding, chiselling or hammering. The patient may not realize that anything ever entered his eye. The doctor too may not see the very small entry wound or the foreign body lying in the eye (*Figs.* 19.4 *and* 19.5).

A corneal or scleral laceration is usually obvious, and uveal tissue often prolapses through the wound. The pupil may be distorted, and the anterior chamber shallow or absent. In any penetrating injury, there is a great risk of

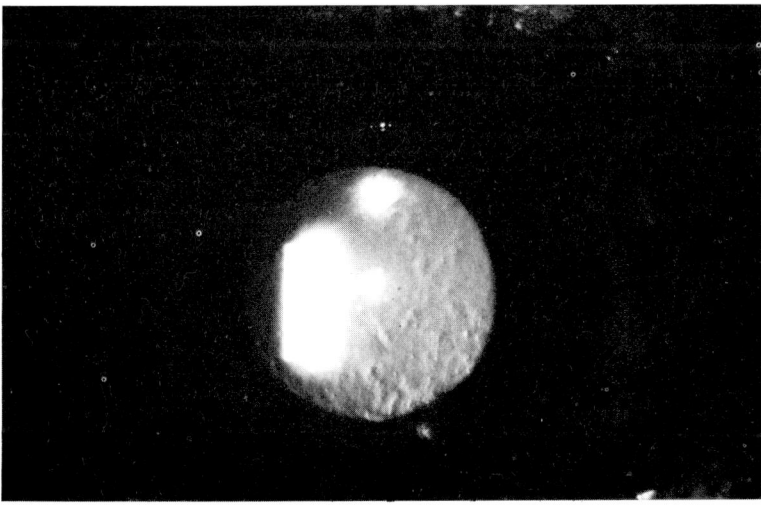

Fig. 19.5 The hole in the iris only becomes obvious when it is seen with an ophthalmoscope.

serious damage to the intraocular structures, and especially to the lens.

The basic treatment for penetrating intraocular injuries is to excise any prolapsed uveal tissue, and suture the wound. However, small puncture wounds are usually self healing, and will not require sutures. If the lens is very badly damaged, it may be best to perform an extracapsular extraction at the same time as suturing the wound.

There are many possible complications from penetrating eye injuries: –
– The entry wound may leave a scar on the cornea.
– Even slight damage to the lens is likely to cause a cataract.
– Intraocular infection is a common complication. It is especially serious if the object which entered the eye was contaminated, and usually results in blindness. For this reason, all penetrating injuries should receive systemic, subconjunctival and local antibiotics to minimise the risk of infection.
– Sympathetic ophthalmitis is a serious but rare complication. Some weeks or months after the injury, the undamaged eye develops uveitis. It is not certain why this should happen, but it may be because the body becomes sensitive to its own uveal tissue. As soon as the immediate danger of infection has passed, it is usual to give fairly intensive local steroid treatment to the injured eye. This will lessen any intraocular inflammation, and reduce the risk of sympathetic ophthalmitis.
– Uveitis, glaucoma and retinal detachment are all possible complications.

It is important to test the vision after any penetrating injury. If there is no perception of light at all, it is safe to assume that the eye will never be able to see. If the eye also looks unattractive, it is much better to remove it, and so avoid lengthy postoperative complications. Any eye which does have projection of light is worth trying to save. However, if it then becomes obvious that there is little chance of useful vision, and if the eye is painful and unattractive, it is again better to remove it.

Sometimes the patient does not come for treatment until many days or even weeks after the injury. If there is still hope of sight in the eye, it is often best to delay surgery until the wound has healed spontaneously and the eye is quiet.

Sometimes small fragments of metal, stone or glass may remain in the eye. Iron fragments should be removed if possible with a magnet because they will rust inside the eye and eventually destroy it. Non-magnetic particles are best left. It is almost impossible to remove them in any case.

Injuries to the eyelids

The eyelids are exposed, and so injuries are frequent. (*Plates* 23e *and* f). However, they have a very good blood supply, and even extensive lacerations will heal well if they are sutured correctly. It is important that no knots or suture ends rub against the cornea. Sometimes, lacerations at the inner end of the eyelids sever the lacrimal canaliculi. It is very difficult to repair a severed canaliculus successfully. It is probably best to suture the lid carefully, and hope that an opening will develop between the conjunctiva and the cut end of the canaliculus.

Bruising and oedema of the eyelids are very common, but usually subside fairly rapidly. Sometimes the eyelids are so swollen that it is impossible to examine the eye. Instill local anaesthetic drops, gently separate the eyelids with a retractor, and then check to see if any intraocular damage has occurred.

Orbital injuries

The front of the orbit is thick, strong bone which protects the eye, and so is quite often injured itself. It is possible to detect serious fractures by feeling the orbital rim beneath the skin, and an X-ray will confirm the diagnosis. However, special treatment is only necessary if the bones are seriously displaced. In such cases, fractures of other facial bones are very likely, and it is usual for a maxillofacial surgeon to reduce and fix them.

Occasionally, a fracture occurs in the very thin floor or walls of the orbit. The injury compresses the orbit, and the thin orbital floor gives way. This is called a 'blowout' fracture and is not in itself important. Sometimes, however, the orbital fat or extraocular muscles are trapped in the fracture site. This limits the movement of the injured eye and causes diplopia. Some damage to the infraorbital nerve is also usual, and numbs the cheek and upper lip. Because the floor and walls of the orbit are so thin, special X-ray techniques are necessary to demonstrate any fractures. If there is any evidence that the movement of the eye is severely limited, it may be advisable to explore the floor of the orbit and free any orbital tissues which are trapped. It may then be necessary to insert an artificial silicone sheet to reconstitute the orbital floor.

Cranial nerve injuries

Cranial nerve injuries are quite common after head injuries. The cranial nerves which supply the eye and which are most likely to be damaged in this way are the II, III, IV and VI nerves.

Damage to the second nerve (optic nerve) is most common after an injury to the temple. The sight in the eye will be affected, and there is usually no pupil response to light. The damage is usually permanent.

The III, IV and VI cranial nerves supply the extraocular muscles, and damage to these will produce diplopia (*see* page 200 for details). Damage to these nerves may gradually recover after a few months, or may be permanent.

20.　Diagnosis of Common Eye Conditions

Diagnosis is the most important step in the care of an individual patient. The purpose of the history and examination is to make the diagnosis, and the purpose of the diagnosis is to give the correct treatment. If the diagnosis is wrong, then the treatment will also be wrong.

Diagnosis is sometimes difficult even for the specialist. It is not surprising that the non-specialist often feels he can only guess the diagnosis. However, a short history and careful examination with a few basic instruments should provide enough information to diagnose most eye patients correctly.

Diagnosis is difficult in the early stages of a disease, but becomes easier as the signs and symptoms become more obvious. This means that diagnosis is sometimes easier in areas where there are few doctors and where patients usually come with advanced disease.

There are two very common diagnostic problems in eye disease: –
– Loss of vision.
– An irritable or painful red eye.

Loss of vision

Loss of vision is the most important symptom of eye disease. The common causes of visual loss can be divided into four groups: –
– Refractive errors in which the patient need spectacles.
– Opacities in the ocular media which prevent the light rays reaching the retina. These patients will have painless loss of vision. An examination with an ophthalmoscope will show either an absent or a poor red fundus reflex.
– Retinal or optic nerve diseases. These patients also have painless loss of vision, but the red reflex is clearly visible with an ophthalmoscope.
– Inflammatory eye disease which causes loss of vision and a painful red eye.
　Table 20.1 (p. 226) summarizes the main features of each of these four groups of disease.

Refractive errors

The pinhole test is a simple test to detect refractive errors (*see* page 22). Often, patients with refractive errors screw up their eyelids to make their own pinhole, and they usually see better in bright light when the pupil constricts.

Refractive errors start at different ages.
– Hypermetropia and astigmatism are present from birth, but young children

can overcome hypermetropia by accomodating.

- Myopia usually starts between 5 and 15 years, but it is occasionally present at birth.
- Presbyopia starts at 40 years, and progresses until 60 years.

Most eyes with refractive errors are otherwise normal. The following are exceptions:—

- Myopic eyes may develop degenerative changes of the macula, and have a higher risk of retinal detachment.
- Children with a refractive error in only one eye may be amblyopic in that eye.
- Some diseases can produce refractive changes. Early lens opacities can alter the refraction, and corneal scars can produce irregular astigmatism.

Opacities in the ocular media

Opacities are very common in the lens, quite common in the cornea, and less common in the vitreous. These opacities are often obvious to the naked eye. However, the best way to assess the density and position of an opacity anywhere in the ocular media is to dilate the pupil, and examine the red fundus reflex with an ophthalmoscope.

- An absent red reflex indicates a dense opacity.
- A shadow or irregularity in the red reflex indicates a slight opacity.

Small opacities which only cast a shadow in the red reflex may be difficult to locate. The best way to locate them is to bring them into focus using a positive lens in the ophthalmoscope.

- An opacity in front of the plane of the iris is probably in the cornea.
- An opacity behind the plane of the iris is probably in the lens.
- An opacity behind the plane of the iris which moves when the eye moves is probably in the vitreous.

It is possible to treat most opacities in the ocular media as long as the retina and optic nerve are healthy. The surgical treatment for lens opacities is fairly easy, but corneal and vitreous opacities require very highly specialized surgery.

One common diagnostic problem is to assess whether there is retinal or optic nerve disease when opacities in the ocular media obscure the fundus (*see also* page 137). The light projection test is a simple test of a normal retina and optic nerve (*see* page 22). The pupil reflexes are also a good test. A brisk pupil reflex indicates a healthy retina and optic nerve. However, there are exceptions:-

- The patient may have used atropine (or some other mydriatic) which dilates the pupil.
- There may be adhesions between the iris and lens.
- There are some very rare diseases which prevent the pupil reacting to light, even though the retina and optic nerve are normal.

A fixed, dilated pupil in a patient who has definitely not had mydriatics is a sign of serious retinal or optic nerve disease.

Diseases of the retina and optic nerve

Loss of vision together with a clear red fundus reflex indicates disease of the retina or optic nerve. If the visual loss comes on suddenly, it usually means there is a vascular disease of the retina or optic nerve, or possibly a retinal detachment.

It is necessary to test the pupil light reflexes before dilating the pupil. Optic nerve disease in particular will cause a loss of the pupil reflex. Unfortunately, it requires a lot of experience to recognize many of the different fundus disorders. However, many of the diseases of the retina and optic nerve are untreatable. This means that making the correct diagnosis is often more important in theory than in practice.

Most retinal and optic nerve diseases are recognized by their appearance. Therefore it is very difficult to make a logical system for diagnosis. However, the following hints may help to identify the more important of these diseases: –

1. Retinal diseases usually produce fairly obvious changes in the appearance of the fundus, but may still leave some useful vision. On the other hand, optic nerve diseases, especially in the acute stage, may produce very few obvious changes to the optic disc, but a severe loss of vision.
2. Hypertension and diabetes are both common causes of retinal diseases, especially haemorrhages and exudates. Always measure the blood pressure, and test the urine for sugar.
3. The most important optic nerve disease to detect is glaucomatous optic atrophy. This is because glaucoma is very common, and early treatment should stop the progress of the disease. Unfortunately, it is difficult for both patient and doctor to recognize glaucoma in its early stages (see page 160). Advanced glaucoma is much easier to detect, but by then is too late to save any useful sight. By the time the patient is first seen, one eye at least is often blind, but the second eye may have useful vision.
4. The retina has no pain fibres. If the eye is uncomfortable and does not appear red or inflamed, then choroiditis or optic neuritis are possible causes of the loss of vision. Choroiditis is often difficult to recognize clinically, but it is usually treatable.
5. Retinal detachments are not common. However, the need for surgical treatment is urgent so that it is very important to recognize them. It helps to remember the three predisposing factors: aphakia, myopia and trauma. It also helps to remember the three warning signs of a retinal detachment: floaters, flashing lights and field defects.
6. If a careful examination of the eye can still not find any cause for the visual loss, it is possible that there is damage to the visual pathways in the brain (see page 159). This will usually cause a homonymous hemianopia.

Inflammatory eye disease

Inflammatory eye disease causing loss of vision and a painful red eye is discussed on the next page.

Defective vision or blindness in children

Defective vision or blindness is a special problem in children. This is because the common causes of blindness are different in children and in adults, and also because the assessment of vision in children is difficult. Young children who are blind in one eye only do not usually complain of poor vision. Even if the disease can be treated, the eye is probably amblyopic, and treatment will not greatly improve the sight.

Nutritional corneal ulceration and its complications are very important causes of child blindness. These complications are: –
– Corneal scarring
– Corneal staphyloma
– Phthisis bulbi
However they are all easy to recognize.

– Cataract is the most common congenital abnormality in children, and it too is fairly easy to recognize. A solid mass behind the lens may look like a cataract. This is a rare, but important cause of blindness (*see* page 152).
– Optic atrophy is quite common in children, and may have many possible causes. It may follow a severe and acute illness, such as meningitis, typhoid fever or measles.
– 'Cortical blindness' occasionally occurs after encephalitis. This means that the child cannot see, but the pupil reactions are normal. The child may not be aware that he is blind.
– Night blindness is usually a sign of vitamin A deficiency, but occasionally it may be caused by retinitis pigmentosa.
– Refractive errors are common in children. The pupil must be dilated with cycloplegic drops in order to measure the refraction of any child with poor vision.
Occasionally, it may be necessary to examine a baby under an anaesthetic in order to see the fundus or to check the intraocular pressure.

The irritable or painful red eye

Any eye injury or foreign body in the conjunctiva or cornea may cause a painful red eye. Therefore the first step is to take the history and make a careful examination so as to exclude this possibility.

There are four common causes for an irritable or painful red eye (*Table* 20.1). Three of them, conjunctivitis, corneal ulcers and iridocyclitis, may occur in any patient, and conjunctivitis is especially common. The fourth, angle closure glaucoma, is uncommon in blacks and patients under 40. (It may be helpful to refer to the pictures of these four diseases in the appropriate chapters).

These four conditions are usually separate diseases, but occasionally, they may occur together. For example, in some types of conjunctivitis there may also be some corneal complications. Some corneal ulcers may develop secondary iridocyclitis, and some cases of iridocyclitis may develop secondary glaucoma. The main clinical features of each of these four diseases are summarised in *Table* 20.2. The details are as follows: –

Pain

The conjunctiva does not have a very rich nerve supply, but the cornea does. Therefore conjunctivitis causes irritation, but a corneal ulcer causes pain and often photophobia also. However, a viral conjunctivitis which also involves the superficial epithelial cells of the cornea may sometimes cause slight pain and photophobia.

The pain of iridocyclitis varies very much.

Table 20.1. Common causes of visual loss

	1. Refractive errors	2. Opacities in the ocular media	3. Diseases of the retina and optic nerve	4. Acute inflammatory disease
Causes	Myopia Hypermetropia Presbyopia Astigmatism	Lens opacities Corneal opacities Vitreous opacities	Retinal degeneration Retinal vascular disease Retinal detachment Optic atrophy Optic neuritis Chronic simple glaucoma Choroiditis	Corneal ulcer Acute iritis Acute glaucoma
Signs and Symptoms	Vision improves with pinhole	Painless quiet eye Absent or poor red reflex	Painless quiet eye Clear red reflex	Painful red eye
Treatment	Spectacles	Surgery or no treatment Not urgent	Often no treatment, sometimes urgent medical or surgical treatment	Urgent medical or surgical treatment

Table 20.2 The common causes of a red, irritable or painful eye

	1. Conjunctivitis	2. Corneal ulcer	3. Iritis	4. Angle closure glaucoma
Pain	Irritation only	Moderate + Photophobia	Moderate	Severe
Vision	Normal	Variable loss	Variable loss	Severe loss
Redness	Diffuse and especially in fornices	Around corneal limbus	Around corneal limbus	Around corneal limbus
Corneal appearance	Normal	Stains with fluorescein	Keratic Precipitates seen with magnification	Oedematous and hazy
Pupil	Normal	Normal or slightly constricted	Constricted and irregular	Half dilated and fixed
Anterior chamber	Normal	Normal or some inflammatory exudate	Inflammatory exudate	Shallow
Special features	Disharge with stickiness often bilateral		Often recurrent and bilateral	Raised pressure
Treatment	Usually antibiotics	Antibiotics antivirals mydriatics steroids usually disastrous	Steroids and mydriatics	Miotics and surgery

In acute angle closure glaucoma, there is usually severe pain. This pain may radiate from the eye to other parts of the head. Sometimes angle closure glaucoma presents less severely, with little or no pain in the eye. If angle closure glaucoma does occur in blacks, it is usually in this less severe form.

Vision

In conjunctivitis, the vision is normal. However, it may be necessary to wipe away discharges and mucus from the eyelids and conjunctival sac.

A corneal ulcer usually causes some blurring of the vision, depending on the size and position of the ulcer.

The visual loss caused by iritis varies very much, according to how severe the disease is.

Angle closure glaucoma causes severe loss of vision, except in very early or less acute cases.

Redness

The eye appears red because the blood vessels are dilated, and are seen against the background of the white sclera.

In conjunctivitis, the superficial conjunctival blood vessels become dilated. The conjunctiva appears red all over, but this redness is often most noticeable towards the fornices and away from the limbus.

Corneal ulcers, iritis and angle closure glaucoma all cause the anterior ciliary vessels to dilate. Therefore the redness is most noticeable around the cornea.

The cornea

In conjunctivitis, the cornea usually appears normal. However, in viral conjunctivitis, the superficial corneal cells may be very slightly involved. This is called 'superficial punctate keratitis', and it is usually only possible to detect it with a slit lamp and fluorescein dye.

Corneal ulcers obviously give the cornea an abnormal appearance. Severe ulcers are visible to the naked eye, but many ulcers only show up with fluorescein dye.

In iritis, the fine keratic precipitates are usually only visible with a slit lamp. However, they may stand out against the red fundus reflex when examined with an ophthalmoscope.

In angle closure glaucoma, the whole cornea looks hazy. This is because the rise in intraocular pressure makes it oedematous.

The pupil and the anterior chamber

In conjunctivitis, the pupil is normal, and the anterior chamber is clear.

In a corneal ulcer, the pupil may be slightly constricted. With severe corneal ulcers, there may be a noticeable inflammatory exudate in the anterior chamber.

In iridocyclitis, the pupil appears constricted and irregular to the naked eye. There is also an inflammatory exudate in the anterior chamber, but this only usually shows up with focal illumination and magnification.

In angle closure glaucoma, the pupil is always half-dilated and non-reactive. The anterior chamber is noticeably shallow.

Other special features

Conjunctivitis typically presents with a muco-purulent discharge, and is often bilateral.

Iridocyclitis is sometimes bilateral and sometimes leads to secondary glaucoma.

In angle closure glaucoma the intraocular pressure is very high, and the eye feels stony hard.

Treatment

The treatment for all four conditions is very different (*Table* 20.2), which shows how important it is to make the correct diagnosis.

Conjunctivitis may have many different causes (*see* pp. 66, 76), but usually the treatment is local antibiotics.

Corneal ulcers may have several different causes (*see* page 102), but usually the treatment is local antibiotics or antiviral agents and mydriatics.

Iridocyclitis may have several different causes, but the treatment to the eye is local steroids and mydriatics.

Angle closure glaucoma is a complete diagnosis in itself. The treatment is miotics, and then surgery.

Disorders at the limbus

The limbus is a common site for pathological changes. Most of these are fairly distinctive, and many of them do not require treatment, but there is often some confusion in recognizing them.

1. Inflammation of the limbus is quite common. It is usually the result of an immune reaction rather than a specific infection, and so usually responds to steroid drops. Some examples are:—
– a phlycten (*see* page 73)
– marginal corneal infiltrates (*see* page 100)
– vernal conjunctivitis (*see* page 70)
– Mooren's ulcer (*see* page 100).

2. Excessive limbal pigmentation is a sign of different conditions in adults and children.
– In adults it is often a sign of previous inflammation. It is also common in severe onchocerciasis.
– In children, vitamin A deficiency and vernal conjunctivitis both produce excessive limbal pigmentation. Vitamin A deficiency also causes a Bitot's spot at the limbus (*see* page 116). Vernal conjunctivitis often causes inflammatory nodules of the limbus.

3. Degenerative changes in older people often occur at the limbus:—
- A pinquecula is a subconjunctival fatty deposit.
- A pterygium is a wedge-shaped opacity that grows over the cornea from the limbus.
- Arcus senilis is another very common degenerative change at the limbus.
4. Other disorders may occur at the limbus: –
- Foreign bodies often come to rest in the shallow groove between the cornea and the sclera.
- Scarring at the limbus will follow any previous inflammation.
- Most conjunctival tumours start at the limbus, but are usually fairly easy to remove.

Index

231